Letts study aids

Revise Nursing RGN

David Parkin BA, SRN, BTA, DN, RNT

Senior Tutor, Musgrove Park Hospital, Taunton

Charles Letts & Co Ltd
London, Edinburgh & New York

First published 1985
by Charles Letts & Co Ltd
Diary House, Borough Road, London SE1 1DW

Reprinted 1986

Editor: Sheila Goater
Design: Ben Sands
Illustrations: Tek-Art

ISBN 0 85097 640 5

Printed by Charles Letts (Scotland) Limited

Preface

It was a privilege to be asked by Charles Letts and Co Ltd to provide a manuscript for Revise Nursing RGN. The task has proved to be both exhilarating and challenging.

Many student nurses have approached me for help in organizing their revision and preparation for examinations and there is obviously a need for guidance on a national scale in view of the cost of failure to individuals and authorities.

Examinations for student nurses present serious problems for some candidates:

1 The scope and depth of the course material is extensive and difficult.
2 Written work has to be completed very quickly in the current examination system.
3 Some candidates have great difficulty interpreting the wording of questions. Many try to learn rote answers to problems, which do not help them to apply themselves to the specific ones on the paper.

This book attempts to provide guide lines for students, mainly in the last year of training, but hopefully also in the earlier parts of the course.

The guide to revision and examinations is intended to generate a sensible and positive approach to them. They need to be respected but not feared.

The précis of the course content in Section 2 is aimed at providing a guide through major conditions and nursing care problems. The 'systems' approach is deliberately traditional. There are moves towards concentration on nursing problems instead of diagnostic conditions, but current examination questions and student queries are 'diagnosis' based. There is, however, an attempt to emphasize the 'nursing responses' throughout. It is anticipated that alternative nursing responses are possible but these are intended as guides rather than rules.

An interesting exercise has been using nursing text books in an average School of Nursing library for source material. A list of sources is included in the introduction to Section 2, but is not inclusive of all the books used. My apologies for any errors gleaned and published. It is the intention of the publishers to revise the book regularly and any errors or suggested inclusions would be gratefully received.

It has been most gratifying to receive so much support from so many sources in compiling the material. My sincere thanks go to the following:

The General Nursing Council for permission to use questions from past final examination papers.

The English National Board for Nursing, Midwifery and Health Visiting for permission to include the examination papers in Sections 4 and 6.

The United Kingdom Central Council for Nursing, Midwifery and Health Visiting for permission to include the Code of Conduct in Section 2.13.

Churchill Livingstone, Publishers, for permission to include the model of nursing from *Essentials of Nursing* by Roper, Logan and Tierney (model A in Section 1).

The Centre for Policy on Ageing for permission to include the 'pressure sore risk scale'.

Mr F. Holden, Professional Adviser (Examinations), English National Board for Nursing, Midwifery and Health Visiting for help with the multiple choice questions in Section 5.

Angela Balchin, Norman Harrison and Steven Pope for their help with diagrams.

My Director of Nurse Education, Miss P. C. Southwell, my colleagues and friends in the Somerset School of Nursing for being so patient, tolerant and supportive.

My thanks also to all the staff of Letts, especially Pat Rowlinson and Karen Sparrock, also to Sheila Goater for helping and editing.

My very special thanks go to my family, Ruth, John and most of all Pam for doing all the typing and still caring!

David Parkin 1984

Contents

Section 1

1.1   Introduction and guide

This book is intended as a guide to student nurses preparing for the final exam
National Board for registration as general nurses. The intention is to cover
that will enable the student to analyse the questions being set and reason for
particular questions. Model answers are not given.

Tutorial staff and clinical staff may also find it a helpful book when assessi
objectives in clinical settings. The core units are written to stimulate nursing r
find other responses in addition to the ones given or indeed contrary, but t
given to the student to consider what nursing actions are necessary and the rea

You are recommended to make use of this book as a framework for yo
imperative that you recognize the need for further reading, accumulating awa
experiences and guidance from your own tutorial staff. The examiners for
Board are nurse tutors and, when you are arranging your revision, regular c
tutor is vital.

A guide to revision and study is included in this section. Many nurses fin
methods as well as their own tried and trusted ones. It is hoped that these

The core units are written to give you ideas about nursing respons
circumstances. The systems approach should enable you to relate your awar
the physical effects of diseases. You will find however that most questions
physical aspects of the disease. They include psychological and social care t
more than one unit to determine a total nursing care approach.

There is no clear separation of 'medical', 'surgical' and 'trauma'. You will
in the system e.g. thoracotomy, fractured ribs and pneumonia are all in the s
the respiratory system.

Following the core units, you will find a selection of final examination que
grouped according to the core units as far as possible. A brief analysis of the
possible approach to planning the answer. Your tutors will probably be abl
analysis and arrange discussions for in-depth analysis that will help you in

Section 6 is a collection of final examination questions. It needs to be stre
you **must** have your work marked by your Tutor. It is important that you lear
carefully. As you approach the examination, you should attempt at least thre
3×35 minutes $= 105$ minutes).

1.2   Examinations for Registered Nurses

The United Kingdom Central Council Training rules state that:
'To qualify as a person who can apply to be registered in Part 1 of the register, the stu
or arranged by a Board which may be in parts, and which shall be designed so as to
practical skills and attitudes and demonstrates her ability to undertake the relevar.
rules'

Relating to the care of the particular type of patient with whom she is likely to come
are required to:

(a) advise on the promotion of health and prevention of illness;
(b) recognize situations that may be detrimental to the health and well being of t
(c) carry out those activities involved when conducting the comprehensive assessr
(d) recognize the significance of the observations made and use these to develop
(e) devise a plan of nursing care based on the assessment with the co-operation of t
   taking into account the medical prescription;
(f) implement the planned programme of nursing care and where appropriate teach
   team who may be responsible for implementing specific aspects of the nursin;
(g) review the effectiveness of the nursing care provided, and where appropriate.
(h) work in a team with other nurses and with medical and para medical staff an
(i) undertake the management of the care of a group of patients over a period of
   services.

1.3   The roles of the Registered Nurse (General)

The roles of a professional nurse may be summarized into six (although c
more).

The staff nurse and ultimately the Ward Sister will be expected to act as
   1 an **assessor** of nursing needs.
   2 a **planner** of nursing care to meet those needs.
   3 a **practitioner** of nursing skills to provide care.

nations of the English
he material required
hemselves answers to

ng the achievement of
sponses. Some would
e stimulus should be
ons for those actions.
ir revision work. It is
eness for your clinical
the English National
onsultation with your

l it helpful to try new
tips will help you.
es to many differing
eness of physiology to
nvolve more than the
oo. Remember to use

find them all included
ction (2.1) relating to

tions which have been
question is given and a
to give you a further
new questions.
ssed emphatically that
n to time your answers
e at each 'sitting' (time

dent shall have passed an examination, held
assess the student's theoretical knowledge,
competencies specified in rule 18 of these
[Rule 19 I.C.]
contact when registered, the competencies

e individual;
ent of a person's nursing requirements;
n initial nursing assessment;
e patient, to the extent that this is possible,

nd co-ordinate other members of the caring
care;
initiate any action that may be required;
social workers;
time and organize the appropriate support

Rule 18 (1)

thers could easily find

adopt a *model of nursing* as
lels for you to choose. Two
luded.

ature

sleep)

t include considerations of
reness of the strictures of

d in written examinations,
n practical skill has scored
uired for a patient with a

Remember that nursing
ogress. For example, you
or two hourly change of
g red.

ments of management in

ful framework based on

1.4   Studying and revising

You will realize from the scope of your nursing experiences and the range of questions, that you cannot do a 'crash revision' course for these examinations. You need to **organize** your studying and revising from very early on in your training.

The first thing you must do is determine that you will enjoy studying and revising. If it becomes a chore to you, no amount of effort will succeed and indeed it could dull the excitement of learning for a long time.

Check

1 *Your concentration time*

Try concentrating on something completely new to your experience and see how soon you have to stop. The times varies from 20–40 minutes in different people. You will need to plan your revision time in periods which fit in with your own concentration time.

2 *Your studying environment*

Some students prefer quiet, some prefer music, some can even study with a television on in the background. This is quite acceptable if you find it works and you enjoy it.

There may be times when you need to be alone, others when a group session is more beneficial. Try doing a 'group test' at some stage. Discuss an answer plan between you and then break off to enable each person to write out the answer. You will be surprised at the differing answers you still get!

3 *Your memory pattern*

Most people need to group material in a particular way to help their memory.

For example, some would learn a list 1 2 3 4 5 6 7 8 9 10

Others would remember better 1 2 3 4   5 6 7 8   9 10

Most people forget about 30–40% of new material in 24 hours and progressively more if they do not revise it. You will need to **revise new material** at least **once** in the following day, to help you retain it better.

Revision

Do not just keep reading over the same material (even your notes). It is far better for you to **do** something with the material.

Try making up your own teaching cards (for use later on). They are cheaper than prepared ones and far more useful to you. The exercise of having to group the information for presentation to a junior nurse and having to focus it on keywords is helpful in itself.

It is also important that you **read around** the subject. You are blessed with a very good nursing press now and publishers are introducing new nursing text books all the time. You must make use of your library to expand and up-date your information.

It is a sobering thought that some of your notes are two to three years old when you are revising and many new strides have been taken in nursing during that time!

You will need to attempt questions as part of your revision. A suggested approach here is to read the question one evening, study the subject(s) that same evening, then, at least two evenings later, sit down and write out your answer to the question in the correct time (35 minutes). As you get more practice, you could do more than one. *Repeat*: you must have them marked by your Tutor!

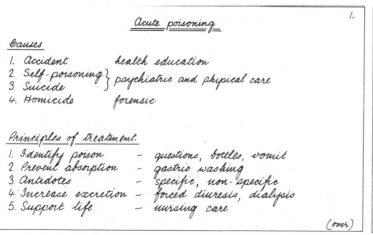

Fig. 1.4.1 A 'teaching' card

1.5   Problem solving and wording of questions

The art of problem solving can be divided into three parts.

The first part is collecting data. In our questions, some information is given to you; you also have your own knowledge to draw upon; you would also gain information from your patient assessment.

The second part is to analyse the relevant data for solving the problem.

The third part is, of course, to suggest solutions to the problems and write them out clearly.

Wording of questions

Instruction in question	Meaning
Give a description of/Describe . . .	Explain the nature, form or function of a particular object or concept, You are rarely asked for diagrams now. They do take time. If you use one, it must be big and clearly labelled in the relevant parts to your answer.
Give an account of . . .	Write an explanatory description
Discuss . . .	Give an account of the various views on a topic
Compare . . .	Put side by side, one or more similarities
Contrast . . .	Put side by side, one or more differences
Explain/Account for . . .	Make known in detail, make understood
State . . .	Present in the form of a concise statement
Define . . .	State precisely and concisely what is meant by
List . . .	Write, one after another, in the form of a catalogue
Write an essay . . .	Write a full account, sub-divided into paragraphs, of the subject
Outline . . .	Write brief notes to describe

1.6   Examination technique

It cannot be stressed enough that the most important factor in examination technique is in your **own mental and physical preparation** before the dreaded day.

You must be as physically fit as possible. You will use a lot of nervous energy in the day and you need to concentrate all through both papers. Only a few have benefited from last minute reading and you are advised to try to have some relaxing activities over the week-end before the day.

Morning paper – essay type

You need to have a plan of action for the three hours. Take a good pen and a pencil. *Golden rule* – pick up pencil first!

Write out (before you read the paper if you wish) your model of nursing, your roles of the nurse and very important – a time schedule.

e.g. 0930–1005 h   1st question
      1005–1040 h   2nd question
      1040–1115 h   3rd question
      1115–1150 h   4th question
      1150–1225 h   5th question

This gives you five minutes reading, alteration or filling in time at the end of the examination.

Read the questions very carefully. Some candidates rewrite them to help them to pick out the essence. Try to analyse the question. **Write out an answer plan** – this will help you sort out the many ideas coming to you. Don't forget to plan the timing according to the weighting of the question. An examiner will expect to see 70% of your writing devoted to that part of the question carrying 70% of the marks. Write as clearly as you can – only a few marks are at stake for bad spelling and grammar, but they could make a difference if you fall on the borderline. **All marks** are at stake if the examiner **cannot read** your work.

Afternoon paper – multiple choice questions

You need to work your way through this carefully. Don't delay over questions where the answer is obvious to you – do them first. Those you find more difficult should be left; go through the whole paper a few times until you are left with those where you really have no idea. You are advised here to take an **intelligent** guess. Go back to your principles of care and trust your judgement. After three years training and experience you will be right in 60 to 70% of cases. You do not lose marks for wrong answers, but none can be given for a blank space.

Book Contents

1.7 Syllabus Guide

	The roles of nurses	Respiratory system	Cardiovascular system	Digestive system	Renal system	Nervous system	Locomotor system	Skin	Endocrine system	Reproductive system	Psychological problems	Social problems	Drugs and treatment	Operating theatre	Needs of children	Needs of elderly patients	Nurse as – manager	– teacher	– health educationalist	– professional person
	1.3	2.1	2.2	2.3	2.4	2.5	2.6	2.7	2.8	2.9	2.10	2.11	2.12	2.13	2.14	2.15	3			
Principles & Practice of nursing																				
General care of ward unit																	●			
General care of patients and nursing procedures		Tested in ward based practical examination →																		
Human behaviour in relation to illness											●	●								
Administration and storage of drugs													●							
Nursing care in the operating theatre														●						
First aid and treatment in emergencies		CORE UNITS →																		
Preparation for professional responsibility	●																			●
Man and his environment		●	●	●	●	●	●	●	●	●	●	●	●		●	●				
The nature and causes of ill health		CORE UNITS →																		
Principles of prevention																		●	●	
Nursing care and treatment of sick people		CORE UNITS →																		
Specification grid for 60 item test (ENB)																				
1 Professional responsibility	●																			●
2 Normal physiological and psychological needs of the individual		CORE UNITS →																		
Care of the individual as a patient with conditions related to:																				
3 Respiration		●																		
4 Digestion				●																
5 Excretion					●															
6 Circulation			●																	
7 Neural						●														
8 Hormonal									●											
9 Locomotion							●													
10 Reproduction										●										
11 Immune response			●												●					
12 Skin								●												
13 Drugs and therapeutic hazards													●							
Examination questions since 1980 (Essay)	3	15	16	26	3	15	16	6	9	10	5	–	4	1	8	8	5	1	1	–

Section 2
Assessing and meeting the needs of patients with specific conditions

Introduction

This section is a composite study through the main areas of the general syllabus. It is written as a guide for your revision and cannot possibly cover all areas in detail.

Sections 2.1 to 2.9 cover the major conditions relating to the systems which you are likely to meet in the examination paper. There is a brief reminder of the functions and structures of the systems, followed by a survey of diseases related. The material is intended to direct you to nursing responses and one must emphasize that your awareness should be of the needs of patients that will be covered by nursing more than anything else.

The pattern of the units will be as follows:

1 Considerations of the normal functions of particular structures
2 Identification of the parts involved
3 A study of the major medical, surgical and traumatic conditions affecting the structures, including causation factors, effects (localized and general), signs and symptoms, investigations and medical or surgical treatment.

Nursing responses will be included at appropriate points to consider aspects of the nurses role which are relevant.

The expressions *Assessment* and *Care* relate to the aspects of nursing process. You could substitute *Problem* or *Potential problem* for *Assessment* and *Care plan* for *Care*. The term *raised metabolic rate* has been used to express the general effects of inflammation. This is a simplification of what really happens, but it has the great advantage in showing the way to the nursing care required.

It is suggested that the material is used in two ways:
1 To direct you to do further 'in depth' reading for the details.
2 To help you to condense even further down to key words for putting on to teaching cards.

The major texts that have been used as source material are:

Anthony & Thibodeau, *Text Book of Anatomy and Physiology* (Mosby)
Lilian Brunner & Doris Suddarth, *Lippincott Manual of Medical–Surgical Nursing* (Harper Row)
Chilman & Thomas, *Understanding Nursing Care* (Churchill Livingstone)
The Essentials of Nursing–Series Edited by Sheila Collins and Edith Parker (Macmillan Press)
Macleod, *Davidsons Principles and Practise of Medicine* (Churchill Livingstone)
McParland, *Basic Clinical Surgery* (Butterworth)
Roper, Logan, Tierney, *The Elements of Nursing* (Churchill Livingstone)
Schafer et al, *Medical–Surgical Nursing* (Mosby)
Tortora and Anagnostakos, *Principles of Anatomy and Physiology* (Harper Row)
Watson, *Medical–Surgical Nursing and Related Physiology* (W. B. Saunders)

2.1 Respiratory conditions

The respiratory system

This system will be considered as follows.
1 **The airway** nasal cavities and air sinuses; pharynx; larynx; trachea; bronchial tree

2 **Lung tissue** alveoli; blood vessels; lymphatics; connective support tissue

3 **Lung surroundings** pleura; chest wall (ribs, intercostal muscles and diaphragm)

1 The airway

Nasal cavities and air sinuses

Functions	Structures involved
1 Opening of the airway	Anterior nares
2 Filtration of air	Hairs, ciliated ephithelial tissue
3 Warming air	Large blood supply, turbinate bones and conchae increase surface area

4 Moistening air	Goblet cells in mucous membrane secrete mucus
5 Protection from irritant inhalants	Mucous membrane sensitive. Smooth muscles cause sneezing
6 Organ of smell	Olfactory apparatus – nerve endings in the ethmoid plate are able to detect subtle smells and taste
7 Drainage of tears	Tear ducts drain into nasal cavities
8 Resonance of voice	Shape of nasal cavities and nasal sinuses
9 Head balance	Nasal sinuses

Pharynx and nasopharynx

Functions	**Structures involved**
1 Continuation of airway	Whole structure
2 Protection from infection	Lymph nodules (adenoids and tonsils) drain to lymph nodes in neck
3 Swallowing	Muscles for swallowing (*Note*: Brain stem lesions may paralyse and cause airway obstruction)
4 Drainage and air balance in middle ear	Tympano – pharyngeal (eustachian) tubes

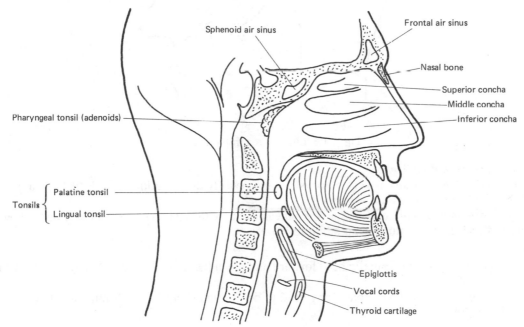

Fig. 2.1.1 The upper respiratory tract

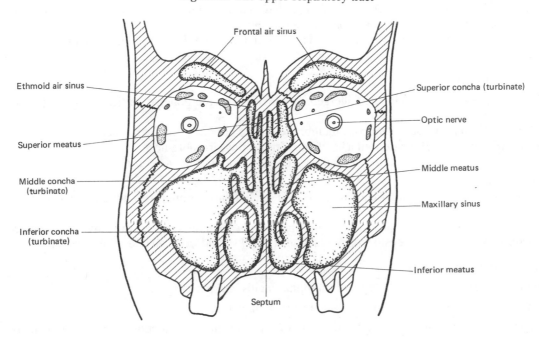

Fig. 2.1.2 Frontal air sinuses

Conditions of the upper respiratory tract

Epistaxis – nose bleeding

Causes

1 Trauma
2 Irritation of the mucosa
3 Nose picking
4 Hypertension
5 Blood dyscrasias e.g. aplastic anaemia, leukaemia

Nursing notes

The nurse may be faced with a patient who is very nonchalant about a nose bleed or one who is over anxious. An individual response is required. It is obviously an incident to report urgently in patients with known hypertension or blood disorders.

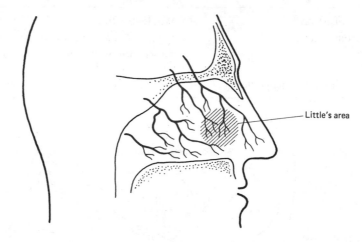

Fig. 2.1.3 Little's area in the nasal cavity

Effects, signs and symptoms

An anterior haemorrhage is very obvious. Note especially that bleeding from Little's area may be quite severe unless pressure is exerted.

A posterior haemorrhage may trickle down the back of the throat and the patient may be swallowing blood which may eventually cause him to vomit.

Treatment

First aid expel the clot, lean the head forward and pinch the nose over Little's area for at least ten minutes.

If bleeding continues a nasal pack may need to be inserted or a Simpson's inflatable bag to apply direct pressure.

Nursing notes

Most ENT departments and Accident Centres have nasal packing materials prepared in advance. Packing is usually done by a specialist surgeon or nurse.

   The patient would be nursed at rest and reassured. Oral fluids help to prevent a dry mouth as the patient breathcs orally.

Allergic rhinitis

Cause Hypersensitivity to inhaled allergens. Main allergens are pollens, particularly grass (though not exclusively).

Effects Inflammation of the mucous membrane due to antibody – antigen reaction.

Signs and symptoms Repeated attacks of sneezing; runny, irritable nose.

Treatment Antihistamine drugs or inhalants. Desensitization 'out of season'.

Nursing notes

The nurse may be able to advise about this condition, but patients are rarely admitted to hospital for care and even Community nurses may have little to do with it.

   One point about desensitization is important. Some patients are known to have anaphylactic reactions when being desensitized. Adrenaline 1:1000 should be available at all times.

Coryza – the common cold

Acute rhinitis, usually associated with nasopharyngitis and pharyngitis.

Cause Rhino viruses and adeno viruses are the main cause.

Cause factors The patient is usually in a state of low resistance to infection – exposure to cold and wetness, malnutrition and fatigue have all been blamed. The main factor is probably close proximity to a victim in a crowded public place.

Nursing notes
Prevention by isolating and protecting vulnerable patients cannot be stressed enough.

Effects, signs and symptoms
 1 *Inflammation of the mucous membrane* due to viral infection leads to red, swollen membranes and excessive mucous production. This leads to a runny, irritable nose with sneezing and loss of smell and to a sore throat – as the air is overheated and dried. Pain receptors in the pharynx are affected which may lead to painful swallowing.

Nursing notes
There are few remedies for the localized inflammation but steam inhalations, gargles and lozenges do help some patients. Increased fluid intake is needed too. Analgesia may be needed for the soreness.
 2 *General effects of inflammation* cause a raised metabolic rate and disturbance of brain functions leading to headache and malaise. A raised metabolic rate will cause a pyrexia, tachycardia and a rapid loss of energy.

Nursing notes
The nurse should respond to a raised metabolic rate by resting her patient until temperature and pulse are returned to normal limits. The temperature may have to be maintained by cooling with light bed clothes and a fan. Energy needs to be restored by giving glucose drinks.

Treatment Rest with palliative measures to reduce the discomfort. Aspirin is helpful not only as an analgesic for the throat and headache, but also as an antipyretic and anti-inflammatory drug. Paracetamol is preferred if allergy to aspirin is known.

Nursing notes
Aspirin and paracetamol both cause profuse sweating. A change of bed clothing may be necessary.

Influenza

Caused by influenza viruses – an infectious disease. Effects may be very similar to coryza, but many patients have a much more generalized fever and debility. Some viral strains may be fatal. Later pneumonia is a dangerous complication. Treatment is as for coryza.

Complications of upper respiratory tract infections

The nurse's main anxieties are about the danger of complications to the upper respiratory tract infections.

Sinusitis Secondary bacterial infection of the sinuses may cause purulent accumulations with severe 'face ache' pain. Needs antibacterial drugs and possible surgical drainage.

Otitis Media Infection may be transmitted to the middle ear, especially in children who have a short tympano – pharyneal tube. The child has severe pain. A young infant may hit the head against a cot side with the agony. There is danger of a ruptured tympanic membrane and further infection including the mastoid air cells and deafness.

Lower respiratory tract infections are dealt with later in this unit.

Nursing notes
Prevention of upper respiratory tract infection can be achieved by avoiding crowds and by separating victims. Early treatment particularly in children is strongly recommended. These infections cannot be treated lightly.

Tonsillitis

Cause Usually viruses, but often bacterial. The most serious is beta haemolytic streptococcal infection which may lead to complications of *acute rheumatism* (rheumatic fever), glomerulonephritis and *Henoch Schonlein syndrone* (rarely).
Cause factors The patient often has a lowered resistance to infection through fatigue and/or malnutrition. Exposure to cold and local irritants may be a factor too. Chronically inflamed or damaged tonsils and adenoids are easily reinfected.

Effects, signs and symptoms
 1 Local inflammation causes redness, swelling and excess secretions from the tonsil and adenoid massess and usually involves all the pharynx. Occasionally, pus may be seen as abscesses form.
   Peritonsillar abscess (quinsy) is a dangerous local effect. Bilateral ones have been known to obstruct the airway and of course rupture would possibly lead to aspiration pneumonia.
   Lymph nodes in the neck become enlarged. The patient complains of a very sore throat, with more acute pain on swallowing (which may be excessive, to cope with the increased volume of secretions). The lymph nodes are tender to touch and may again add to the difficulty of swallowing.

Suggested nursing response

Assessment	Care
A direct view of the tonsils is obtained by using a tongue spatula and asking the patient to say 'ah'. A throat swab will be taken before antiseptic gargles or antibacterial agents are given.	Mild antiseptic gargles and lozenges may soothe the throat. Analgesia will be required. Aspirin mucilage may be swallowed. Children may have 'Aspergum' (aspirin in chewing gum).

2 General effects of inflammation in tonsillitis often cause the metabolic rate to be markedly raised, particularly in children. The patient complains of malaise, headache and may be shivery alternating with feeling hot. The face is flushed. The patient may have difficulty in concentrating for long and become tired easily. Dehydration will occur rapidly.

Suggested nursing response

Assessment	Care
1 Pyrexia and tachycardia – observe continually and record at least 4 hourly. *2* Children may present with abdominal pain and vomiting – they need careful observations to confirm diagnosis.	Rest in bed until pyrexia and tachycardia are controlled. Apply general cooling methods to maintain temperature. Give plenty of fluids with added glucose for energy. Give prescribed antipyretic agent – paracetamol or aspirin. Give prescribed antibacterial agent (particularly for streptococcal infection) – usually one of the penicillins.

Tonsillectomy

Is performed to remove chronically enlarged tonsils which have become prone to infection.

Suggested nursing response For surgery the following need to be considered:
1 Pre operative nursing assessment and care.
2 Nursing care in the surgery itself.
3 Post operative nursing assessment and care both immediately after surgery and during the convalescent period.
Only specific care will be given – general surgical care may need to be added in a total nursing management question.

1 *Pre operative nursing assessment and care*
 1 Identify the age and anxieties of the patient.
 2 Ensure that they are free from infection and have been for a minimum of three weeks.
 3 Note any indications of blood dyscrasias that could result in an interference with the blood clotting mechanism.
 4 The main elements of care are psychological reassurance and ensuring an empty stomach prior to surgery.
Many children have loose teeth prior to surgery. These should be reported. The surgeon will decide if they should be extracted and when.

2 *Nursing care in the surgery* The nurse's rôle is to care for the patient prior to anaesthetic – especially a child. Parents should be encouraged to help as much as possible, but do check their own fears first.
Surgery needs' to be done efficiently and the theatre nurse needs to be aware of the order that instruments may be needed.

3 *Post operative nursing assessment and care*

Immediate Assessment and care of the airway.
Assess for reactionary haemorrhage – direct view is not easy, but excessive swallowing would indicate possible bleeding. Note also indications of restlessness. Pulse and blood pressure are good indications but blood pressure may not change until a lot of blood has been lost. Some give ice to suck, but others prefer to return to theatre quickly.

Convalescent Assess for indications of infection (see tonsillitis) which may lead to the problem of secondary haemorrhage later. Care is as for acute tonsillitis.
Assess for swallowing ability and gradually progress to normal diet as soon as possible.

At home Avoid contact with upper respiratory tract infections and infectious diseases for at least a month if possible.

Larynx

Functions	Structures involved
1 Continuation of the airway	Thyroid and cricoid cartilages maintain tube structure
2 Protection of the airway	Epiglottis is attached to inner surface of anterior part of thyroid cartilage. As thyroid rises, epiglottis closes airway
1 when swallowing	
2 from particles	Ciliated epithelium moves mucous towards pharynx. Cough reflex protects the larynx
3 Voice production	Vocal cords are attached to inner surface of thyroid cartilage in front and the arytenoid cartilages at the rear. Muscle movement of the arytenoid cartilages causes movement of the cords. They are controlled by impulses through the recurrent laryngeal nerve

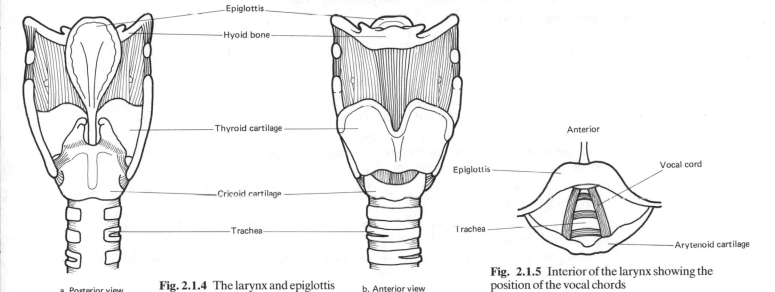

a. Posterior view   **Fig. 2.1.4** The larynx and epiglottis   b. Anterior view

Fig. 2.1.5 Interior of the larynx showing the position of the vocal chords

Conditions of the larynx

Laryngitis

Cause Usually viral, associated with pharyngitis and tracheitis. It may be bacterial, occasionally caused by mycobacterium tuberculosis.

Effects, signs and symptoms
1 *Local inflammation of the mucous membrane* (which also covers the cords) leads to loss of voice (aphonia). Lymph nodes are usually enlarged and with the associated pharyngitis, there may be considerable pain and difficulty in swallowing (dysphagia).

Suggested nursing response

Aphonia Try to keep the patient quiet – 'silence for a week' helps to provide local rest for the cords.

Dysphagia Ensure soft, easily swallowed food. Give prescribed analgesia before meals.

2 *General effects of inflammation* usually cause a raised metabolic rate but severity depends on · total condition.

Suggested nursing response
1 Rest the patient in bed until pyrexia and tachycardia are controlled.
2 Give extra glucose fluids for restoration of energy.
3 If bacterial, give prescribed antibacterial agents.

Note: If mycobacterium tuberculosis are found, the care and treatment are as for pulmonary tuberculosis, including barrier nursing.

Laryngo – tracheitis

In infants is known as **croup**. Spasm of the vocal cords produces a characteristic 'croup' sound on inspiration. It may lead to severe stridor and, fortunately rarely, airway obstruction.

Suggested nursing response
Parents are often very distressed as well as their children. A calm assuring manner is essential.

Moistening of the air often reduces the spasm – the child is nursed in a 'croupette' tent or with a nebulizer directing cool steam at the child. Steam kettles are not used in modern units but a mother may be advised to boil a kettle in a child's sick room at home as a temporary measure – she must be advised not to leave the child.

In hospital, a tracheostomy set should be ready in case of obstruction.

Carcinoma of larynx

Cause The cause has not been identified but the main factor appears to be cigarette smoking.

Effects, signs and symptoms
1 *Early* The tumour may originate on one cord or may infiltrate quickly to involve both and other laryngeal structures. The patient complains of a hoarse voice which persists.

Nursing notes
The rôle of the nurse here is as a health educationalist. If diagnosed early, surgical excision or radiotherapy may be very successful without laryngectomy. Advice about early consultation is very important. If a hoarse voice persists for three weeks, an early appointment is essential.

2 *Late* If infiltration has occurred, then **laryngectomy** is indicated.

Suggested nursing response
Pre operative assessment and preparation includes assisting with a laryngoscopy to confirm diagnosis and ensuring that the patient is free from infection. The patient (and his family) needs a full explanation of the implications of surgery. Acceptance of a permanent tracheostomy and oesophageal speech will need to be carefully taught.

Surgery involves dissection of the larynx leaving the permanent tracheostomy. Most surgeons would leave a nasogastric tube in place for early feeding as oedema of the oesophagus may occur.

Post operative assessment and care should include:
1 Observation and maintenance of the airway through good tracheostomy care. Intensive care is needed for the first few hours.

2 Observations for and prevention of infection through aseptic technique for dressings and tracheal suction.

3 Maintaining good communications with the patient through the provision of a bell and a pad for writing until oesophageal speech is developed.

4 Providing adequate nutrition in the form of glucose and proteins from the early stages. Nitrogen loss does occur in such major surgery and can affect healing.

5 Providing sensitive psychological care for the patient and his family. It is not unusual for them to be quite depressed after the surgery.
Eventually the patient is taught self care of the tracheostomy.

Tracheostomy

This is a surgical opening into the trachea below the level of the larynx. It may be temporary or permanent.

Indications for tracheostomy

Temporary
1 Obstruction of the airway due to facial injuries, burns, pharyngeal muscle paralysis or pharyngo tracheitis.
2 To shorten the airway for patients who are too weak to move their tidal volume effectively.
3 To enable tracheal aspiration of excessive secretions when the patient cannot cough.
4 For attachment to intermittent positive pressure ventilators. (Some surgeons prefer to use endotracheal intubation in the early stages.)
Permanent Laryngectomy – usually for malignancy

Suggested nursing response
Pre operative assessment and care includes recognition of the patients fear and giving a careful explanation of the procedure.

Surgery The incision is made beneath the ring of the cricoid cartilage and isthmus of the thyroid gland. Either a silver tube with an inner tube or a plastic tube will be inserted and secured by taper. Modern cuffed tubes have a low pressure 'floppy' cuff and do not need to be deflated as previously.

Post operative assessment and care involves:
1 Maintenance of the airway by tracheal suction. This is important in the early stages as any bleeding may cause clots which can obstruct the tube. Inner tubes may need to be removed and cleaned to remove deposits. A replacement tube is left at the bedside with a pair of tracheal dilators. If a tube should fall out, the replacement must be introduced immediately.

2 Prevention of infection by aseptic technique for dressings and aspiration.

3 Ensuring good communication with the patient with a call bell, pad and pencil or indicator card. In the early stages the patient should not be left, but later the patient with a permanent tracheostomy will be taught to care for it himself.

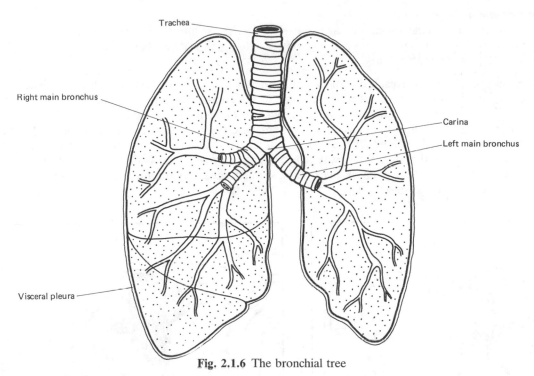

Fig. 2.1.6 The bronchial tree

Bronchial tree

Functions	Structure involved
1 Continuation of the airway	Cartilage rings in walls prevent collapse
2 Continual filtering and moistening of the air	Ciliated epithelial mucous membrane
3 Protection of alveoli from physical and chemical irritants	Mucous secretions and sensitive membranes cause coughing. Smooth muscles cause bronchospasm if continually irritated
4 Controlling the partial pressure of gases, especially carbon dioxide and oxygen in alveoli	Smooth muscle dilates on inspiration, constricts on expiration

Note: Air is not sterile – a large lymphatic drainage is provided in the airway. Bronchioles (the terminal ends of the tree) do not have cartilage in the walls. In children with bronchiolitis, they may collapse and obstruct – still causing asphyxia.

Conditions of the bronchial tree

Acute bronchitis

Should really be considered with the upper respiratory tract infections – see coryza etc.

Special effects Inflammation of the bronchi causes a cough which is initially dry and irritating but later there is tenacious mucoid or muco-purulent sputum.

Nursing notes
It is tempting to try to suppress the cough in the early stages with a linctus. This should be avoided. A sweet syrup or honey will have the effect of soothing the cough and giving more energy without suppressing respirations (would lead to sputum retention and pneumonia).
All other care is as for upper respiratory tract infections.

Chronic bronchitis (chronic obstructive airway disease)

This is a distinctive disease from acute bronchitis. There are chronic inflammatory changes in the bronchial tree.

Cause factors The main cause factors are:
1 *Irritants* Air pollution cigarette smoking, dust particles, sulphur dioxide
2 *Infections* Usually recurrent childhood infections and as a complication of measles
3 *Industry* For example: the effects of silica on quarry workers (silicosis), coal dust in coal miners (pneumoconiosis)

Effects, signs and symptoms

1 *Early changes* Inflammation of the mucous membrane leads to excessive mucus formation, irritation and possible bronchospasm. The patient complains of a cough with sputum, usually early in the morning. Cilia are damaged by cigarette smoke and cannot move the mucus while the patient is sleeping. There may be wheezing due to bronchospasm.

Suggested nursing response
The patient rarely seeks much help at this early stage. Important health education points are:
  1 there is no such thing as a normal morning cough.   *2* the effects on a marriage?
Advice at all stages – *stop smoking*.

2 *Progressive changes* Resolution of the inflammation is rarely complete and chronic thickening of the mucous membrane leads to the danger of infections. The main organisms involved are *streptococcus pneumoniae* and *haemophilus influenza*, but others may be involved.

There is also danger of the formation of micro-abscesses in the tissues. The patient will have a more persistent cough with either flecks of pus or larger quantities in the sputum. Bronchospasm may be more marked and as the airway may be quite narrow, there is increased dyspnoea.

Fever will occur with pyrexia, tachycardia, loss of energy, dehydration and mood changes. The leucocyte count will be raised.

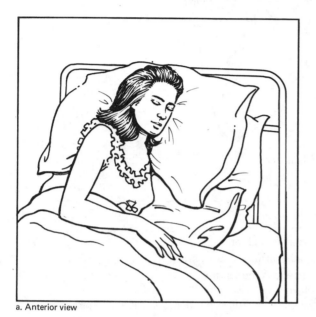
a. Anterior view
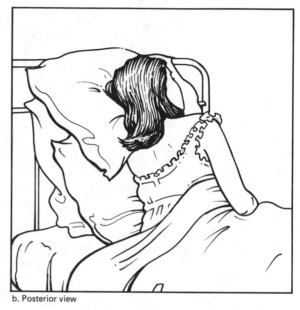
b. Posterior view

Fig. 2.1.7 High side lying position for patients with dyspnoea

Suggested nursing response

Assessment	Care
1 Observe sputum and dyspnoea	Collect specimens before antibacterial drugs commence.
	Provide disposable sputum pots and handkerchiefs.
	Help with physiotherapy – breathing and coughing exercises.
	Assist expectoration of sputum with mucolytic agents (e.g. steam inhalations).
	Expectorants (a cup of tea works well!).
	Do not give a linctus or any drug which may suppress breathing or coughing.
	Orthopnoeic or high side lying position
2 Assess fever	
1 tachycardia – pulse recorded 4 hourly	Rest in bed. Careful positioning
2 pyrexia – temperature recorded 4 hourly	Maintain temperature with light clothing and fan cooling
3 loss of energy ⎫ *4* dehydration ⎭	Give extra fluids with glucose added for energy

Drug administration
1 Antibacterial drugs may be given in high doses for first 48 hours. Give most 30 minutes before meals for good blood levels.
2 May need intravenous antispasmodic drugs. Nurse may need to assist doctor, observe puncture sites, and for desired and undesired effects.
3 Inhalants may be given via a nebulizer – mucolytic agents and antispasmodics can be given this way.

Development and effects of emphysema

Chronic fibrosis will progressively lead to airway narrowing and obstruction. The partial pressure of gases in the alveoli is altered and leads to changes in the blood. Carbon dioxide retention is the early problem.

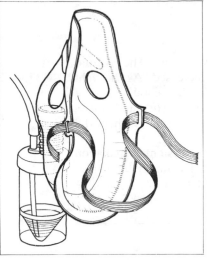

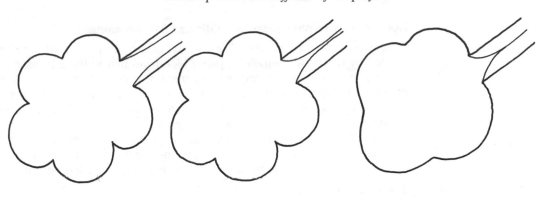

Normal – inspiration

Thickening of bronchiole membrane narrows lumen. During expiration the pressure in the alveolus increases. Carbon dioxide is retained.

Airway obstruction complete. Alveolus destroyed and bulla formed. No gas exchange → hypoxia.

Fig. 2.1.8 Inhalation nebulizer

Fig. 2.1.9 Diagrammatic representation for emphysema bulla formation

Later destruction of the alveoli is due to a combination of air trapping, inflammation and possibly an effect of cigarette smoke in encouraging catabolism of proteins. The alveoli destroyed are functionless and no gas exchange can take place in them – this will lead to an increasing hypoxia as more are destroyed. *Emphysema* is the trapping of the air and individual swellings are known as *bullae*.

The patient has increasing dyspnoea with the use of the accessory muscles of respiration. The lungs are hyper inflated, causing a flat diaphragm, narrow mediastinum on chest X-ray and the typical 'barrel chest' appearance. There is a progressive loss of energy with hypoxia and many can no longer work – they may be registered as disabled with emphysema.

The nurse should try to imagine the effects of this disease process on a patient's family – consider the changes of esteem for the victim, the loss of earnings and ultimately the home care that will be needed.

Retention of carbon dioxide leads to changes in the control of respiration in the medulla of the brain. Stimulus for increased ventilation is through the hypoxia recorded in the carotid sinus chemoreceptors. Carbon dioxide levels may continue to rise as the disease progresses and also if the patient gets pneumonia in non damaged lung tissue. Carbon dioxide then acts as a narcotic, depresses the nervous system, makes the patient become drowsy and may lead to a coma.

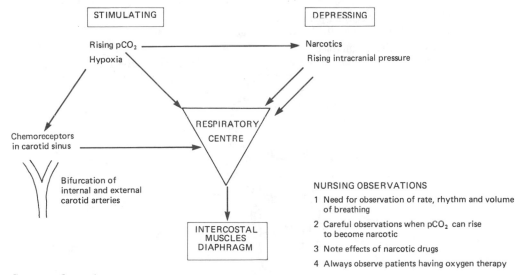

Fig. 2.1.10 The action of blood gases on the respiratory centre

Suggested nursing response

Assessment	Care
1 Observations of breathing – rate, rhythm and volume	Assist with physiotherapy. Use effort exhaling through pursed lips.
2 Observe for hypoxia	Oxygen therapy 24–28% maximum
3 Observe for drowsiness	If still becoming drowsy, doctor informed. Difficult problem for the doctor ? ventilation, ? respiratory stimulants
4 Assess effects of identity loss and social effects	Careful psychological support. May need economic help. Some home nursing may be needed

Development of pulmonary heart disease (cor pulmonale)

Progressive destruction of alveoli leads to damage to the pulmonary capillary network. The pressure needed by the right ventricle to pump blood through to the left heart is increased. As the right ventricle works harder, it begins to enlarge but eventually it will fail to take the venous return of blood adequately. This leads to pressure changes in the systemic capillary network and causes widespread oedema. Neck veins are distended, the liver becomes engorged and with portal interference, dyspepsia and ascites may occur.

Remember that the blood supply to the pleura in the lungs is through the systemic circulation and that a pleural effusion can occur – making breathing even more difficult. The nurse should also realize that the toxaemia from pneumonia may cause the left ventricle to fail too.

Suggested nursing response

Assessment	Care

1 Degree and effects of oedema
  1 examine legs and sacrum
  2 breathlessness from effusion
  3 fluid balance
  4 sodium retention
2 Undesired effects of drugs
  1 digoxin (pulse and apex beats)
  2 diuretics (effects of potassium loss)
	Care of pressure areas. Careful positioning of the patient. Stress good lifting techniques. Drainage of fluid e.g. chest aspiration. Reduced sodium diet.

Complications

Broncho pneumonia (p 20); *Pneumothorax* (p 25); *Polycythaemia* – chronic hypoxia causes excessive production of erythrocytes leading to an increased blood viscosity.

Danger for our patient – *deep vein thrombosis* and *pulmonary embolism*.

Nurse's role in specific investigations

Investigation	Nurse's role
1 Chest X-rays	The patient needs to be able to sit up straight for a good view; assess before going to department or arrange portable X-ray
2 Sputum	Culture and sensitivity specimens needed before antibacterial drugs are given. Specimens for histology are usually taken

3 Lung function tests
  1 vitalograph
  2 peak-flow meter
	
	Assess that patient can co-operate
	Operate apparatus correctly. Record accurately

4 Blood gas analysis	No problems if re-breathing technique. If arterial puncture, exert digital pressure for 5-10 minutes and observe for 24 hours

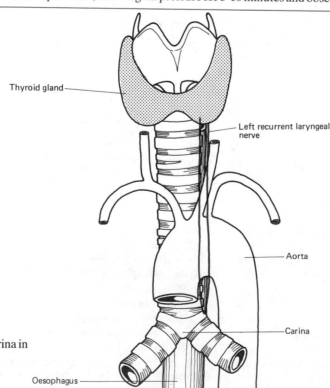

Fig. 2.1.11 The carina in relationship to the recurrent laryngeal nerve

Thyroid gland

Left recurrent laryngeal nerve

Aorta

Carina

Oesophagus

Carcinoma of the bronchus

The most common malignant condition in Britain.

Cause factors

1 The main cause factor is cigarette smoking.
2 Other cause factors are working with asbestos, nickel and chromium.
3 Air pollution has been blamed, but one of the highest incidences is the Channel Islands!

Effects, signs and symptoms Most tumours occur within 4 cm of the carina. Infiltration of the mucous membrane causes irritation. The patient has a cough which he usually ignores.

Further infiltration will cause inflammation of the mucous membrane. Occlusion of a bronchus may occur leading to collapse of lung tissue behind the obstruction (atelactesis). This causes even further inflammation and infection (pneumonitis). The patient may feel unwell and have all the signs and symptoms of a chest infection, but it does not readily respond to treatment.

Suggested nursing response is as for chest infection.
Local infiltration may cause erosion through the sub mucous coat and a blood vessel may rupture leading to haemoptysis (coughing of blood). This is a frightening experience for the patient. It usually causes him to seek medical help.

Suggested nursing response

Assessment	Care
1 Blood loss (measured in sputum pot)	Prepare for possible blood transfusion
2 Degree of tear	Give assurance and support
3 If cough persists	A cough suppressant – even a narcotic may be prescribed

Local infiltration near to the carina may involve the recurrent laryngeal nerve and cause paralysis of the vocal cords. The patient complains of a husky voice at first, but it may go on to produce a very distressing *laryngeal stridor.*

Suggested nursing response
The patient is very alarmed and self conscious about his noisy breathing. He may withdraw and wish to be nursed in isolation. Relatives find it distressing too. Tracheostomy may be needed. Sedation is often required.
The pleura may be involved (note the proximity of the pleura in the hilum of the lung) and a large *pleural effusion* may occur.
The patient complains of dyspnoea – 'as if a band were round my chest, nurse'.

Suggested nursing response
Prepare for chest aspiration
1 Position the patient carefully.
2 Assist the doctor and observe the patient. Warn if he wishes to cough.
3 Aseptic technique and dressing applied.
4 Observe site and patient for indications of recurrence or collapse from air embolism (rare).

If the brachial plexus is infiltrated, severe pain in the neck and arms will result. Strong analgesia is indicated.

Lymphatic metastases

Spread of the tumour cells to lymph nodes is fairly rapid. The scalene nodes in the root of the neck or the hilar nodes are involved. Gross enlargement can cause compression and occlusion of a bronchus leading to atelactesis. The enlargement may also compress the superior vena cava – an ominous development *superior vena caval obstruction.*

The patient complains of a tight collar, swelling of the neck and face, headache and also swollen arms.

Prognosis is very poor at this stage.

Suggested nursing response

Assessment	Care
1 Swelling of neck, face and arms – possibly measuring	Use loose clothing around neck
2 Enquire if headache	Analgesia as prescribed

Note: *Radiotherapy* may be used to treat superior vena caval obstruction
1 Nursing care of the skin irradiated.
2 May have difficulty in swallowing as oesophagus may be inflamed.

Haemorrhagic metastases

The main sites for secondary tumours spread by the blood stream are

1 *The brain* This causes severe headaches, behavioural changes, epilepsy, meningism, ultimately coma and death.

Suggested nursing response – see *care of brain tumours*, p 112.
Principles

1 Analgesia for headaches
2 Understanding of behavioural changes
3 Anticonvulsants for epilepsy
4 Care of unconscious patient

2 *The bones* – notably the spinal column. These cause severe pain and possibly paraplegia.

Suggested nursing response Very difficult nursing problems here:

1 to give strong analgesics depresses respirations and causes pneumonia.
2 spinal lesions require the patient to be nursed flat, but our patient has breathing difficulty. Agreement with the patient on his most comfortable position and regime would seem to be an intelligent approach, but it has to be an individual approach.

3 *The liver* – which may produce jaundice and liver failure

Suggested nursing response

1 Skin care is important
2 Liver failure may alter action of drugs.

General disease

There is a pattern of rapidly progressing cachexia (debility) with weight loss, weakness, sallow complexion and a lowered resistance to infection.

Diagnosis is made by examining sputum for malignant cells, examining pleural fluid for cells, possibly a pleural biopsy, bronchoscopy and biopsy.

Bronchoscopy

Suggested nursing response
Pre operative assessment and preparation

1 Check that the patient understands
2 Check for indications of infection
3 Nil by mouth for 4–6 hours

Bronchoscopy is usually carried out under local anaesthetic to the throat. Even if a general anaesthetic is used, some anaesthetists will still apply a local anaesthetic to the throat.

Biopsy is done through the endoscope.

Post operative assessment and care

1 Until swallow reflex has returned (careful testing after about 4 hours) nil by mouth to prevent inhalation of fluid.
2 Nurse in semi prone position to prevent inhalation of vomit. Observe carefully.
3 Observe for haemoptysis or indications of internal haemorrhage.

Treatment for carcinoma of bronchus

1 Surgical
   1 Lobectomy
   2 Pneumonectomy   } But only 5% survive 5 years.
2 Radiotherapy – some successes recorded.
3 Cytotoxic drugs – some successes but note the danger of infection if leucopenia occurs.

Prognosis for carcinoma of bronchus is still very poor.

Suggested nursing response

1 Health educationalist – prevention by discouraging cigarette smoking is vital.
2 Care of the terminally ill and dying patient. This is a condition that you should apply your total nursing care assessment and care plan to (see 1.3).

Bronchial asthma

Cause Hypersensitivity of the bronchial tree to various stimuli including antigens (known as allergens). The allergens may be grouped as:

1 *Animal*	furs, feathers, dust (mainly shed keratin from skin), house dust mites
2 *Vegetable*	pollens, spores from various plants e.g. grasses, flowers
3 *Fungi*	certain moulds (particularly dangerous – aspergillus)
4 *Minerals*	talcum powder, cosmetics
5 *Other stimuli*	micro-organisms (infection), drugs (see especially aspirin, penicillin), cold air.

There is debate about two other factors

6 *Exercise* Some find that strenuous exercise may bring on an attack, but some top athletes are known to have asthma.

7 *Psychological* There is a clear relationship, in many patients, with stress, emotions and their asthmatic attacks, It is difficult to know which came first though – asthma itself causes stress.

Suggested nursing response

Assessment	Care
1 Presence and reaction to allergens or other stimuli	Nursing environment should be free from possible allergens (e.g. avoid feather pillows, vacuum bedding for mites)
2 Psychological reactions	A calm, confident approach – firm but understanding attitude is important

Effects, signs and symptoms Inflammatory response of mucous membranes causes oedema and narrowing of the airway and an increase in sputum content. The sputum is thick and tenacious making it difficult to expectorate. Fungi may form casts which may appear in the sputum. The inflammatory response also causes severe, spasmodic contractions of the smooth muscles, causing even further narrowing, especially as the patient exhales. This causes the characteristic 'wheezing' and acute 'tightness of the chest'. There may be alteration of blood gases, with carbon dioxide retention, and hypoxia may eventually cause cyanosis.

Status asthmaticus is the condition when the attack is persistent. The patient becomes progressively agitated and distressed.

Suggested nursing response

Assessment	Care
1 Cough and sputum for casts or pus	Provide sputum pot and handkerchiefs. Help patient to cough effectively
2 Observe	
1 respiration rate, rhythm and volume	Assist with physiotherapy (concentrate on exhaling)
2 for indications of carbon dioxide retention	Give prescribed oxygen with great care (24–28% concentration – remove if the patient becomes drowsy)
3 for indications of hypoxia	

Status asthmaticus is a medical emergency. Drugs may be needed intravenously and the nurse needs to ensure that they are available immediately.

Management

1 Ensure a calm efficient atmosphere. Staff need to be aware of needs and the positive approach. A team approach with physiotherapists is ideal.

2 Drugs
  1 *Antispasmodics* Aminophyline or salbutamol intravenously for acute attack. Salbutamol inhalations for less acute attack.
  2 *Anti-inflammatory* Hydrocortisone intravenously followed by oral steroids.
  3 *Antibacterial agents* if evidence of bacterial infection.

3 Oxygen therapy is not always tolerated by the patient with asthma. It is only vital if signs of hypoxia occur.

Desensitization

Patients who are hypersensitive to specific allergens may be desensitized. A series of graduated, increasing challenges of the allergens are made under controlled conditions. It may be done in a specialist out-patient clinic or some general practitioners may do it in their own surgery.

Suggested nursing response
The nurse might be involved either in out-patients or as a Community nurse helping the general practitioner. The important danger is anaphylactic shock. Adrenaline 1:1000 should be available for immediate use.

Prophylaxis

Some patients find benefit from inhalations of sodium cromoglycate to prevent the antibody/antigen response. Not all physicians are happy with its use however.

Bronchiectasis

Is a condition in which there are distensions of the terminal bronchi.

Cause The cause is thought to be plugs of thick mucus causing an obstruction, or obstructions, from outside the lumen in infants by enlarged lymph nodes. One common cause was whooping cough. It may be associated with cystic fibrosis.

Nursing notes
This condition emphasizes the need for early and effective treatment of chest infections and the health education need for information about vaccination as well as treatment.

Effects, signs and symptoms The dilated sacs in the bronchi become traps for mucus and infected material. There can be quite constant purulent sputum being expectorated. Occasionally, the infection causes erosion through a blood vessel and haemoptysis may occur. If not treated effectively, there is progressive loss of energy and weight due to chronic inflammation.

Suggested nursing response

Assessment	Care
Observations of	
1 sputum for infection	Sputum collection
2 pyrexia and tachycardia	Rest in bed. Cooling. Energy foods
3 evidence of haemoptysis	Reassurance and (rarely) blood transfusion

Treatment
Medical Antibacterial drugs for infection. Postural drainage of sputum.

Nursing notes
The nurse needs to give drugs as prescribed. Observe for undesired effects of antibacterial agents. Assistance with postural drainage and encouragement is important.

Surgery If bronchiectasis is confined then surgical removal may be indicated. See lobectomy or pneumonectomy.

2 Lung tissue

Functions	Structures involved
1 Release of carbon dioxide from the blood	Alveoli – collection of air sacs terminal to the bronchioles of the bronchial tree
2 Perfusion of oxygen into haemoglobin of erythrocytes in the blood	Blood vessels – pulmonary arteries, arterioles, capillaries around alveoli, venules and pulmonary veins, reticular connective tissues

Conditions of the lung tissue

Pneumonia – pneumonitis

Causes Inflammation of lung tissue is usually caused by micro-organisms (infection) but may be caused by inhaled toxins too. The main micro-organisms involved are:

1 Viruses
2 Haemophilus influenzae
3 Streptococcus pneumoniae (pneumococcus)
4 Eschericia coli (more rarely)
5 Staphylococci (note the serious danger of profound toxaemia from exotoxins)

The classification of pneumonias varies in different text books.

The useful classification from a nursing needs point of view is
1 *Broncho pneumonia* when there are multiple foci of infection at the ends of the bronchi.
2 *Lobar pneumonia* when one or more lobes of lung tissue are inflamed including the associated visceral pleura.

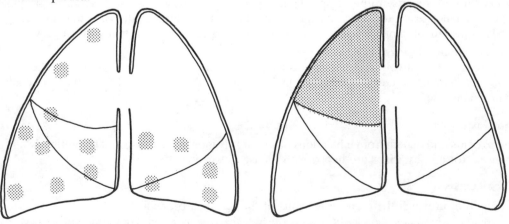

a. Broncho pneumonia   b. Right upper lobe pneumonia

Fig. 2.1.12 Lung field appearances on X-ray plates

Effects, signs and symptoms

1 *Local* Inflamed lung tissue is engorged with blood and is described as consolidated. It appears opaque on a chest X-ray.

Broncho pneumonia appearances are 'like fluffy ball patches' of consolidation. There is less pain in broncho pneumonia, but there is usually associated bronchitis causing the patient to have a cough. Sputum eventually appears and may be muco-purulent or purulent, sometimes containing flecks of blood which gives a characteristic rusty coloured appearance. The cough is exhausting to the patient and may cause considerable soreness in the thorax.

Lobar pneumonia appearance is a distinct opaqueness of the lobe(s) involved. There is considerable pain due to pleurisy as the visceral pleura is inflamed. The pain is most acute on inhalation (pleuritic pain). The cough and sputum may be similar in effect to broncho pneumonia.

Suggested nursing response

Assessment	Care
1 Observe type and degree of pain	There are difficulties in controlling acute pain. Strong analgesia would depress respirations and cause more hypoxia. Local heat applications (Kaolin poultice) may be effective
2 Observe cough and sputum appearances (as patient becomes more exhausted, it is more difficult to expectorate)	May need assistance with expectoration

2 *Hypoxia and carbon dioxide retention* Inflammation of lung tissue causes a failure of gas exchange in the alveoli leading to carbon dioxide retention and low oxygen concentrations in the blood (hypoxia).

The patient experiences difficulty in breathing. The respirations become rapid and shallow. He may find difficulty thinking at first, may become confused, and exhaustion will increase. Tachycardia will occur. *Cyanosis* is a late sign of hypoxia and needs urgent care.

Carbon dioxide retention will eventually cause a depression of the nervous system (narcosis) making the patient more drowsy and respirations even more shallow. Coma may occur.

Suggested nursing response

Assessment	Care
1 Indications of hypoxia	Give prescribed oxygen therapy, normal 40–50%, patient
2 Observe respiratory rate, rhythm and volume	with chronic lung disease 24–28%
3 Observe behaviour	If drowsy, inform doctor
4 Observe for cyanosis	
5 Observe effects of oxygen therapy	Support in orthopnoeic or high side lying position. Remember – the patient is exhausted

3 *Severe toxaemia*

There is a marked rise in the metabolic rate in both types of pneumonia.

Pyrexia The temperature may rise over 40°C and rigors may occur (febrile convulsions in children). 'Swinging' of temperatures may be demonstrated on charts.

Tachycardia There is an acute increase in heart rate with a reduction of the refractory period of the cardiac cycle. Cardiac arrhythmias may occur and heart failure may be the cause of death.

Energy resources (glucose and glycogen stores) will be used up rapidly, increasing the exhaustion. As energy stores are depleted, proteins may be used with subsequent muscle weakness and wasting.

Dehydration will occur due to excess water loss from sweating and metabolic processes.

Toxaemia produces behavioural changes such as confusion and delirium.

The patient will feel alternatively hot or cold (shivery). He will be very tired and weak. He may experience palpitations and can collapse.

The mouth will be dry and coated. Some patients get herpes around the lips which can be very irritating and sore.

Staphylococcal pneumonia

May lead to a profound toxaemia due to the release of exotoxins. 'Toxic shock' describes the condition when blood pressure can no longer be maintained.

Pneumonia is still a very dangerous condition and patients are in danger of dying.

Suggested nursing response

Assessment	Care
1 Indications of toxaemia	
2 Observe temperature (record at least 4 hourly)	Cooling techniques. Light clothing and a fan. (Tepid sponging can tire the patient even more)
3 Observe pulse rate, rhythm and volume (frequency of recording depends on condition)	Complete bed rest
4 Note weakness and exhaustion	Glucose drinks, protein in convalescent stage
5 Observe dehydration	Fluids, mouth care frequently
6 Observe behavioural changes	Protect the patient in delirium and confusion

Note: In children, the vomiting centre may be affected and great care is needed to prevent inhalation of vomit. This is a condition where you do need to apply your own model for a total patient care plan. Remember the problems of communication and fear of dying.

Nurse's role in specific investigations

Investigation	Nurse's role
1 Chest X-rays	The patient who is exhausted may need physical support whilst X-rays are taken. Protective aprons must be worn
2 Sputum	Save all early specimens of sputum. Culture and sensitivity can only be done on specimens taken before antibacterial drugs are given. Inform the doctor of pathology results
3 Blood gases	Assist the doctor to obtain samples. If arterial sample is taken apply digital pressure for 5–10 minutes and observe for 12–24 hours. Report results
4 Drugs	Antibacterial drugs. Blood levels need to be kept high, especially in first 24–48 hours. Drugs may be given intravenously with great care. Observe for undesired effects of drugs – especially hypersensitivity

Prognosis Although a dangerous condition, modern treatment and nursing has reduced mortality greatly and patients can be reasonably reassured of complete recovery.

Pulmonary tuberculosis

Is caused by the bacillus mycobacterium tuberculosis. Factors affecting development of the disease are malnutrition, overcrowding and poverty. It is a notifiable infectious disease and although the incidence rate has fallen dramatically since 1960, recent outbreaks and immigrant cases have given cause for concern. Spread of infection is by droplet infection from the patients coughing or contact through articles used by the patient.

Nursing notes
Isolation is still indicated, although the danger of cross infection is minimal in modern general wards. All sputum pots and handkerchiefs are incinerated and cutlery sterilized.

Nursing staff need to be reminded about their own health, BCG vaccination and the need for chest X-ray if in contact with cases.

Effects, signs and symptoms
1 *The Primary complex*
A small focus of infection occurs in the lung tissue (Ghon focus). The lymph vessels draining the part may be inflamed (lymphangitis) and the lymph node may be involved (lymphadenitis).
Primary complex = Ghon focus + lymphangitis + lymphadenitis.
This complex often resolves with very few indications of disease but complications that may arise are:

1 an enlarged lymph node may compress a young bronchus and, by occlusion, cause atelectasis (collapse of lung tissue). The child would present with indications of a chest infection.

2 spread of infection through the blood stream may cause miliary tuberculosis, with multiple areas of inflammation in the lungs and other organs including the meninges and kidneys.
The formation of antibodies will be stimulated by this first attack. This may provide active acquired immunity against a further invasion.
The Heaf and Mantoux tests determine the presence of the antibodies.

Nursing notes
A positive Heaf or Mantoux test would indicate either
1 infection is present at the time of the test, or
2 antibodies were formed some time before the test.

2 *Post Primary disease*
Local Infection tends to begin in the upper lobes of the lungs. Inflammation leads to the formation of a tubercular abscess containing the characteristic 'cheese like' pus (caseation). The pus is then

expectorated leaving behind a cavity with a thick fibrosed wall around it. Unfortunately bacilli remain to continue the process and the cavities may enlarge. Widespread lung damage develops and there is danger of erosion through a blood vessel.

In the early stages, there are few signs and symptoms and progress is insidious. There may be an irritating cough with increasing amounts of sputum. Involvement of the pleura may cause chest pain and rupture of a cavity into the pleura would cause a pneumothorax. Erosion of a blood vessel leads to haemoptysis.

General As the metabolic rate increases, the patient becomes more tired, apathetic and listless. Loss of weight will be due to extensive protein breakdown (both in the lung tissue and to provide energy). There is a classical 'swinging' temperature. Pyrexia in the evening is followed by profuse night sweats and a subnormal temperature in the morning.

Occasionally, there is a rash known as erythema nodosum – patches of inflammation on the skin which are thought to be an allergic reaction to a tuberculotoxin.

Complications
1 Miliary tuberculosis
2 TB laryngitis
3 Fistula in ano. Mycobacterium tuberculosis are not killed by gastric juice and may lodge in the rectal wall after passage through the alimentary tract, the subsequent lesion can be infected by coliform organisms too.

Suggested nursing response

Assessment	Care
1 Cough	Assist with coughing
2 Sputum	Care of sputum pots and handkerchiefs. Collect early morning specimens for culture and sensitivity (or gastric washings)
3 Haemoptysis	Give reassurance to the patient. May need sedation and possible blood transfusion if there is severe loss
4 Raised metabolic rate: pyrexia; tachycardia	Rest in bed according to temperature and pulse rate. Give glucose drinks. Change bed clothing if night sweats
5 Weight loss and muscle wasting	Increased protein in the diet

Complications
1 *Miliary* Observe for deterioration, care and treatment are the same
2 *Meningitis* Observe for loss of consciousness, care of coma patient should be included
3 *Kidney* Observe for haematuria
4 *TB laryngitis* See care of laryngitis
5 *Fistula in ano* May require analgesics, dressings and possible surgery

Treatment The modern treatment of tuberculosis is in two phases:

1 *The initial phase* makes use of at least three antituberculous drugs e.g. daily doses of isoniazid + rifampicin with either ethambutol or streptomycin – continued for at least eight weeks or until the results of drug sensitivity testing. (Colonies grow very slowly – culture and sensitivity may be as much as twelve weeks.)

2 *The continuation phase* uses two drugs, usually isoniazid and rifampicin, ethambutol or streptomycin – continued for about nine months.

Nursing notes
Long term treatment It is very important to gain co-operation of the patient or ensure correct administration of drugs under supervision, to prevent the development of drug resistant organisms.

Undesired effects of drugs See the British National Formulary

Note:
1 Streptomycin – prevent sensitization of staff (wear mask and gloves).
  Beware of vestibular disturbance, especially in elderly patients.
2 Ethambutol beware of visual disturbances.
3 Rifampicin – may damage the liver.

Prevention Prevention is mainly through improved social conditions, education and immunization by BCG (Bacille, Calmette-Guerin) vaccine.

Nursing notes
The nurse's role as a health educator is vital here.

BCG can only be given following a Mantoux or Heaf test which should be negative. A careful explanation to parents and children should be given (children have been known to play truant to avoid the '6 needles'!).

Pulmonary embolism

Causes

1 A clot, or fragment of clot, detached from a deep vein thrombosis travels through the venous return, the right ventricle, pulmonary trunk and a pulmonary artery.
2 A clot may detach from the wall of the right side of the heart following myocardial infarction (mural thrombus).
3 An air bubble may enter a vein and travel through the venous return and pulmonary trunk.
4 A fat globule may enter the venous return following a fracture (fat embolism).
5 Pus may enter the venous return.

Effects, signs and symptoms

The size of the obstruction will determine the amount of lung tissue involved and the effects on the patient.

Large infarction This is one of the few medical causes of *sudden death* – due to acute and profound hypoxia and heart failure. There may be no warning, but occasionally the patient may describe a sudden 'urge to pass stools' just before the event. Some will have a severe chest pain and present in a state of shock. They may be saved by emergency thoractomy and embolectomy.

Smaller infarction Inflammation will occur around the infarcted tissue. The patient experiences pleuritic pain as the pleura is involved. Indications of general inflammation vary in individual patients. Occasionally, pieces of clot and blood get into the airway and haemoptysis will be seen.

Suggested nursing response

Assessment	Care
1 Degree of pain	Position according to blood pressure recording
2 Pain	Analgesia
	(Possibly preparation for emergency thoractomy)
3 Raised metabolic rate with general inflammation	Rest, maintain temperature
4 Haemoptysis	Reassurance, possible sedation required

Treatment Many patients would be given anticoagulant therapy to prevent further clot formation.

Nursing notes

Observe carefully all patients having anticoagulants for indications of haemorrhage. Aspirin cannot be used for analgesia if anticoagulants are used.

Thrombolytic drugs may be used occasionally to encourage the breakdown of a persistent clot.

3 Lung surroundings

Pleura, ribs, intercostal muscles and diaphragm

Functions	Structures involved
1 Breathing (ventilation of lung tissue)	
1 Inhalation	Intercostal muscles contract. Diaphragm flattens as muscles contract. Parietal pleura attached to inner side of ribs, muscles and diaphragm exerts pull on the visceral pleura (two moist surfaces) causing lungs to expand and draw air in through the airway
2 Exhalation	Intercostal muscles relax. Diaphragm returns to dome shape as muscles relax. Elasticity of lung tissue will cause lungs to contract and push air out of the airway
Control of breathing rate, rhythm and volume is through activity of the respiratory centre in the medulla of the brain stem. Breathing may be controlled by the will, but is normally a subconscious activity, dependent on blood gas concentrations.	
2 Protection of the contents of the thoracic cavity	Ribs and chest wall provide some protection from injury

Conditions of the surroundings of the lungs

Pleurisy – inflammation of the pleura

Causes

1 Infection (also associated with lobal pneumonia)
2 Irritants in the pleural space
3 Infarcted lung tissue (see pulmonary embolism)
4 Infiltration by neoplasms

Effects, signs and symptoms

1 *Local* The inflamed pleura causes the patient to become aware of his breathing action. Receptors on the parietal pleura cause acute pain on inspiration. The patient tends to breathe less deeply to avoid the pain but may subsequently have more hypoxia.

Nursing notes

It is important to give prescribed analgesia to enable the patient to breathe more freely. Local heat application may help too. Pain relief should be followed up by breathing exercises and physiotherapy.

Later, there may be excessive production of serous fluid leading to a pleural effusion. The patient experiences increasing 'tightness' in his chest and dyspnoea.

Suggested nursing response

It will be necessary for the nurse to prepare the patient (and a trolley) for chest aspirations.

Procedure

1 Local anaesthetic
2 Drainage through an aspiration needle attached to a syringe via a two way tap
3 Aseptic dressing

Nursing points

▶ Upright position with arms over a table
▶ Aseptic technique
▶ Observe and reassure the patient
▶ Warning if he wishes to cough

▶ Record fluid colour and amount
▶ Save specimens and label carefully
▶ Observe site and patient for possible infection or pneumothorax

2 *General* Pleurisy will again lead to an increased metabolic rate as general response to inflammation.

Nursing note

See *care of lobar pneumonia*, p 21.

Empyema is a collection of pus in the pleural cavity. It is comparatively rare in modern medicine. Thoracic surgery is required for drainage and decortication. Long term dressings may be required.

Pneumothorax – air in the pleural space

Causes

1 *Trauma* Fractured ribs and stab wounds may allow air to enter the space from outside. Penetration of the visceral pleura will cause air from the lungs to enter the space.

2 *Congenital* Small blebs on the visceral pleura may be due to congenital weakness. They are called bullae and may rupture when the patient coughs, breathes in suddenly or is engaged in vigorous exercise (referred to as *spontaneous*).

3 *Chronic bronchitis and emphysema* A bulla near to the visceral pleura may rupture – usually when the patient coughs.

4 *Pulmonary tuberculosis* A cavity may rupture through the visceral pleura.

5 *Thoracotomy* Surgery in the thoracic cavity usually leaves a pneumothorax.

Effects, signs and symptoms Loss of continuous contact of the two wet surfaces of the pleura prevents expansion of the lung tissue on inhalation and the underlying lung will collapse due to its own elasticity. Three stages may be considered but a patient can proceed from one stage to the next quite quickly.

Stage 1 As the lung begins to deflate, the perforation may close and leave only a 'shallow' pneumothorax with minimal lung collapse. The patient at this stage may have few signs and symptoms. There may be slight chest pain and shortness of breath on effort. Some may not even seek medical advice.

Suggested nursing response

Assessment	Care
1 Observations for the chest pain persisting and increasing shortness of breath	Mild analgesia may be prescribed
2 Visual inspection of the exposed chest will allow the nurse to see unevenness of expansion (asymmetrical breathing)	Rest in bed or in a chair may be sufficient
3 Observe for indications of fear	A confident approach is important

Stage 2 There is a progressive collapse of lung tissue until it is completely deflated, with progressive decrease in oxygenation. The patient becomes much more short of breath, even at rest, and may begin to show signs of hypoxia – loss of concentration, restlessness, tachycardia and eventually cyanosis.

Suggested nursing response

1 Continual observations for hypoxia are important. Cyanosis is a **late** sign.
2 Give prescribed oxygen concentration.
3 Prepare for insertion of intercostal drain (see overpage).

Stage 3 Some patients develop a pneumothorax with a valve like hole or flap of tissue. As the patient inhales, air passes through the flap into the pleural space. When he exhales the air is trapped in the space as the flap closes. Pressure of air will increase in the pleural space (*tension pneumothorax*) and will eventually cause the mediastinum to shift towards the opposite side. The venous return of blood to the heart is impeded, heart action is embarrassed and heart failure will occur.

The patient becomes distressed with severe tachycardia (palpitations) increasing cyanosis and fears that he is dying.

Suggested nursing response

This is an emergency needing quick action. A doctor may wish to insert a long, hollow needle into the chest immediately in order to relieve the tension, before proceeding with the insertion of the intercostal drain.

Assessment and preparation

1 Check the patient's understanding of the procedure and explain carefully.
2 Position the patient – usually sitting upright
  1 anterior site – lying against the pillows,
  2 posterior site – leaning forward over bed table.

Procedure

1 Local anaesthetic is given.
2 Small incision may be made.
3 Intercostal tube introduced with a trocar which is then removed.
4 Connect to long length of tubing which is attached to the long tube of the underwater seal – the end being under the fluid in the drainage bottle (fluid depends on doctor – normal saline is popular).
5 Intercostal tube may be attached to a Heimlich valve.
6 The tube is retained with an anchor suture.
7 The long tubing may be anchored to the bed clothes.

The nurse needs to assist the doctor and at the same time continue her observations of the patient throughout the procedure.

Assessment	Care
1 The patient for pain or breathlessness	Analgesia may be needed
2 The puncture site for inflammation or surgical emphysema	Aseptic dressing technique
3 The tubing for blockage by kinking or fluid	Report – may need resiting of tube. Move and 'milk' the tube carefully
4 The drainage apparatus. Note if bubbles or not and the presence of 'swing' (corresponds with breathing)	Report. Maintain position below the patient's chest to prevent syphoning. If drainage is stopped or broken, apply clamps to intercostal tube immediately. Apart from this, the tube should only be clamped on doctor's orders

Removal (when ordered by the doctor)
1 Prepare the patient with explanation and give analgesia before starting.
2 Check the position of the tube by looking at the chest X-ray.
3 Prepare occlusive dressing, free the tube and remove very quickly. (This prevents air entering through side holes.) It sometimes helps easy removal if the patient breathes in deeply before the tube is pulled.

The prognosis for a patient with pneumothorax is usually very good.

Patients who have a persistent pneumothorax despite drainage, or have had a previous one on the opposite side, may need a pleurectomy.

Thoracotomy

The only operations dealt with here are lobectomy and pneumonectomy. The principles are similar for other thoracic operations.

Indications for surgery

1 Trauma of lung tissue
2 Neoplasms – mainly carcinoma of the bronchus
3 More rarely now, bronchiectasis and pulmonary tuberculosis

Pre operative assessment and preparation

1 Respiratory functions
2 Physiotherapy
3 Many patients are given anticoagulants

Suggested nursing response

Assessment	Care
1 Respiration rate, rhythm and volume	Help with breathing exercises and coughing
2 Help with lung function tests	
3 State of cardio vascular system	
1 pulse, blood pressure	Rest and calm approach by staff
2 evidence of anaemia	Possible blood transfusion before surgery
3 temperature (in case of chest infection)	
4 Anxiety (relatives too!)	Reassurance
5 Skin condition	Washing and shaving

If anticoagulants are given – nursing observations for bleeding

Operation

Anaesthesia Very important **not** to use inflammable gases as diathermy will be used in close proximity. Endotracheal tube has to extend beyond the carina.

Position Lateral position of extension.

Incision Very long sub scapular, through the rib bed after eversion of periosteum.

Lobectomy Two drainage tubes – apical and basal.

Pneumonectomy Some do not insert a drain, some put in a clamped drain to be released hourly or on doctor's orders.

Post operative care is as in general surgery but some dangers to be aware of are:

  1 Obstruction of a bronchus with sputum (sometimes forms a thick plug) leading to atelactesis and infection.

Suggested nursing response

Breathing exercises and assistance with coughing need to be started as soon as possible. Both are obviously painful, but analgesics must be given in doses to avoid respiratory depression. The art is to use the effectiveness of the analgesic, by following up with exercises after the drug administration.

  2 Obstruction of intercostal drainage tubes or breakage of the under water seal.

Suggested nursing response

There needs to be continual observation of the site, the tubing and the bottle. Some surgeons would apply light suction to the drainage – this would eliminate any 'swing' in the tubing. Gentle, skilled 'milking' of the tube will assist drainage. If system breaks – apply 2 clamps immediately. Careful measurement of blood loss through chest drains can be balanced by controlling the blood transfusion rate.

  3 Development of a fistula through the bronchial stump if infection interferes with healing. (Infected fluid could enter the remaining healthy lung tissue.)

Suggested nursing response

The patient may be nursed towards the affected side to prevent this, to encourage drainage and to ventilate the unaffected lung. (Some schools do not incline patients in the early stages, but maintain good posture for total ventilation.)
All other care is really as for general surgery

Drains are removed on the surgeons instructions after chest X-rays (see removal of intercostal drains)
Sutures are removed as for general surgery
Mobilization Sit out the next day. Leg exercises as well as breathing and coughing

Trauma

Chest wall injuries are very painful. Even bruising may cause a serious inhibition of breathing with the danger of hypostatic pneumonia.

Suggested nursing response

Always observe respiration rate, rhythm and **volume**. Encourage deep breathing exercises following the administration of a prescribed analgesic. Careful posturing of the patient is important for good ventilation. The chest should **not** be bound unless expressly indicated by a doctor.

Fractured ribs

There are two dangerous effects of fractured ribs, apart from the shock of pain and possible haemorrhage.

  1 *Pneumothorax* Often a haemopneumothorax with blood and air in the pleural cavity.

2 *'Flail chest'* A segment of the chest wall can move paradoxically to the rest because a number of ribs are broken in two places. The tidal movement of air in the thoracic cavity instead of through the airways leads to progressive hypoxia.

Both should be treated as emergencies. They will need intercostal drainage, possibly the assistance of an Intermittent Positive Pressure Ventilator and will need intensive nursing care.

Suggested nursing response
The priorities of care here are:
1 Treatment for shock due to pain, haemorrhage and fear of dying.
2 Ensuring and maintaining a clear airway.
3 Prevention of chest infections and treatment if they should occur.

2.2   Cardiovascular conditions

Cardiovascular system

The major parts to be considered are as follows.
1 **The blood**   3 **The heart and circulations**
2 **The blood vessels**   4 **The lymphatic system**
   arteries; veins; capillaries   lymph capillaries and vessels; lymph nodes; spleen

1 The blood

Functions	Structures involved
1 Homeostasis	
1 Carriage of oxygen	Erythrocytes containing haemoglobin
2 Carriage of carbon dioxide	Plasma – bicarbonate ions and plasma proteins
3 Carriage of nutrients – glucose, amino acids, lipids, vitamins and salts	Plasma
4 Carriage of waste products of metabolism – creatinine, urea and carbon dioxide	Plasma
5 Carriage of drugs	Mainly plasma proteins
6 Acid/base (pH) balance	Plasma proteins, electrolytes
7 Temperature balance	Whole blood
2 Immunity	
1 Phagocytosis (ingestion of micro organisms)	Leucocytes (polymorphonuclei and monocytes)
2 Formation and carriage of antibodies	Lymphocytes. Immunoglobulins (plasma proteins)
3 Maintaining its own volume	
1 Blood clotting	Fibrinogen, prothrombin, calcium, platelets and clotting factors (see diagram)
2 Osmotic pressure draws fluids into capillaries	Plasma proteins – especially albumin

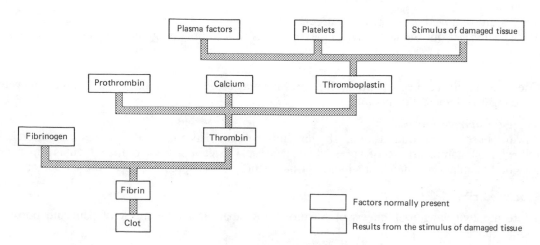

Fig. 2.2.1 Blood clotting

Production of red blood cells (erythropoiesis)

Manufacture takes place in the myeloid tissue (red bone marrow) at the rate of over 100 million per minute.

Factors
1 Kidney secretes the hormone **erythropoietin** – increased production follows blood loss or chronic hypoxia.
2 Erythropoietin stimulates the **myeloid tissue** to produce red cells.

Development

Pro **erythroblast** – large nucleated cells

↓

Normoblasts – smaller nucleated cells

↓

Reticulocytes – contain reticulin in the cytoplasm

  – leave bone marrow and enter blood stream at this stage

  – they already contain haemoglobin

↓

Erythrocytes 5×10^{15} per litre

Factors in development – from diet and body stores
1 Vitamin C   *4* Iron
2 Folic acid   *5* Vitamin B_{12} (absorption needs intrinsic factor in the stomach)
3 Amino acids

Blood groups and blood transfusion

These are determined by the presence of antigens on the cell membranes of erythrocytes. Reactions occur if the antigen meets a specific antibody in the plasma

	Antigen	Antibody
O	none	Anti A Anti B
A	A	Anti B
B	B	Anti A
AB	AB	none
Rhesus positive	D	none
Rhesus negative	d	normally none

Introduction of factor D into a patient who is rhesus negative through a blood transfusion, or in a mother through her carrying a baby with rhesus positive blood stimulates the production of anti D antibody which could threaten the life of a subsequent baby.

Golden rule Never introduce an antigen that is not there already. Universal donor is **O Rhesus negative**.

Incompatibility reactions
1 *Agglutination* – red cells sticking together.
2 *Haemolysis* – red cells breaking open, releasing haemoglobin.

Both may cause acute renal failure (see 2.4).

Other major reactions from blood transfusion
1 Other antigens in the donor blood may cause a reaction similar to a hypersensitivity.
2 Infection may be introduced.
3 Excessive tranfusion may cause pulmonary congestion and heart failure.
4 Phlebitis and cellulitis through inflamed infusion site.

Modern laboratory techniques and checking procedures have made reactions rare these days, but the nurse needs to retain her vigilance in observation and care.

Suggested nursing response

Assessment	Care

1 Incompatibility
  1 the main indicator is loin pain or tenderness indicating renal damage
  2 oliguria (diminished urine production) or anuria (absence of urine production) may occur
	Stop the infusion immediately. Send for medical help. Reassure the patient. Prepare to treat renal failure. Retain blood and giving set

continued overleaf

continued from previous page

Assessment	Care
2 Hypersensitivity reactions; urticarial rash, mucous membrane swollen, anaphylactic shock (rarely)	Stop the infusion. Send for medical help. Prepare adrenaline or antihistamine. Retain blood and giving set
3 Infection; raised metabolic rate, tachycardia, pyrexia	Send for medical help. Decision to stop infusion by doctor unless local decision to stop
4 Pulmonary congestion and heart failure; shortness of breath, cough with sputum, 'bubbling' sounds in the chest (vulnerable patients are given packed cells now)	Slow infusion down. Send for medical help. Sit the patient up and help with expectoration
5 Phlebitis and cellulitis; local inflammation	Infusion may need to be resited. Local application of heat (e.g. kaolin poultice)

Conditions of the blood

Anaemia

Is defined as a reduction in the oxygen carrying capacity of the blood.

Causes
1 Inadequate production of mature red cells (erythrocytes)
2 Excessive loss of red cells
3 Excessive break down of red cells

Anaemias due to inadequate production of erythrocytes may be caused by:

1 Renal failure – due to lack of erythropoietin
2 Leukaemia
3 Aplastic anaemia
4 Pernicious anaemia
5 Folic acid deficiency
6 Malnutrition
7 Iron deficiency

Aplastic anaemia

Causes There is a group of patients who get this for no apparent reason (idiopathic). The main causes are, however, drugs (e.g. phenylbutazone, chloramphenicol, sulphonamides) and radiation.

Nursing note
It is important to note drugs that contain sulphonamides, e.g. co-trimoxazole is a combination of trimethorpin and sulphamethoxazole.

Effects The bone marrow becomes atrophied (reduced in amount and activity) and all cells normally produced are decreased. As well as the effects of anaemia, there is a loss of immunity to infection and blood clotting is impaired.

Nursing note
Very careful observations for sore throats, chest or urinary tract infection is important. Make careful note of bruising as well as obvious bleeding.

Treatment Is aimed at removing the cause (e.g. stopping the prescribed drug) and using blood transfusions for the anaemia, antibacterial drugs for infection and controlling bleeding.
The prognosis is not always very good and a lot of support therapy is needed.

Pernicious anaemia

Is an insidious condition in which there is failure to produce the intrinsic factor in the stomach. It is associated with a lack of hydrochloric acid production (achlorhydria). Lack of intrinsic factor makes it impossible to absorb vitamin B_{12} from the diet (see chart of erythropoiesis, p 28). The result is the release into the blood stream of large cells which do contain haemoglobin. The anaemia is described as:

1 Macrocytic – large cells   *2* Hyperchromic – too much colour

The cause is unknown. The major suspicion is that it is due to an auto immune reaction in the gastric mucosa.

Effects Vitamin B_{12} and folic acid are essential for the production of DNA. Bone marrow activity demands a large supply. The liver stores a considerable amount and, therefore, the anaemia does not always present itself obviously, but when the stores have been used, the fall in haemoglobin may be quite profound. The anaemia produces serious weakness, pallor (sometimes ashen colour) with a pale lemon jaundice. There is usually a red, inflamed tongue which may be quite sore. Heart failure may occur.

Nursing notes
Very careful observation is important to assess the degree of anaemia. Community nurses may be the ones who notice it, particularly in the elderly, living alone. Night nurses should note how many severely anaemic patients sleep with their mouth open.

Vitamin B_{12} deficiency also affects the metabolism of the myelin sheath in nerve cells. The main ones affected are in the spinal cord. The condition is known as *sub acute combined degeneration of the cord*. The patient will complain of periphereal sensation impairment – particularly on the hands and feet (glove and stocking parasthesia). There may also be a toxic confusional state leading to eventual dementia.

Nursing note
These effects may occur from middle age onwards and should be reported quickly as treatment is so efficient.

Diagnosis – investigations The clinical features will be reinforced by specific tests

Nurse's role in specific investigations

Investigation	Nurse's role
1 Full blood count	Blood from the correct patient. Observe venepuncture sites
2 Bone marrow biopsy – from sternum or iliac crest	Explanation understood by the patient. Preparation of equipment, bed and patient. Assist medical staff. Observe the patient during and after the procedure. Aseptic dressing to the site and possibly analgesia following
3 Schilling test	Explanation to the patient. *Procedure* Fasting period of at least 6 hours. Oral dose of radioactive labelled vitamin B_{12}. Intra muscular 1000 micrograms cyanocobalamin. 24 hour specimen of urine to estimate the amount of radioactive vitamin excreted

Note: Low amounts of radioactive vitamin in the urine would indicate lack of intrinsic factor unless a disorder of intestinal tract had interfered with absorption

Treatment
1 If haemoglobin is very low (e.g. below 4 g per 100 ml) a blood transfusion, usually of packed cells would be given.
2 Replacement of vitamin B_{12} (cobalamin) by giving hydroxocobalamin intramuscularly
Initial dose   1mg repeated 5 times at intervals of 2-3 days
Maintenance   1mg every 2-3 months
May also need increased iron in the form of ferrous sulphate.

Suggested nursing response

Assessment	Care
1 Effects of anaemia: tachycardia, fatigue, skin pallor, loss of concentration, irritability, restlessness and insomnia	Rest – could be in a comfortable chair unless severe tachycardia and fatigue. Careful use of make up for ladies. Careful psychological approach – individual may need sedation and help for sleeping
2 Degeneration of the cord	Careful protection of feet and hands if pareasthesia. Care of confused patient. Reassurance about recovery
3 Response to treatment	Encourage as it will be necessary to continue for life

Note: Nursing care of patients having blood transfusion (particularly elderly) – danger of lung congestion, agglutination and anaphylaxis. Increased red cell production increases the need for protein and iron in the diet – not always easy in elderly patients.

Folic acid deficiency

Is usually due to inadequate intake of folic acid in the diet.

Malnutrition

Serious lack of protein, vitamin C, vitamin B_{12}, folic acid and iron in the diet may lead to a dangerous anaemia, sometimes similar to pernicious anaemia, sometimes similar to aplastic anaemia with loss of resistance to infection, haemorrhages and weakness.

Nursing notes
These types of anaemia are usually treated with a careful restoration of a well balanced diet which then needs to be maintained. This may be difficult if people cannot afford some of the foods or have problems digesting them.
Foods which are high in:
Vitamin C   – fresh fruit, salads and vegetables
Vitamin B_{12} – meats (particularly liver)
Folic acid and iron – green vegetables
The dietician may need to advise further.

Iron deficiency anaemia

Causes

1 Inadequate dietary intake (although normal intake is only small).
2 Achlorhydria (lack of hydrochloric acid in the gastric juice) may cause a failure to absorb iron in the diet.
3 Chronic excessive loss of red blood cells (most common).

Anaemia due to excessive loss of red blood cells can be caused by:

1 Excessive menstrual flow (menorrhagia).
2 Insidious bleeding in the oesophagus (hiatus hernia), stomach (erosion from alcohol, erosion from aspirin, peptic ulcers and tumours), rectum and anus (haemorrhoids and tumours) and urinary tract lesions.

Effects, signs and symptoms
Red blood cells are formed in the bone marrow but are short of haemoglobin (needs iron) and cannot, therefore, carry sufficient oxygen to the tissues.

The patient complains of increasing fatigue, particularly after effort and at the end of the day. They may be restless and irritable. The skin and mucous membranes are pale. The patient may feel cold. There is increasing tachycardia, breathlessness on effort and the patient may have angina pectoris (chest pain on effort). Ultimately, heart failure may occur.

Nursing notes
Many of the effects are quite insidious. A nurse may notice them when a patient is admitted, but could miss them in patients on long stay wards.

Notice the behaviour changes and altered sleep patterns that may occur.

Associated effects

Glossitis   – inflammation of the tongue
Stomatitis   – inflammation of the corners of the mouth.
Koilonychia – spoon-shaped, thin and brittle finger and toe nails.
Dysphagia   – difficulty in swallowing.

Plummer Vinson or *Paterson-Brown Kelly syndrome*   Anaemia + achlorhydria + associated effects

Diagnosis and investigations

1 Clinical history and examination
2 Examination of blood for haemoglobin level and red cells which are usually small (microcytic) and pale (hypochromic)
3 Extensive search to find the site of haemorrhage

Treatment

1 Correction of the anaemia by:
   1 Packed blood cell transfusion (severely anaemic)
   2 Iron preparations – ferrous sulphate, ferrous gluconate
   3 Intramuscular or intravenous iron preparations (rarely used now)
2 Treating the haemorrhage according to the site

Suggested nursing response

Assessment	Care
1 Effects of hypoxia; fatigue, behaviour changes, tachycardia, angina, heart failure	Rest in a chair or in bed. Calm atmosphere. Analgesia for pain, but avoid effort. Care of heart failure
2 Associated effects	
1 Glossitis and stomatitis (irritating and difficult to treat)	Gentle mouth care at least four hourly and after meals
2 Koilonychia	Care of nails – filing and trimming
3 Effects of iron preparations	
1 Gastric erosion	Give iron preparations after meals
2 Stool discolouration (may disguise blood in the stool)	Reassurance
3 Staining of skin when injected intramuscularly	Deep intramuscular injection, retracting the skin over the injection site first

Iron tablets are extremely dangerous if taken by children. Strong advice and warning for safe storage of drugs is very important (see 2.12).

Haemolytic anaemia

An anaemia due to excessive breakdown of red blood cells.

Causes

1 Idiopathic – there may be no obvious reason
2 Abnormal red cells e.g. sickle cell anaemia
3 The effects of some drugs

Effects, signs and symptoms These are the same as for iron deficiency anaemia. In addition, excessive breakdown increases the amount of pigment released as bilirubin. The patient has a pale jaundice which may be alarming and irritable.

Diagnosis – investigations
1 Clinical history and examination
2 Blood for serum biliribum
3 Exclude other causes of jaundice

Treatment As for iron deficiency anaemia and care of jaundice.
Drug prescriptions need review.

Nursing notes
When taking a nursing history, past evidence of living in areas where 'sickling' occurs (those where malaria and the mosquito are found) will help. Note any past drug therapy too. Assessment and care are as for anaemia plus the care of mild jaundice.

Leukaemia

A malignant condition in which there is excessive production of abnormal white cells in haemopoietic tissues.
1 Myeloid leukaemia affects the bone marrow production of granulocytes.
2 Lymphatic or lymphoid leukaemia affect the production of lymphocytes.

Cause The cause is unknown, but factors that have been suggested are:
1 exposure to excessive radiation
2 possibly viral or chemical changes affecting DNA
Both types, myeloid and lymphatic are then classified into acute and chronic. The effects and needs of patients are almost identical in the acute disease.

Acute leukaemia

Effects, signs and symptoms Usually children, adolescents or young adults are affected. The onset is rapid and the effects can be considered with the change of the whole blood picture.
1 *Deficiency of normal white cells* makes the patient prone to acute infections.
  High fever, sore throat which persists and the patient deteriorates with a rising metabolic rate.
2 *Deficiency of platelets* causes faulty blood clotting, with haemorrhages.
  The usual sites are bleeding of the gums, nose and lungs. The slightest knock may produce large haematoma in joints.

Nursing notes
Haemorrhage is a particularly alarming feature of the disease, causing distress to the parents, almost more than the child. Calm reassurance is needed.
3 *Deficiency of erythrocytes* causes a severe anaemia, with profound loss of energy and possibly heart effects of anaemia may be noted (see iron deficiency anaemia).

Diagnosis – investigations
This is made by examination of blood cells and the bone marrow biopsy.

See *pernicious anaemia* for nursing roles for these.

Suggested nursing response – problems

Assessment	Care
1 Low resistance to infection	Reverse barrier nursing
1 presence of infection	Nurse at rest. Glucose for energy. Maintain body temperature
2 raised metabolic rate; pyrexia, tachycardia, fatigue	
Note: Cytotoxic drugs reduce leucocyte count even more	
2 Poor blood clotting	Very careful handling to prevent bruising. Mouth care applied
1 observe for haemorrhage	gently for bleeding gums
2 observe for fear in patient and relatives	Nursing staff and medical staff should agree on communications to relatives and the patient. Avoid 'the conspiracy of silence' and conflicting explanations
3 Severe effects of anaemia – note how easily fatigued even when infection or haemorrhage are not occurring	The pulse rate is a guide to what the child can do – if rapid, rest is needed, if slower, allow a little more play activity and teaching

Remissions do occur in acute leukaemia and some make spectacular recovery. The nurse must maintain a positive approach at all times. There is, however, a large mortality rate and the nurse in charge may have the difficult task of helping junior staff to cope with the death of a child. Emotional involvement is inevitable. Professional control is best demonstrated by example.

Chronic myeloid leukaemia

Effects, signs and symptoms More commonly affects people in early adult life and middle age. The main effects are those of anaemia. The spleen and liver may become grossly enlarged causing dyspepsia and abdominal tenderness. There may be bouts of fever. The tendency to bleed usually occurs during an acute exacerbation or prior to death which usually occurs within 2–3 years.

Chronic lymphatic leukaemia

Effects, signs and symptoms Most commonly affects men in later middle age. The anaemia produces a slowly progressing tiredness. The spleen, liver and lymph nodes are enlarged producing discomfort and tenderness. There is a large increase in the number of lymphocytes in the blood. Progress is slower and patients have lived for 10 years or more before finally succumbing.

Chemotherapy Cytotoxic drugs may be used in combinations and in periodic intervals according to different centres for treatment. All cytotoxic drugs, at present, have depressant effects on bone marrow and monitoring of cell counts is essential. Reverse barrier nursing may be indicated. See *British National Formulary* for details of individual drugs used.

The blood vessels

Functions	Structures
1 The transport of blood to the tissues from the left ventricle of the heart	Systemic arteries, arterioles and capillaries
Factors affecting blood flow in systemic arteries are: *1* the blood pressure exerted by the left ventricle of the heart *2* the patency of the vessels and the smooth (anticoagulant) endothelium *3* the lumen of the arterioles which is controlled by the autonomic nervous system and the vaso dilator and vaso constrictor substances	
2 The transport of blood from the tissues towards the right side of the heart	Capillaries, systemic venules and systemic veins
Factors affecting blood flow in systemic veins are: *1* the arterial blood pressure *2* the presence of valves in veins *3* the pumping action of limb muscles with walking and using hands and arms *4* the action of breathing produces a suction pressure on blood flow in large veins	
3 Maintaining the balance of tissue fluid	Systemic arteries, capillaries and systemic veins. Plasma proteins in blood

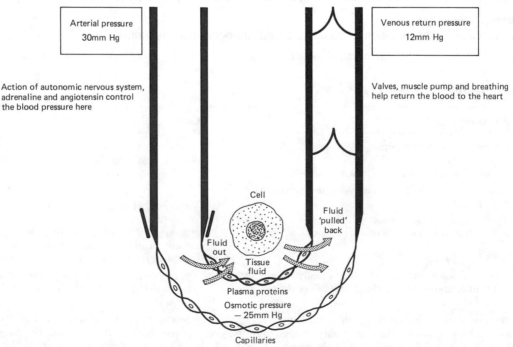

Arterial pressure 30mm Hg

Venous return pressure 12mm Hg

Action of autonomic nervous system, adrenaline and angiotensin control the blood pressure here

Valves, muscle pump and breathing help return the blood to the heart

Cell

Fluid 'pulled' back

Fluid out

Tissue fluid

Plasma proteins
Osmotic pressure – 25mm Hg

Capillaries

Fig. 2.2.2 'The loop'–maintenance of tissue fluid in the systemic circulation   *continued next page*

4 Maintaining the blood flow through the lungs for oxygenation and carbon dioxide release

Pulmonary arteries, arterioles, capillaries, venules and pulmonary veins. Plasma proteins

Factors affecting blood flow through the lungs are:
1 right ventricular blood pressure on systole (contraction)
2 patency and smooth flow through the vessels
3 the ability of the left side of the heart to receive the blood flow

5 Maintaining the blood flow to the heart muscle (myocardium)

Coronary arteries and capillaries. Coronary sinus

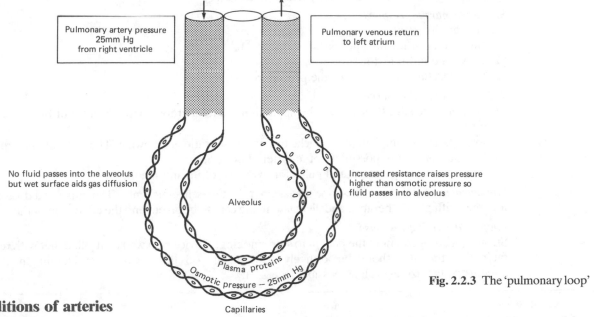

Pulmonary artery pressure 25mm Hg from right ventricle

Pulmonary venous return to left atrium

No fluid passes into the alveolus but wet surface aids gas diffusion

Increased resistance raises pressure higher than osmotic pressure so fluid passes into alveolus

Alveolus

Plasma proteins
Osmotic pressure – 25mm Hg

Capillaries

Fig. 2.2.3 The 'pulmonary loop'

Conditions of arteries

Arteriosclerosis

This is a degenerative disease of the arteries known as *hardening of the arteries*. It is a feature of the ageing process and patients with diabetes mellitus.

Atherosclerosis is described separately by some authors, but others consider it as the same condition, but mainly affecting the aorta, large arteries, coronary and cerebral arteries. Atherosclerosis specifically involves the laying down of *atheroma* – fatty plaques – in the wall of the artery. Atheroma plaques have been found even in teenagers.

Factors leading to atheroma formation are
 1 Cigarette smoking
 2 Hypertension
 3 Hyperlipidaemia – now thought to be a problem of total fat intake, not specifically cholesterol and animal fats.

The effects of both conditions is to narrow the lumen of the artery and diminish the blood supply to the affected tissues – ischaemia.
Cerebral ischaemia – see nervous system 2.5
Coronary ischaemia – see coronary thrombosis p 47

Peripheral vascular disease

Effects, signs and symptoms Poor oxygenation of the muscles leads to the build up of lactic acid causing pain on exercise which is relieved with rest – *intermittent claudication*. Poor blood flow leads to cold extremities which can again be very uncomfortable and even painful. An already diminished blood supply may be obliterated if inflammation occurs. This will cause necrosis (death of tissue) leading to gangrene and ulceration.

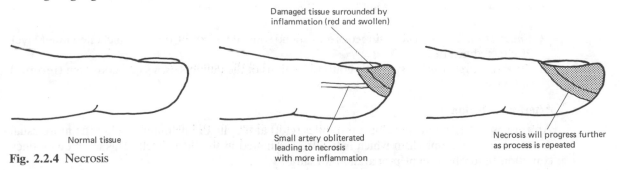

Damaged tissue surrounded by inflammation (red and swollen)

Normal tissue

Small artery obliterated leading to necrosis with more inflammation

Necrosis will progress further as process is repeated

Fig. 2.2.4 Necrosis

Nursing note
Patients with peripheral neuropathy (e.g. diabetes mellitus) may have a loss of sensation and be unaware of injury and inflammation.

Diagnosis – investigations
1 Clinical examination
2 Arteriogram – the injection of a radio opaque fluid into an artery followed by a series of rapid X-ray films. The injection may be either
   1 directly into the artery, or
   2 through an arterial catheter (Seldinger catheter)

Suggested nursing response
Before the procedure
1 Nil by mouth for 4–5 hours
2 Shave the groin as for surgery
3 Very careful explanation of the procedure

The nurse should observe
1 the puncture site. Pressure will be applied in the radiography department, but blood may leak for some time.
2 some patients complain of headache or burning sensations following. These should be reported.
3 foot pulses for the possibility of an arterial occlusion.
4 four hourly temperature and pulse for evidence of inflammation.

Management It is better to describe management of the ischaemic limbs. The nurse and doctor work together with physiotherapist and dieticians in the care to be given, and the education of the patient.

Suggested nursing response
Strong encouragement to the patient to stop smoking. Advice on a well controlled diet with reduced fat intake – the nurse should be positively encouraging foods that **can** be eaten. Helping the diabetic patient to stabilize as well as possible (see 2.8).

Assessment	Care
1 Patient's perception of pain	Advice about rest. Prescribed analgesia
2 Condition of skin, particularly of the feet, including nails	Washing and drying carefully. Treatment of minor lesions (e.g. blisters). Professional chiropody for nail and foot care. Treatment of fungal infections (e.g. athlete's foot)
3 Limb temperature	Avoid extremes of heat and cold (Overheating increases metabolic needs of tissues. Excess cooling causes more vaso constriction)

Blood supply may be improved by
   1 Reflex dilation Applying heat to the trunk, warms the blood and stimulates the vaso motor centre of the brain to cause dilation of peripheral arterioles.

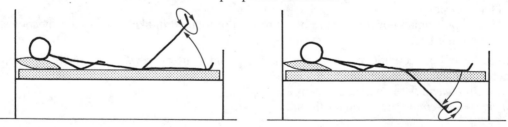

Fig. 2.2.5 Buerger-Allen exercises

   2 Buerger-Allen exercises The patient is taught by the physiotherapist and the nurse encourages the patient to alternately elevate and lower the legs while lying at the edge of the bed. Elevation is about 45 degrees and one minute in each position, while at the same time exercising the feet.

Surgical intervention
   1 *Lumbar sympathectomy* Division of the sympathetic nerve supply causes more or less permanent vaso dilation.
   2 *Endarterectomy* Specialist surgeons may spend some time 'coring out' the thickened inner layer of affected arteries.
   3 *'By pass' surgery* using synthetic grafts or sections of the patients own saphenous vein (reversed of course).

Arterial occlusion

Any diseased artery may develop a thrombus (clot) at the site of inflammation, but the more usual danger is from an embolism which may have originated in the heart itself. This is an emergency condition requiring urgent preparation for surgery.

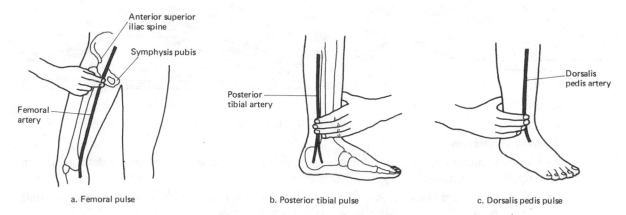

Fig. 2.2.6 Detecting arterial pulses in the lower limb

Suggested nursing response

1 *Observations* by the nurse are vital for sudden onset of pain, coldness and numbness of the limb, loss of colour and absence of pulses (e.g. foot pulses if femoral embolism).

2 *Care of the limb* Rest the limb at room temperature – a bed cradle with an open end will allow air to circulate and the nurse may observe more. Reflex dilation may be tried. Anticoagulants may be prescribed. Carefully clean and shave ready for surgery.

3 *Psychology* Firm reassurance is needed to calm a frightened patient.

Embolectomy may be carried out under local anaesthetic

A saddle embolus is one which has lodged over the bifurcation of the abdominal aorta (very rarely they may lodge over the arch of the aorta). Both limbs may be occluded. Removal is by use of a Fogarty catheter.

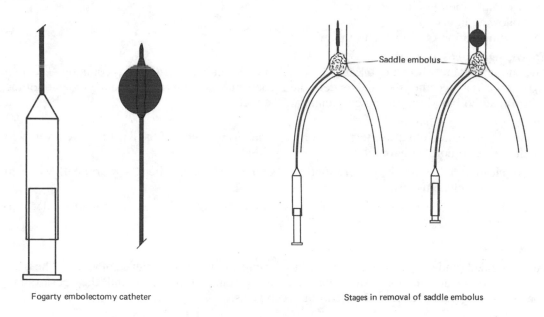

Fig. 2.2.7 Removal of saddle embolus using a Fogarty catheter

Amputation of a limb may be necessary if severe ischaemia persists. See locomotor system 2.6

Inflammation of arteries

A number of conditions may cause inflammation giving similar effects to arteriosclerosis. Only a brief mention can be made here.

Arteritis

Rheumatoid arthritis (see 2.6)

Buerger's disease usually affects men who are cigarette smokers. Despite a lot of advice and care, a number unfortunately need multiple amputations before their demise.

Syphilis – tertiary (third stage) syphilis may cause severe damage to arteries, particularly the aorta.

Aneurysm is a dilation of a vessel. Arterial aneurysms are due to weakness in the area. They may be saccular, fusiform or dissecting. The cause may be arteriosclerosis, inflammation or congenital.

Treatment is surgical. The main problem is the sudden rupture of an aneurysm with subsequent major haemorrhage and collapse.

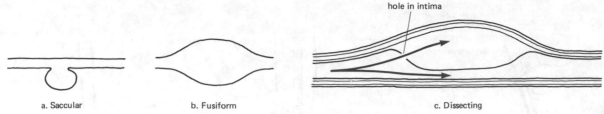

a. Saccular　　　　　　b. Fusiform　　　　　　hole in intima　　c. Dissecting

Fig. 2.2.8 Aneurysms

Trauma to arteries

Are usually due to lacerations, fractures, crush injuries or may be due to damage during investigations or surgery.

Effects Haemorrhage is usually very severe and collapse due to loss of blood pressure may be rapid. A severed radial artery may cause death within a few minutes.

Treatment

1 Blood tranfusion to restore blood volume　　2 Ligation of the bleeding points

Suggested nursing response – first aid

1 Apply direct pressure with a pad and bandage
2 Rest the limb
3 Urgent transfer to Accident Centre

Many crash teams carry intravenous sets and plasma.

Conditions of veins

Phlebitis (thrombo phlebitis)

Is inflammation of the veins, usually the superficial ones.

Cause factors

1 A complication of varicose veins
2 Following injury
3 A complication of intravenous therapy

Effects, signs and symptoms

The endothelial layer becomes thickened and narrow. Thrombosis formation is common. The area around the vein becomes red, and tender – the redness may be seen tracking along the path of the vein. Impaired blood return causes swelling of the feet.

Suggested nursing response

1 Strict observation of intravenous infusion sites and an awareness of the line of the vein will help the nurse to note early onset.

2 Application of heat is usually very soothing – kaolin poultice may help. A warm bath will help those with phlebitis in the legs.

3 Anti-inflammatory drugs and analgesics may help. Rest with the legs elevated is advisable. (See care of varicose veins.)

Varicose veins

Are distended (and often distorted) veins which result from the incompetence of valves. The main problems occur in the long and short saphenous veins in the legs and the 'perforating' communicating veins between them and the deep veins.

Cause factors

1 There appears to be a familial tendency
2 People with occupations involving standing for long periods (it is an occupational hazard of nursing!)
3 Pelvic tumours
4 Pregnancy
5 Congestion of venous return to the heart

Nursing note

The nurse can act as an adviser to vulnerable groups, including practical matters like sitting for feeding patients, and continual foot exercises when having to stand for long periods.

Effects, signs and symptoms As stated, the veins may appear dilated and tortuous, causing considerable cosmetic embarrassment. Poor venous return causes oedema of the ankles and feet, particularly towards the end of the day and after long journeys sitting down.

There is considerable discomfort and aching in the legs and the skin over the lower leg particularly becomes irritable, eczema develops and eventually ulceration. The dilated veins may easily be ruptured by minor injury or even spontaneously. Considerable blood loss may occur.

Thrombophlebitis often occurs in the superficial veins damaged by the varicositis.

Diagnosis Clinical history and examination for the position of incompetent valves:
1 patient's foot elevated, distended veins emptied
2 patient stands – observe for filling from above (instead of below)
3 repeat, using a rubber tourniquet as artificial valve to detect site of valve damage – mark with skin pencil

Suggested nursing response

The nurse may need to care for patients with varicose veins before treatment and education to sufferers is helpful.
1 Assist superficial venous drainage by spending periods with legs elevated, wearing correctly measured supporting hosiery and doing walking exercises to use the muscle pump.
2 Care for the skin over drainage areas by washing, drying and application of counter irritants.
3 Advice to prevent injury and rupture
First aid for rupture

1 Lie the patient down – treat for shock.	**3** Elevate the limb.
2 Pad and bandage – firm but not too tight.	**4** Urgent transfer to Accident Centre

Treatment

Surgery
1 Ligation and stripping of the long saphenous vein
2 Ligation of perforating veins (Lockett's procedure)

Suggested nursing response

Pre operative assessment and care (specific)
1 Note evidence of phlebitis, eczema.
2 Thoroughly wash and dry, shave the groin for stripping and the affected leg.

Surgery Incisions may be needed at various sites for ligation and insertion of stripper.

Post operative assessment and care
1 Observe for haemorrhage and inflammation.
2 Legs elevated for first day, but early mobilization with support bandaging.

This has become an operation done in short stay wards and it may be the community nurse who needs to assess that the home environment and the patient's understanding of post operative care is clear. Sutures may be soluble or removed in the home or at the health centre.

Compression sclerotherapy (usually in out-patients)

A sclerosing agent is injected into the veins and a pad is used to compress them. A firm support bandage is applied. A 'sterile' phlebitis causes the two inner surfaces of the vein to fibrose together.

Eczema and varicose ulcer – see 2.7 for conditions of the skin

Deep vein thrombosis

Cause factors
1 Tissue damage (see chart for blood clotting p 28)
2 Immobilization – operating table; bed rest
3 Poor venous return – pregnancy; chronic chest conditions
4 Changes in blood clotting factors and blood viscosity e.g. polycythaemia, effects of drugs (contraceptive hormones)

Nursing notes
Nurses are well aware of the danger, and measures to prevent are taught from the introductory course onwards. Points to remember:
1 Many surgeons use anticoagulants prophylactically but early breathing exercises and mobilization are still very important.
2 All patients whose mobility is impaired are vulnerable and those who are too weak or unconscious may need repeated passive exercises.

Effects, signs and symptoms Obstruction in the deep venous return may occasionally be painless and asymptomless, but usually the leg is painful and swollen. The calf is tender to touch. When the toes of the foot are bent upwards (dorsiflexion) there is often pain in the calf (Homan's sign).

Swelling may be considerable and the leg may be discoloured. Pallor produces the classic *white leg* in the early stages of a major thrombus. The most severe form may produce cyanosis and gross swelling as there is stasis of blood and even limitation of the arterial supply.

Inflammation increases the metabolic rate and a low pyrexia may occur with tachycardia and malaise. The first indication may, in fact, be the complication of pulmonary embolism (see 2.1).

Treatment
1 Preventing the clot extending – anticoagulant therapy
2 Dissolution of the clot – thrombolytic therapy

Suggested nursing response

Assessment	Care
1 Observations of the legs (do not wait for the patient to complain) for tenderness, pain, swelling and discolouration. Calf may be measured	Early information for medical staff. Rest under bed cradle. Prescribed analgesia for pain.
2 Raised metabolic rate – pyrexia, tachycardia	Rest in bed
3 Indications of pulmonary embolism	See p 24 in 2.1

4 Anticoagulant therapy
  1 Heparin acts immediately
  2 Warfarin action delayed, but lasts for five days
  3 Observe for bruising and bleeding
  4 Care if previous lesions
  5 Test urine daily – observe all specimens
	Prevention of injury. Take care with shaving. Care of intravenous injections. Careful drug administration – see prothrombin times

5 Thrombolytic therapy
  1 Streptokinase
  2 Danger of bleeding and inflammatory reaction (Cannot be used in the immediate post operative period)
	Very careful drug administration – intravenous rate has to be constantly regulated

Some consultants prefer to simply apply support bandages and rest the leg in an elevated position.

3 The heart and circulations

Functions	Structures involved
1 **Left heart** The maintenance of the arterial blood pressure and the supply of oxygen and nutrients to the capillaries for diffusion to the cells	Left ventricle contracts – systolic pressure opens the aortic valve, mitral valve should be closed. Volume – approx. 70 ml on each beat. Pressure 120 mm Hg. Force – contraction of thick myocardium
2 **Right heart** The flow of blood through the pulmonary circulation for the diffusion of carbon dioxide and oxygen	Right ventricle contracts – systolic pressure opens the pulmonary valve, tricuspid valve should be closed. Volume – approx. 70 ml on each beat. Pressure 25 mm Hg.
3 Controlled rhythmic contractions of atria to complete filling of ventricles to maintain cardiac output	Nerve supply to the sino atrial node, atrial walls, atrio ventricular node, bundle of His and ventricular walls
4 Provision of its own blood supply and drainage	Coronary arteries, capillaries and veins. Coronary sinus in the right atrium
5 Smooth, concentrated contraction but limited expansion	Parietal pericardium of connective tissue. Visceral pericardium of serous membrane
6 Smooth flow of blood through the inside of the heart	Endocardium of squamous epithelium

Conditions of the heart
Heart failure(s)

It is useful to consider heart failure(s) as caused by conditions in the *reverse order* of the blood flow – left ventricular failure first, followed by right. The individual conditions will then be considered separately.

Left ventricular failure

Causes

1 *Hypertension* Peripheral resistance in the arterioles means that the left ventricle has to work too hard, enlarges (hypertrophies) and fails.
2 *Aortic valve stenosis* due to rheumatic fever usually, causes resistance to ventricular contraction.
3 *Myocardial infarction* Part of the left ventricular wall necrosed and also the rhythm affected.
4 *Mitral valve incompetence* Some blood regurgitating on ventricular contraction lowers cardiac output, ventricle works quicker and harder to compensate.

Effects, signs and symptoms

Cardiogenic shock There is a fall in the cardiac output, blood pressure and oxygen levels to all tissues. Death may occur very quickly. The patient may collapse and lose consciousness, or become distressed and restless.

Pulmonary oedema As the left side of the heart cannot receive the pulmonary venous return, there is serious congestion of blood in the lungs, with fluid pouring into the alveolar spaces. In very acute cases, blood cells may enter the alveoli.

    The patient becomes acutely short of breath, develops a cough with frothy sputum which may be pink or flecked with blood. Hypoxia is made worse and cyanosis often occurs. Confusion may occur. In order to reduce the pulmonary congestion, many patients will reduce the venous return to the

right side of the heart by putting their legs down – often over the side of the bed. There is a great sense of impending death which will add fear to make the shock more profound. Myocardial infarction will also cause severe pain.

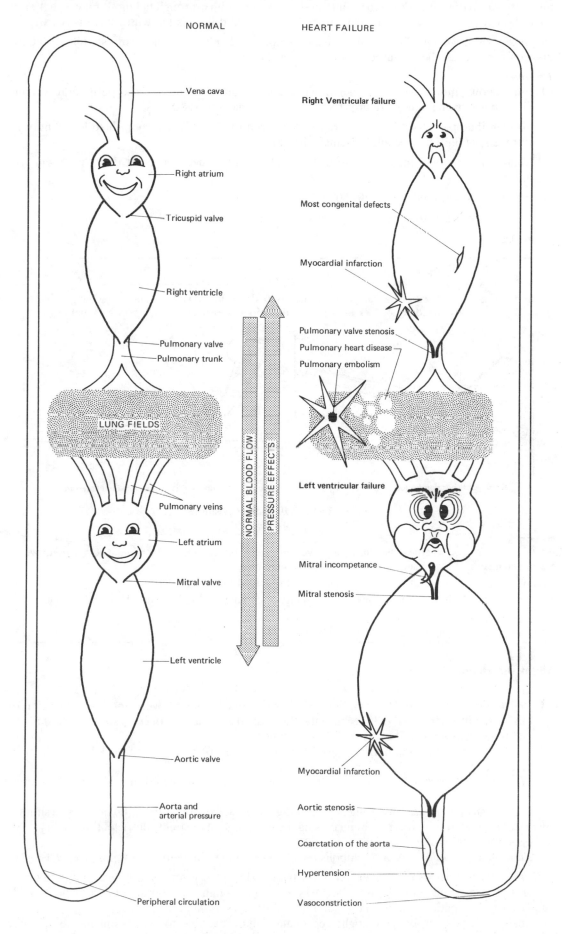

Fig. 2.2.9 Blood flow and heart failure

Nursing notes
This is a major emergency and the nursing team must work quickly and efficiently as soon as it occurs. It often occurs at night time – paroxysmal nocturnal dyspnoea. There is a tendency for nurses to scoop the patient's legs back into bed, to prevent injury through falling. It may be better to have the bed low enough for the patient to feel the ground if he is known to have attacks.

Diagnosis – investigations The clinical examination and electrocardiogram should establish diagnosis, but it can be confused with acute bronchospasm.

Treatment

1 Intravenous morphine (or a derivative) relieves anxiety and causes peripheral venous dilation – reducing venous return. (Not used if chronic airways disease.)

2 Oxygen therapy – 40–50% concentrations (reduced to 24–28% if carbon dioxide retention)

3 Intravenous diuretic – usually frusemide 10–20 mg

   Nursing note: works quickly – have urinal ready or a wet bed and great embarrassment will follow!

4 Intravenous aminophyline – 250–500 mg given slowly

   Nursing note: if given quickly, may cause vomiting

Suggested nursing response

Assessment	Care
1 Low cardiac output and falling blood pressure	Position the patient according to blood pressure. If very low, raise feet but great care needed (see Jack-knife position). If blood pressure normal, legs down is better

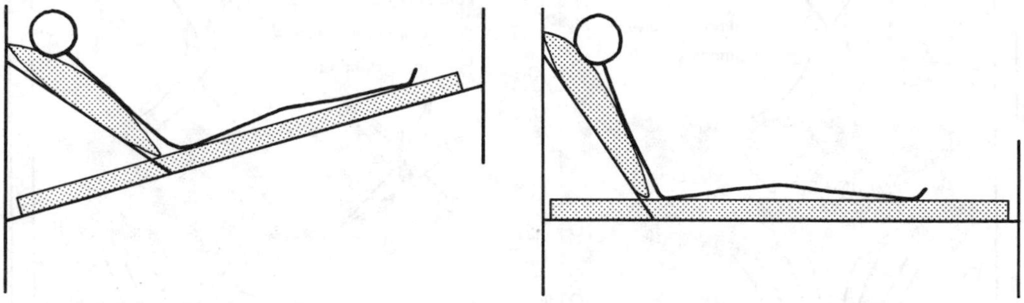

a. Jack-knife position for low blood pressure   b. Good position for normal blood pressure

Fig. 2.2.10 Patient positions

2 Pulmonary congestion	
1 cough, sputum	Sit the patient up to improve lung expansion and ventricular filling. Oxygen therapy.
2 hypoxia – behaviour changes	Assist with the giving of intravenous drugs
3 Acute anxiety – fear of dying	Sensitive reassurance needed. Prescribed narcotic is helpful

Following the attack, the patient will be hot and sweaty (may need a change of clothing) and feel exhausted (nourishment in a drink will help).

There will be further treatment and care according to the cause of the heart failure.

Right ventricular failure

Causes

1 *Left ventricular failure* The right ventricle has to work harder to overcome the congestion of blood. It will enlarge and fail. Technically, this is the true definition of *congestive cardiac failure*. A similar syndrome will occur with mitral stenosis.

2 *Chronic lung disease* Pulmonary heart disease (see 2.1, p 16) increases the work load of the right ventricle

3 *Myocardial infarction* Part of the right ventricular wall in necrosed and abnormal rhythms affect filling

4 *Congenital heart disease* involving the 'shunting' of blood from one side to the other. The shunt is invariably from left to right, thereby increasing the work load of the right ventricle. Pulmonary valve stenosis also causes more resistance.

5 *Pulmonary embolism* A large embolism will cause acute right ventricular failure (see 2.1, p 24)

Effects, signs and symptoms Remember many patients have left ventricular failure with pulmonary congestion or chronic lung disease. Shortness of breath, cough with sputum and possible hypoxia may occur. The patient 'cannot breathe' unless sitting up – *orthopnoea*.

   Specifically, the problems of right ventricular failure are due to congestion in the systemic venous return – seen by the raised jugular venous pressure.

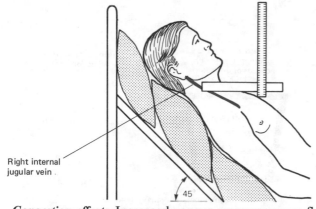

Right internal
jugular vein

Fig. 2.2.11
Measuring jugular venous pressure

Congestion effects Increased venous pressure causes fluid retention in intercelluar spaces.
1 *Pleural effusion* There is a **systemic** circulation to the lungs and pleura as well as the pulmonary. The patient's shortness of breath is increased and there is a sensation of trying to breathe with a 'band around the chest'. Hypoxia may cause behavioural changes and eventually cyanosis.

2 *Liver engorgement and portal hypertension* The patient may have an enlarged, tender liver. Portal hypertension causes increased pressure in:
  1 gastric vein–may cause dyspepsia.
  2 splenic vein–splenomegaly (enlargement of spleen) with tenderness.
  3 mesenteric veins–ascites and haemorrhoids.

3 *Poor venous drainage from dependent parts* will lead to oedema of the legs and sacral area–especially when the patient is immobile or in bed.
4 *Poor left ventricular flow* reduces flow to kidneys–oliguria will occur.

Nursing notes
Right ventricular failure is usually gradual in onset rather than acute. Observation of vulnerable patients (see causes) may help to note the effects before signs and symptoms become more distressing.

Diagnosis – investigations
1 Clinical examination   2 Tests for causes may be needed later

Treatment
1 Diuretics–usually a thiazide or loop diuretic such as frusemide may be given orally. Potassium supplements will be needed.
2 Digoxin–not used by some physicians now but the nurse should be aware of the undesired effects (see nursing response).
3 Treatment for the underlying cause of the failure.
4 Oxygen if hypoxia is present.

Suggested nursing response

Assessment	Care
1 Increasing shortness of breath and dyspnoea	Reassurance. Nurse in orthopnoeic position, high side lying position, or sitting in a comfortable armchair
2 Indications of hypoxia; increasing pulse rate, mood or behavioural changes, cyanosis	Oxygen therapy–40–50% (24–28% if chronic lung disease). Possibly chest aspiration for pleural effusion
3 Abdominal discomfort, tenderness and distension with ascites	Comfortable positioning. Prescribed analgesia or antacid. Very light diet. Prescribed diuretics. Possibly drainage of the ascites (paracentesis abdominus)
4 Oedema of legs and sacral area – the skin is tense and shiny, very vulnerable to breakage from the slightest injury. Observe pressure areas hourly.	Careful positioning. Gentle movement and physiotherapy. Avoid friction–good lifting technique. (Drainage of the oedema in legs is very rare but possible using silver Southey's tubes)
5 Observe urine output for oliguria. Poor renal flow increases salt and water retention, making the oedema even worse	Reduced sodium diet. Salt free diets are not used so strictly, but avoid added salt and very salty foods
6 Effects of drugs *Diuretics* Urine output and duration of diuresis. Daily weighing. Evidence of potassium depletion–apathy, muscle weakness, mental confusion	The choice, dosage and timing of diuretics could be determined individually–especially for patients at home. Prescribed potassium drugs or potassium containing drinks (try tomato juice)
Digoxin Apex beat or pulse for bradycardia, coupling of beats or ectopic beats if the patient is monitored with a cardioscope. Anorexia, nausea, vomiting. Rarely visual disturbance such as xanthopsia–seeing colours–yellow or brown are most common: 'like looking through coloured paper'.	Delay drug administration until seen by physician as excretion period is long, and accumulation occurs. Some doctors suggest a day off a week

Hypertension – high diastolic blood pressure

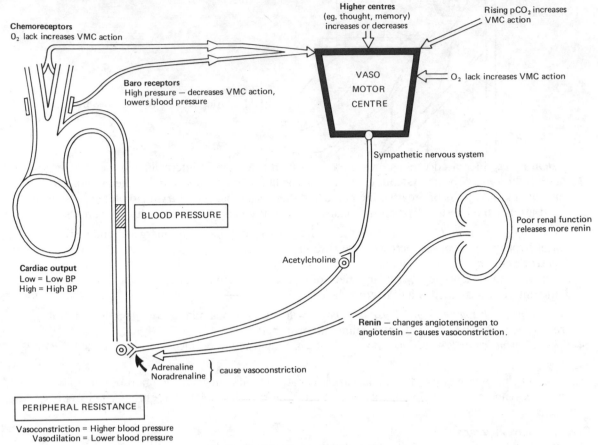

Fig. 2.2.12 Control of blood pressure

Cause factors

1 *Essential* The majority of cases are in this category and the cause is not known (idiopathic). Research is going on to confirm the associations with stress, and salt intake.
2 *Renal disease* Some authorities say about 30% of cases, others think even more, may be associated with kidney damage (see 2.4). See Fig. 2.12.
3 *Hormonal*
    1 Excessive corticosteroids – Cushing's syndrome (see 2.8)
    2 Adrenaline secreting tumours – phaeochromocytoma
4 *Coarctation of the aorta* Congenital narrowing of a portion of aorta, increases pressure at the cardiac side of the narrowing

Obesity does not cause hypertension but will increase the work of the heart in the hypertensive patient.

Effects, signs and symptoms
Cardio vascular effects
1 Causes left ventricular failure and ultimately congestive cardiac failure.
2 Contributes to the development of atherosclerosis which may lead to coronary artery disease – angina and myocardial infarction.

Neurological effects
1 Produces pathological changes in the eye – papilloedema and retinopathy. The patient may have rapidly failing eye sight.
2 Produces headaches and may produce pathological changes in the brain – encephalopathy. The patient may undergo serious behavioural changes and some have been admitted for psychiatric care.
3 Atherosclerosis may cause cerebral thrombosis.
4 Cerebral haemorrhage may occur.

Renal effects Increased blood pressure will damage the glomerulus of the kidney, increasing the release of renin which in due course increases blood pressure. Renal failure may be the sequel (see 2.4). This is probably the mechanism known as malignant hypertension.

Nursing note
Remember when teaching junior nurses how to take blood pressure to stress the importance of accuracy and reporting – including the **diastolic** pressure.

Diagnosis – investigations

The diagnosis is obvious, but the investigations needed are extensive to determine both the cause and effects of hypertension.

Major tests include:
1 Evidence of stress factors
2 Dietary patterns
3 Renal function tests – urine testing
    1 24 hour urine specimens – creatinine clearance test; catecholamines; ketosteroids
    2 Intravenous urogram
4 Blood for serum urea; creatinine
5 Cardiology – electrocardiogram; possible angiography
6 Cerebral – angiography; electro encephalogram; examination of eyes; neurological examinations

Suggested nursing response

The nurse's role in these tests can be quite demanding. They may take some time before treatment is commenced and the waiting increases the patient's frustration and stress.
1 Assessment of the patient before the test – careful explanations for understanding
2 Organizing ward tests (e.g. 24 hour urine specimens), visits to departments and preparation for tests (e.g. IVP)
3 Supervising and performing ward tests
4 Careful recording and reporting of the results

Treatment

1 Counselling to relieve stress factors, alter life style and eating habits.
2 Hypotensive drugs
    1 Some physicians use diuretics to reduce blood volume and control mild hypertension.
    2 Sedatives and tranquilizers may control some patients.
    3 Beta adrenoreceptor blocking drugs (e.g. Propanalol) are used extensively but cannot be used if the patient is in heart failure or has a history of asthma.
    4 Methyldopa is the main specific hypotensive drug used.
    5 Bethanidine and guancthidine cause postural hypotension.
    (Lying and standing blood pressure recordings may be needed)

Accelerated hypertension (in malignant hypertension) is a crisis in which the blood pressure rises quickly and progressively. Strong hypotensive drugs such as diazoxide or hydralazine will be given – possibly intravenously. Careful monitoring of blood pressure is needed.

Suggested nursing response

Assessment	Care
1 Evidence of stress factors – some may have more stress if they cannot work	Calm atmosphere. Discuss visiting and work
2 Evidence of weight problems	Discuss with dietician. Acceptable reducing diet
3 Effects of drugs – monitoring of blood pressure	
4 Some drugs may cause failure of ejaculation – impotence	Careful counselling may be needed
5 Observe for complications: heart failure; stroke; blindness; renal failure	Send for medical help

Advice to patients with hypertension needs to be discussed between nurses, physicians and relatives to ensure that it is realistic. To be told to stop doing too many things or eating favourite foods may increase stress factors.

Rheumatic heart disease

Acute rheumatism or rheumatic fever

Cause An abnormal immune response to infection by Group A haemolytic streptococci – usually pharyngitis

Effects, signs and symptoms There may be a period of 7–21 days after the sore throat before acute rheumatism occurs.

The metabolic rate is increased. In children this may be quite high. Pyrexia and tachycardia may be pronounced. The patient feels very weak and ill, may have a headache and feel shivery. Rigors may occur.

There is a polyarthritis (inflammation of more than one joint) but also, single joints may be affected. There is a typical 'flitting' of inflammation from one joint to the other. The joints are swollen, hot and tender to touch, with pain on movement. There is a typical rash – erythema marginatum – patches of red with well defined edges.

The most serious effect is carditis and most young children are vulnerable to heart damage with this condition.

Pericarditis Inflammation of the pericardium causes a retrosternal soreness. A pericardial effusion may occur which causes cardiac embarrassment when the patient moves or coughs.

Myocarditis may cause severe tachycardia, abnormal heart rhythms, enlargement of the heart and heart failure.

Endocarditis Inflammation of the cusps of the valves. The problem is mainly on resolution when the edges may be fused together by fibrosis (occasionally calcification) and cause a narrowing of the valve (stenosis). Later, tears may develop, allowing blood to flow back through the valve (incompetence).

Nursing notes

Although acute rheumatism is less common than previously, it can be seen that the consequences are very serious. The nurse should advise all parents that a sore throat in a child is an indication for medical attention. Throat swabs should be taken.

Diagnosis – investigations

The clinical examination and history should be enough and the patient treated for acute rheumatism until proved otherwise.

Tests: Electrocardiogram; Chest X-ray (for heart size); Blood for erythrocyte sedimentation rate (increased) and antistreptolysin 'O' (high following streptococcal infection); Throat swab

Treatment

1 Complete rest
2 Salicylate for the inflammation – aspirin is analgesic, antipyretic and anti-inflammatory
3 Corticosteroid drugs to prevent fibrosis and act as anti-inflammatory drug
4 Penicillin – intramuscularly followed later by oral

Suggested nursing response

Assessment	Care
1 Raised metabolic rate: pyrexia, tachycardia, dehydration	Complete bed rest. Cooling with fans and light clothing. Glucose drinks for energy. Fluids. Mouth care needed
2 Joint pains – inspect all joints regularly	Handle very gently. Warm wool wrapping. Passive physiotherapy. Prescribed analgesia
3 Indications of heart involvement – increased tachycardia, arrhythmias, chest pain, breathlessness	Continue complete bed rest until resolved – difficult at times with young children – involve the parents

The course of the disease varies from a short period, to a very long period (months) and great support is needed to maintain development. Schooling and play are very important.

Mitral valve stenosis

May occur alone or with incompetence.

Effects, signs and symptoms Narrowing of the mitral valve causes the pressure in the left atrium to rise and there is *congestion* in the pulmonary veins and alveoli. The patient complains of a progressive shortness of breath – first on effort, but later at rest. Congestion may eventually cause orthopnoea and acute pulmonary oedema may lead to paroxysmal nocturnal dyspnoea. The patient has a distressing breathlessness, frothy sputum (which may be blood stained) similar to acute left ventricular failure. Eventually, right ventricular failure will occur. The 'moist' lungs are prone to infection.

Atrial fibrillation may occur at any time. Instead of the regular wave impulse going through the atrial wall, the atrial walls tremble and contract rapidly and irregularly. The atrio ventricular node cannot send regular impulses to the ventricles and there is a subsequent irregularity of ventricular contractions. Not all the contractions are effective because filling of the ventricles is incomplete. Effective contractions may be felt at the radial pulse, non-effective ones will not. The apex beat will therefore be quicker than the radial pulse – pulse deficit. The patient complains of palpitations and is usually restless and unable to sleep as cardiac output is reduced.

The combination of mitral stenosis and atrial fibrillation may cause stasis of blood in the left atrium which may coagulate. This clot may dislodge, pass through an incompetent or relaxed valve and lead to *embolism* – cerebral, mesenteric, renal or limbs.

Aortic valve stenosis

This is usually rheumatic but may also be congenital or occasionally the third stage of syphilis – again, incompetence may be present.

Effects, signs and symptoms The narrowed aortic valve increases the work of the left ventricle. It becomes enlarged and will eventually fail. Whilst enlarging, the coronary artery supply is insufficient and the patient may complain of angina (pain on effort). The first indications may, however, be those of left ventricular failure followed by right ventricular failure (congestive heart failure). Sudden death may occur.

Some authorities give a prognosis of only two years from the onset of symptoms unless treatment is given.

Rheumatic fever may also, more rarely, cause damage to the tricuspid and pulmonary valve and some patients may in fact have damage to all four valves together!

Diagnosis – investigations
1 Clinical examination and history
2 Chest X-ray
3 Electrocardiography
4 Cardiac catheterization – obstructions and pressure changes may be detected.

Cardiac catheterization is done in specialist units and cannot be dealt with here in detail. The techniques involve:
1 Catheter passed through cephalic vein to the right side of the heart.
2 Catheter passed through an arterial puncture (usually femoral) for the left side of the heart.

Nursing points – dangers
1 Haemorrhage from puncture sites
2 Infection into puncture sites
3 Abnormal rhythms may occur if the catheter causes a further lesion on the wall of the heart

Treatment
Cardiac surgery is indicated for valve disease. Most units now employ open heart surgery using a pump oxygenator in cardio pulmonary by-pass. Mechanical or biological valves may be introduced.

Nursing notes
Details of heart surgery nursing cannot be given in a book of this nature. It is obviously extensive. The general nurse may be involved in explaining surgery to anxious patients and relatives before transfer for operation. Although the success rate is much better, the technical difficulties (e.g. suturing myocardium that has been damaged by rheumatic disease) are considerable and the risks are serious.

Coronary artery disease

Arteriosclerosis – ageing degeneration; diabetes mellitus
Atherosclerosis – cigarette smoking; hyperlipidaemia; hypertension

Both conditions may cause narrowing and eventual occlusion of the coronary arteries.

Ischaemic heart disease (Ischaemia – diminished blood supply)

May cause *angina pectoris* (chest pain on effort) and *heart failure*.

Angina pectoris

There is a typical chest pain in which the patient clasps the fist over the heart. It may radiate into the neck, arms or abdomen. It is often overlooked as indigestion. The pain is relieved by resting.

Nursing note
The patient needs advice to attend his doctor and will need thorough investigations.

Treatment Glyceryl trinitrate tablets taken sublingually work quickly but the effect is only for 20 30 minutes. Beta blocking drugs (e.g. propanalol) may be used for long term care.

Nursing note
Patients should normally be allowed glyceryl trinitrate at the bed side, but the nurse should still endeavour to report all incidents of chest pain and any persistence of pain.

Coronary thrombosis

The formation of a clot in a coronary artery which occludes the flow to the myocardium – *myocardial infarction*. The result is necrosis (death of tissue) of that piece of heart muscle.

Effects, signs and symptoms
1 *Sudden death*
    1 Cardiac arrest – the heart stops beating completely (asystole).
    2 Ventricular fibrillation – the lesion in the ventricle wall causes it to 'tremble' rather than contract. Cardiac output is virtually nil.

These both cause sudden death – some authorities quote as many as 25% of patients die at the first attack.

Nursing note
External cardiac compression ('heart massage') may be successful in restarting the heart for the patient to be transferred to a coronary care unit.

2 *Acute heart failure* The damaged myocardium cannot work hard enough for ventricular contraction and acute heart failure will occur – usually left ventricular failure. As with heart failure, the patient will be acutely short of breath, have very low blood pressure (cardiogenic shock), and will be afraid of dying.

3 *Arrhythmias* The lesions in the myocardium lead to alteration of the wave contraction rhythm in the heart. Spontaneous contractions may occur (especially in the ventricular walls) – known as ectopic beats. The patient may have palpitations or a sensation of the heart having stopped for a moment. It may increase the anxiety and cause restlessness.

Damage in the septum of the heart will interfere with impulses going through the bundle of His. The ventricles may then contract independently – usually much slower than normal. This is known as 'heart block'. The cardiac output may be seriously diminished. The patient will again be anxious and restless and have occasional 'blackouts' (syncope) as the blood supply to the brain is insufficient to maintain consciousness. (Known as *Stokes-Adams syndrome*.)

4 *Angina pain* Spasmodic contractions of the coronary vessel to try to get blood through the obstruction causes excruciating pain which is severe enough to cause shock (neurogenic) with a low blood pressure. The pain radiates – often down the arm, sometimes the neck, sometimes abdominal pain.

Nursing note

Shock is cardiogenic, neurogenic and also emotional (fear of dying) and urgent steps are needed to assess and treat it.

5 *Inflammation* All necrosed tissue causes inflammation around it. If the infarction is affecting the full thickness of the myocardium, there will be pericarditis and endocarditis as well as myocarditis. Metabolic rate will be increased. The patient may have a persistent soreness in the pericardium. Pyrexia may be noted. The major problems concerning the inflammation are the complications that may occur:

1 A full thickness infarction may be suddenly pushed out as the ventricular contraction tears the scar tissue edges – rupture of the heart. The patient collapses and dies about 7–14 days or more after the original attack.

2 Endocarditis may cause clot formation on the inside wall of the heart – mural thrombus. Separation of this clot may lead to pulmonary embolism from the right side or systemic embolism from the left.

6 *Further thrombus formation* Clotting mechanisms have been initiated by the damaged tissue. Deep vein thrombosis is a hazard for the patient on bed rest.

Diagnosis – investigations

1 Clinical examination and history
2 Electrocardiogram monitoring
3 Blood – serum transaminases will be increased (not specific to myocardial infarction)

Treatment

1 *Emergency resuscitation* External cardiac compression; expired air resuscitation; intubation with endotracheal tube; defibrillation; intracardiac adrenaline; intravenous – sodium bicarbonate for acidosis and lignocaine for arrhythmias.

2 *Treat for shock* Diamorphine (or morphine derivative) – an analgesia, a sedative and treats left ventricular failure

3 *Treat heart failure* Diuretics – digoxin may *not* be used as it excites the ventricle wall and may cause more ectopic beats

4 *Treat arrhythmias* Initially intravenous lignocaine, later oral drugs (e.g. procainamide, quinidine) or Beta blocking agents. For heart block – atropine sulphate

5 *Prevent further thrombosis* Anticoagulants – heparin initially and warfarin later. Some physicians are now using aspirin as a prophylactic (preventive) agent for clot formation.

Suggested nursing response

Assessment	Care
1 Recognition of cardiac arrest: sudden collapse and loss of consciousness; no femoral or carotid pulse; dilating pupils	Cardiac arrest drill
2 Indications of shock and heart failure: ashen colour; 'thready' pulse; low blood pressure; restlessness and anxiety; shortness of breath	Prescribed drugs – diamorphine is a controlled drug. Position patient according to his condition. If blood pressure low – use Jack-knife position (see heart failure). Calm reassurance for the patient and relatives. Complete bed rest
3 Recognition of cardiac arrhythmias and the effect of anti arrhythmia drugs: attach to electrocardiogram; monitor (cardioscope); recognize changes	Care of intravenous infusion. Placement and care of ECG leads. Careful explanation to the patient and relatives.
4 Observe for the effects of anticoagulants	Careful moving to avoid bruising. Avoid cuts

See also nursing responses for heart failure and the complications such as pulmonary embolism.

Coronary care units Some doctors prefer to treat patients at home unless serious arrhythmias are detected. There are often serious psychological effects of patients having been in high dependency care and then moved out to wards and finally home.

Nursing note
The nurse should be aware of this and warn patients and relatives of the increased anxiety when moves are made.

Memory and revision aid

See how many A's you can associate with coronary artery disease.
e.g.

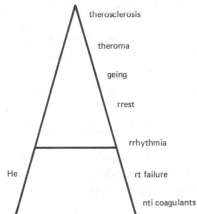

- therosclerosis
- theroma
- geing
- rrest
- rrhythmia
- He — rt failure
- nti coagulants

Congenital heart disease

Cause factors
1 *Genetic* Some children may have heart defects as part of other conditions e.g. trisomy 21 (Down's) syndrome.
2 *Rubella* The most common cause is rubella during pregnancy. Rubella vaccine should reduce this number.

Nursing notes
It is very rare for more than one child in a family to have a congenital heart lesion but parents may like to have genetic counselling if the first baby is affected. Remember the nurse's role as a health educationalist in advocating vaccination for rubella.

Effects, signs and symptoms The changes affect the embryonic development of the heart and the completion closures that should normally take place when the baby is born.

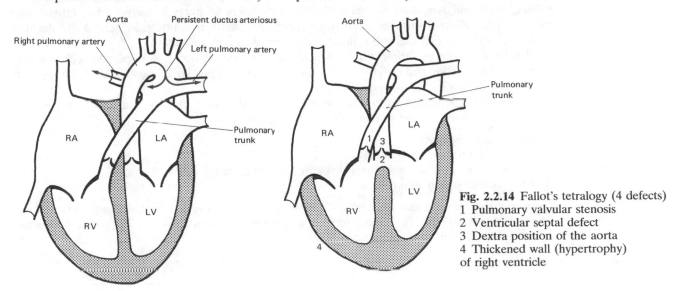

Fig. 2.2.14 Fallot's tetralogy (4 defects)
1 Pulmonary valvular stenosis
2 Ventricular septal defect
3 Dextra position of the aorta
4 Thickened wall (hypertrophy) of right ventricle

Fig. 2.2.13 Patent or persistent ductus anteriosus

Patent or persistent ductus arteriosus Shunting of blood from the aorta to the pulmonary arteries may lead to pulmonary hypertension. The main effect is breathlessness, including feeding dyspnoea which may lead to a failure to thrive.
Atrial septal defect Similar effects but often much later in life (some are undetected). (Shunt is not so severe.)
Ventricular septal defect Again, left to right shunt. The effects are often more severe and the child may go into heart failure.
Tetralogy of Fallot One error of development that leads to four defects

1 Pulmonary valve stenosis
2 Ventricular septal defect
3 Dextra position (moved to the right) of the aorta
4 Hypertrophy (over growth) of the right ventricle

One can see that there will be very poor oxygenation of blood in this condition and the baby is cyanosed ('blue baby') as well as breathless and usually retarded in growth. They are in serious danger from heart failure, chest infections and endocarditis.

The signs of congenital heart disease are through heart murmurs heard on early examination of new born babies.

Nursing notes

Children with heart lesions are often very precious to the family and are often very affectionate themselves. The establishment of an understood relationship with the nurse, the child and the parents is important.

Exercise tolerance is variable and children often find their own level of activity. An interesting phenomenon is to note the child 'squatting' to reduce the venous return after exercise.

Diagnosis – investigations

1 Clinical examination for heart murmurs   2 Cardiac catheterization

Treatment Heart surgery is indicated.
Patent ductus arteriosus may be ligated through a thoracotomy. Other lesions usually require cardio pulmonary by-pass.
Tetralogy of Fallot – there may be two stages:
1 Pulmonary valvotomy as soon as possible.
2 Correction of defects when more developed.

Suggested nursing response

Apply – the *care of 'precious children'* (see 2.14), the *care of heart failure* (see p 42), the *care of chest infection* (see 2.1), and possibly the *care of endocarditis* (see p 51).
Details of paediatric cardiac surgery will not be covered in this book.

Pericarditis–inflammation of the pericardium

Causes

1 *Viruses* – may follow upper respiratory tract infection
2 *Rheumatic* – see acute rheumatism p 45
3 *Myocardial infarction*
4 *Uraemia* – see chronic renal failure 2.4
5 *Tuberculosis* – rare in this country now
6 *Neoplasms* – the pericardial sac is occasionally infiltrated by a bronchial carcinoma

Effects, signs and symptoms Raised metabolic rate leads to pyrexia, tachycardia, fatigue and malaise. The inflamed surfaces cause pain – typically a sharp, irritating pain behind the sternum (retrosternal). A pericardial rub is heard by the physician on auscultation.

Whenever serous membranes are involved, an effusion may occur. A pericardial effusion may embarrass heart action and lead to breathlessness and a raised jugular venous pressure. The effect is increased if the patient is moved quickly.

Tuberculous pericarditis resolves leaving a calcified fibrosis ('stony heart') which becomes 'constrictive' – again leading to embarrassment of heart action.

Diagnosis – investigations

1 Clinical history and examination
2 Chest X-ray – may show a pericardial effusion and certainly calcified lesions
3 Electrocardiograph changes

Treatment Rest in bed – may need to be 2–3 weeks. Corticosteroid drugs relieve pain and fever, but will not prevent effusion. Aspiration of a pericardial effusion is dangerous but may be necessary if a large effusion is affecting heart action.

Suggested nursing response

Assessment	Care
1 Raised metabolic rate: pyrexia; tachycardia (4 hourly observations)	Rest in bed. Control temperature with fans
2 Pain – note the position and nature of pain	Prescribed analgesia and corticosteroid drugs. Reassurance – the patient may think of a heart attack
3 Indications of effusion: tachycardia; abnormal heart rhythms (cardiac monitoring); raised jugular venous pressure	Careful lifting and moving of the patient. Prepare for drainage of the effusion – needle and syringe used. Patient must be observed throughout the procedure – two nurses should assist the doctor – one to observe

Endocarditis–inflammation of the endocardium

Causes
1 Mainly bacterial
 1 Acute bacterial endocarditis may be a complication of septicaemia.
 2 Sub acute bacterial endocarditis is usually caused by streptococcus viridans which is a normal inhabitant (commensal) bacteria in the mouth, but may enter the blood stream in dental caries (tooth decay) or following dental care.

Nursing notes
All patients with known heart lesions need advice about dental hygiene and care. They should be seen by a professional hygienist. Prophylactic antibacterial drugs are given before dental treatment.

2 Myocardial infarction–see p 42   3 Rheumatic–see acute rheumatism p 45

Sub acute bacterial endocarditis

Effects, signs and symptoms Inflammation only occurs on a previously damaged heart and the valves are the most vulnerable. Previous damage may be rheumatic or congenital. There is a raised metabolic rate and a prolonged fever with pyrexia and tachycardia, weakness, tiredness and malaise.

The patient is anaemic, often with a pale brown discolouration under the skin. The complexion is known as 'cafe au lait' (milky coffee). There may be small haemorrhages under the skin – petechial spots may appear. Under the nails, they are seen as 'splinter' haemorrhages. 'Vegetations' on the valves are loosely bound and fragments may break away leading to emboli. Small emboli may cause tender, red swellings on finger and toe pads–known as *Osler's nodes*. Emboli may lodge in the glomeruli of the kidney and lead to a progressive renal damage. Red cells may escape into the urine through the glomerulo nephritis.

Further infection of the valves will cause more damage and heart failure will eventually develop.

Diagnosis – investigations
1 Clinical history and examination
2 Blood cultures–specimens of blood should be placed in warm containers and will be examined as quickly as possible in the laboratory
3 Blood–for haemoglobin, leucocytes and erythrocyte sedimentation rate
4 Examination of the mouth for lesions
5 Throat swabs

Treatment
1 Long term rest in bed
2 Antibacterial agents–benzyl penicillin is given, usually with gentamicin, for at least 4 weeks and may be given intravenously or intramuscularly in large doses
3 Valve replacement may be indicated even in a very ill patient as a life saving measure

Suggested nursing response
This is a very serious consequence of heart disease and measures to prevent it by good mouth care must be stressed again.

Assessment	Care
1 Raised metabolic rate: 4 hourly observations for pyrexia and tachycardia	Rest in bed – long term. Temperature control. Often very weak and tired – need a lot of careful moving, hygiene and care of pressure areas
2 Observations for emboli: look for Osler's nodes; regular urine observation and testing for blood	Local and general pain relief is required. Care of ischaemic areas
3 Indications of heart failure	Careful positioning. Oxygen therapy. Chemotherapy

Drugs Observations and care of intravenous infusion line for a long period.
 1 Check bags and additives carefully
 2 Check the giving set and should be replaced every 24 hours
 3 Check the site for cellulitis or phlebitis
See the *British National Formulary* for undesired effects of drugs being used in large doses.

Shock

Shock is a sudden failure of the circulatory system to supply enough oxygen (blood) for the cells, characterized by a serious fall in the blood pressure.

Causes
1 *Cardiogenic*–failure of the left ventricle to maintain blood pressure. Usually follows myocardial infarction.
2 *Hypovolaemia*–gross loss of blood volume due to haemorrhage or plasma loss in burns.
3 *Neurogenic*–extreme pain causes a fall in blood pressure (moderate pain usually increases it).
4 *Toxic or septic*–extensive vaso dilation as part of the inflammatory response.

5 *Anaphylactic*–extreme reaction to antibody/antigen response (may happen with drugs e.g. penicillin).

6 *Emotional*–extreme fear may cause a fall in blood pressure.

Nursing notes

It should be recognized that a combination of causes may be present, contributing to the depth of shock that occurs. Urgent recognition of blood loss, pain and fear will often help to save a patient's life.

Effects, signs and symptoms Profound shock will kill a patient within minutes due to lack of oxygen to brain cells. Shortage of oxygen to brain cells may cause rapid loss of consciousness or the patient may be anxious and restless. Some have shown quite bizarre behaviour after accidents such as walking for many miles from the scene. Amnesia is possible without apparent loss of consciousness. Nausea and vomiting may occur as the vomiting centre is affected.

Lack of oxygen to periphery The skin is pale, cold to touch and is clammy as evaporation of sweat ceases. Patients complain of feeling cold and shivery.

Lack of blood pressure to the kidneys leads to a failure of the glomerular filter and leads to acute renal failure (see 2.4). There is a diminished urine output (oliguria) and may even be a complete failure of production (anuria)

Nursing notes

Observation of actual urine output may delay the finding and it may be necessary to regularly palpate the bladder. Catheterization may help but there is danger in putting a catheter into an empty bladder. Post operative observations for urine output are mainly looking for oliguria (suppression) rather than retention.

Poor blood flow to the lungs may cause changes in the alveolar membranes, leading to further hypoxia and a danger of inflammatory changes. The patient will be short of breath with a 'bubbly' chest sound.

Diagnosis Very low blood pressure and patient collapse. There is little time for detailed investigations.

Treatment Depends on the cause

1 *Cardiogenic* In itself difficult to treat (see coronary thrombosis p 47)

2 *Hypovolaemic* Rapid replacement of blood volume with blood (O Rhesus negative may be used) plasma or Dextran. Arresting bleeding

3 *Neurogenic* Strong analgesia may be given intravenously if peripheral circulation is poor

4 *Toxic/septic* Intravenous antibacterial agents

5 *Anaphylactic* Adrenaline 1:1000(IM) or hydrocortisone 100 mg(IV) are given urgently

6 *Emotional* Sensitive reassurance will help

Suggested nursing response

The word *shock* demands rapid action by the whole nursing team. Discuss roles beforehand if possible–one nurse will need to be with the patient constantly until recovery has started.

Assessment	Care
1 Loss of consciousness	Semi prone position. Protect the airway. Nil by mouth
2 Blood pressure levels: pulse is rapid and feeble–observe frequently, record at least every 15 minutes if below 80 mm Hg systolic (or on doctor's orders)	Legs raised to increase venous return. Jack-knife position if conscious. Nurse needed constantly
3 Blood or fluid loss: restlessness; tachycardia; obvious haemorrhage	Intravenous infusion trolley prepared – 2 IV lines needed. Assist doctor. Rapid administration. (Blood may need to be warmed if rapid infusion)
4 Central venous pressure line for recording venous pressure (CVP)	Infusion rate adjusted according to CVP recording
5 Pain	Prescribed analgesia
6 Nausea and vomiting	Possibly antiemetic
7 Suppression of urine: palpation of bladder, catheter drainage	Treat renal failure (see 2.4)

Note: Rising serum potassium levels (hyperkalaemia) may cause cardiac arrest. Acidosis will occur and sodium bicarbonate IV may be required.

8 Anxiety levels: defence mechanisms to hide fear (inappropriate responses)	Reassurance in words and confident approach to the patient

Patients with lung affects may need to have intermittent positive pressure ventilation through an endotracheal tube. Transfer to an intensive care unit should be arranged.

Haemorrhage (bleeding)

Usually classified according to the vessels damaged or the occasion of onset.

Arterial Blood from an artery – bright red in colour – ejected in spurts corresponding to the pulse wave. Major arteries severed will lead to death from shock in a few minutes. Smaller arteries may retract and stop bleeding – until blood pressure is restored. Punctures in the wall of an artery may bleed for many hours.

Venous Blood from a vein – dark red in colour – seepage may go on for some time and shock may be delayed.

Capillary No real characteristics in the blood, often regarded as trivial, but death can result if there is a wide area damaged or if clotting factors are inadequate.

Primary Immediately following injury or surgery.

Reactionary Bleeding which occurs as blood pressure is restored (post operative danger).

Secondary When a lesion has been infected, the clot may break away and cause bleeding 7–10 days after injury

Treatment
1 Arrest bleeding   2 Replace blood if severe loss

Suggested nursing response

Assess the injury by exposing the wound. Observe for indications of internal bleeding (restlessness, rising pulse rate and falling blood pressure, air hunger).

Care Apply sterile pads and bandages (do not remove large foreign bodies) until controlled. Treat the patient for shock. Transfer to Accident Centre urgently.

Haematoma (bruise)

Blood in tissues may form a haematoma which may resolve over a few days. They will cause inflammation though and may become infected, with abscess formation.

Nursing note

Careful observations of bruising itself and for evidence of a rising metabolic rate are needed. Persistent ones may occasionally need surgical treatment.

4 The lymphatic system

may be considered a subsidiary part of the cardio vascular system

Functions	Structures involved
1 Drainage of intercellular fluid – permeable to proteins, micro organisms (living and dead) and even small particles	Lymph capillaries, lymph vessels – structures similar to veins but finer. Valves give the 'beaded' appearance
2 Filtration of lymph and phagocytosis (destruction of micro organisms by ingestion)	Lymph nodes – reticulo endothelial cells remove micro organisms, particles and cells (including malignant ones!). Superficial nodes and deep nodes are present
3 Manufacture of lymphocytes, monocytes and antibodies	Lymphoid tissue in the nodes, thymus gland in infancy and the spleen
4 Transportation of lipids (digested fats) following absorption	Lymph capillaries in the intestinal villi drain into lymph vessels known as lacteals (appear milky white after a fatty meal)
5 Breakdown of red blood cells (erythrocytes) and platelets (thrombocytes). pigments go to the liver; iron goes to bone marrow (but some is stored)	Spleen (and other reticulo endothelial cells in the liver and lymph nodes)

Lymphoid tissue is also found in areas without a confining capsule. They are referred to as nodules. Main sites are: tonsils and adenoids; intestines – Peyer's patches; vermiform appendix.

Conditions of the lymphatic system

Lymphangitis

Inflammation of the lymph vessels. It is usually a sequel to a localized infection such as an abscess. Superficial vessels can be observed as red lines when inflamed.
Treatment is for the infection, but is an indication for using antibacterial agents.

Lymphadenitis

Inflammation of the lymph nodes follows lymphangitis. The nodes may be tender to touch. Again, antibacterial drugs are indicated. The metabolic rate rises and general care of the patient with inflammation as well as localized care to the infected lesion are necessary.

Nursing note
Observations for early lymphangitis may help to speed up the treatment of an infection.
Lymph nodes are sites for secondary malignant tumours (metastases). See, especially, bronchial carcinoma and the hilar nodes, breast carcinoma and the axillary nodes.

Glandular fever (infectious mononucleosis)

Cause Epstein Barr (EB) virus. Mildly infectious, often spread by oral contact (sometimes called the kissing disease). Mainly affects children and young people. Incubation period (period between contact and appearance of symptoms) is 5–10 days.

Effects, signs and symptoms Raised metabolic rate in fever. The patient is progressively tired, feels ill, loses the appetite. Pyrexia and tachycardia appear.

Lymph nodes become enlarged and there is often a sore throat with an exudate. Enlarged cervical glands and the sore throat may cause difficulties in swallowing and even breathing may be difficult in rare cases. The spleen may enlarge (splenomegaly) and cause abdominal discomfort. Some patients may feel ill and depressed for many weeks or months with occasional feverish attacks.

Diagnosis – investigations
1 Clinical examination and history
2 Paul-Bunnell agglutination test of blood (not always positive)

Treatment
1 Rest in bed if high fever.   2 Treat the symptoms.

Nursing notes
This condition has affected many nurses themselves. Admission to hospital is rarely needed. Care at home is that of a patient with a raised metabolic rate and careful understanding of the later depression that occurs.

Hodgkin's disease

A malignant disease of the lymph nodes, but often involves lymphoid tissue outside the nodes too.

Cause Not known

Effects, signs and symptoms It is thought that Hodgkin's disease starts in one area and spreads to the others. The nodes are initially swollen but painless. Cervical ones may be more obvious but some are discrete. There may be bouts of fever, but in some cases fever does not present until the terminal stages. Pressure by enlarged glands may cause dysphagia, dyspnoea, jaundice or even paraplegia. If adjacent tissues are infiltrated, other symptoms may occur, e.g. mediastinal spread may cause an irritating cough.

There are four stages of Hodgkin's disease classified:
1 Involvement of a single node region.
2 Two or more regions, or 1 region + site outside lymph nodes on the same side.
3 Involvement of regions on both sides of the diaphragm.
4 Wide involvement of lymph nodes and tissues outside the lymphatics.

Diagnosis – investigations
1 Clinical examination
2 Biopsy of affected node(s) – for assessment purposes, this may involve multiple procedures, including laparotomy before treatment is commenced
3 Lymphangiography – X-rays using radio opaque dyes in the lymphatics
4 Chest X-ray – for mediastinal involvement

Nursing notes
Investigation procedures may be very prolonged and the nurse will need to support patients psychologically as well as physically assisting in them. A careful assessment of the patient's reaction to 'cancer' and a sensitive discussion with all the health team, relatives and the patient, emphasizing the optimism of treatment may be the best way of obtaining co-operation.

Treatment Localized disease responds well to radiotherapy. More widespread disease needs extensive radiotherapy combined with the use of cytotoxic drugs – given in combinations and at intervals to prevent profound bone marrow depression.

Suggested nursing response

Assessment	Care
1 Effects of radiotherapy and cytotoxic drugs:	
1 on skin	Skin care
2 nausea and vomiting	Antiemetic drugs
3 bone marrow depression	Possible reverse barrier nursing if white cell count is very low

continued next page

4 epilation (hair falling out) — Reassurance – it usually grows again

2 Evidence of rising metabolic rate; pyrexia, tachycardia, fatigue — Rest in bed. Maintain body temperature. Glucose drinks

Many patients feel tired for a long time. Sleep is often lost during cytotoxic treatment periods. Depression may become quite serious. The nurse needs to warn the relatives of this.

Rupture of the spleen

Cause

1 The normal spleen may be ruptured by severe violence such as road traffic accidents, heavy fall across an obstruction or kicking.
2 An enlarged spleen (due to disease) may be ruptured by quite a minor blow.

Effects, signs and symptoms

Severe damage – torn from its pedicle or fragmented. There is obviously massive blood loss, with profound shock and death occurs before resuscitation is possible.

Rupture of the capsule leads to haemorrhage into the upper abdomen, spreading through the peritoneum. Signs of haemorrhage include restlessness, increasing pallor, rising pulse rate, falling blood pressure and sighing respirations ('air hunger'). Signs of haemo-peritoneum include generalized tenderness and guarding, tenderness on rectal examination, abdominal distension and loss of peristalsis.

Haematoma due to laceration inside the capsule may expand and rupture through the capsule (may be up to 10 days later). Signs of haemorrhage and haemo-peritoneum.

Diagnosis – investigations

1 Clinical history and examination
2 Careful observations up to every 15 minutes
3 Chest X-ray and abdominal X-ray
4 Aspiration through abdominal wall
5 May not be confirmed until laparotomy

Nursing note

As haemorrhage is progressive and the patient may be very weak, great care and support may be needed for X-ray examinations.

Treatment

1 Rapid blood tranfusion before surgery – vast quantities may be needed for surgery too.
2 Laparotomy and splenectomy

Suggested nursing response

Assessment	Care
1 Shock and haemorrhage: restlessness and anxiety; tachycardia (increasing rate); hypotension (systolic falling); air hunger, pallor and cyanosis; pain; fear; central venous pressure	Reassurance by speech, body language and efficient care. Rest in Jack-knife position or semi prone if loss of consciousness. Prepare for rapid blood transfusion, including bath for warming blood. Analgesia may be part of pre medication for surgery
2 Effects on peritoneum: *1* abdominal tenderness	Careful positioning of the patient
2 abdominal distension (girth measurements) *3* loss of peristalsis (no bowel sounds) – may lead to vomiting, fluid and electrolyte imbalance	May need nasogastric aspiration. Nutrients may need to be given intravenously – especially protein and glucose to maintain the nitrogen balance and restore energy loss

Splenectomy may also be needed for other pathological conditions

Pre operative assessment and care
1 Circulation (may need blood before surgery)
2 Skin – hygiene and shaving

Surgery All splenic tissue needs to be removed. In trauma, there is often severe blood loss as the laparotomy incision is made. Drain usually left in the bed of the spleen.

Post operative assessment and care
1 Observations and care of the airway
2 Observations and care of the wound and drains
3 Continue the care of a shocked patient – remains very ill
4 Nasogastric aspiration and intravenous nutrition until peristalsis is restored
5 Complications: dilation of the stomach; paralytic ileus persisting; subphrenic abscess (infection); splenic or portal vein thrombosis

2.3 Digestive conditions

The digestive system

This system will be considered as follows.

1 The alimentary tract   3 The pancreas
2 The liver and gall bladder   4 The abdominal wall – hernias

The alimentary tract is then divided into:

1 The mouth and pharynx   *4* The small intestine
2 The oesophagus   *5* The large intestine, rectum and anus
3 The stomach

1 The alimentary tract

The mouth and pharynx

Functions	Structures involved
1 The ingestion of food for nutrition	Mouth opened by the action of the lower jaw (mandible) by facial muscles
2 The mechanical digestion of food begins in the mouth	Teeth – incisors cut the food, pre-molar and molar teeth grind the food to increase the surface area for the enzyme action. Mastication (chewing) is brought about by the action of the lower jaw and muscles. Bolus formation is by the mechanical action of the tongue against the hard palate
3 Chemical digestion of food begins in the mouth	Salivary amylase changes starch into maltose in the alkaline medium of saliva. Saliva is secreted by the three pairs of salivary glands – paratoid, sublingual, sub-mandibular
4 Tasting of food – provides pleasure and also stimulates the production of gastric juice in preparation for swallowing	Taste buds on the tongue send sensory stimuli along the facial and the glosso-pharyngeal nerve (cranial nerves)
5 Voice production – speech, laughter and singing are influenced by the mouth structures	Action of the tongue, teeth, facial muscles, mandible and lips
6 Self cleansing and control of micro-organisms	Saliva is cleansing as is mucus from mucous membranes. Commensal bacteria inhibit fungal growths – streptococcus viridans. Large lymphatic drainage to tonsils
7 Kissing	Lips

Conditions of the mouth (see 2.1 for Pharynx)

Dental caries – tooth decay

Cause
1 Poor dental hygiene – micro organisms and food debris form plaques in the pits or crevices of the teeth
2 Refined sugars combine with the plaque to produce lactic acid which is thought to erode tooth enamel

Effects, signs and symptoms May be undetected for some time until erosion reaches the pulp on the inside. Sensitivity to cold and heat is the first symptom. Toothache is the usual symptom that leads to treatment. Infection may enter and lead to more serious conditions such as sub acute bacterial endocarditis

Suggested nursing response
The nurse is a health educationalist in all aspects and can advise on:
1 Prevention of tooth decay by giving guidance on teeth cleaning, the use of dental floss and reducing or eliminating sugars from the diet
2 Early dental treatment for toothache and repeated inspection

Remember to examine the mouths of patients for evidence of dental caries.

Inflammation of the mouth

Stomatitis inflammation of the oral mucosa
Gingivitis inflammation of the gums
Glossitis inflammation of the tongue

Causes
1 Trauma – biting of the cheek, badly fitting dentures, irritants such as alcohol or hot, spicy food

2 Infections – may be bacterial, such as streptococcal, gonococcal or syphilitic, or fungal – *Candida albicans* causes *moniliasis* (oral thrush)
3 Vitamin deficiencies – scurvy is vitamin C deficiency and may be seen in elderly patients
4 Poisoning by heavy metals – mercury or lead
5 Undesired effects of some drugs

Effects, signs and symptoms Local signs of inflammation – hot, swollen, red tissues. The patient complains of soreness, particularly when trying to eat. Inflammatory changes may cause mouth odours that are offensive to the patient and relatives and alter the taste of food, lowering the appetite. Metabolic rate may be increased and the patient may have a fever with pyrexia, tachycardia and feel very ill and miserable.

Moniliasis produces white spots. Syphilis produces chancre – an open sore.

Treatment
1 Intensive but gentle mouth care
2 Antibacterial agents if organism identified
Moniliasis – amphoteracin B or nystatin (more rare but still effective is to paint with Gentian violet!)
Syphilis – the chancre is infectious. See care for Syphilis in 2.9

Suggested nursing response

Assessment	Care
1 Careful examination of the mouth, tongue and gums	Gentle mouth care. Use mouth washes frequently – 2–3 hourly. Involve a professional dental hygienist
2 Assess for raised metabolic rate – pyrexia, tachycardia	Rest in bed or in a chair. Note the problem of giving oral energy foods
3 Abject misery	Reassurance that the mouth has good healing properties
4 Review drug therapy – especially broad spectrum antibacterial drugs	Withhold drugs until the patient has been examined

Inflammation of salivary glands – parotitis

Cause
1 *Non specific* – may be a complication of stomatitis or due to severe dehydration. Poor mouth and dental care
2 *Specific* – mumps virus

Effects signs and symptoms The glands become swollen and tender. Fever will occur with pyrexia, tachycardia and malaise.

Complications
Non specific type May form pus (suppurate) which drains into the mouth. Obstruction and calculus (stone) formation may occur – the gland becomes grossly swollen and may need surgical drainage and probing.

Mumps Infectious disease with incubation period of 21 days or more. Post puberty there is a danger of orchitis in boys (sterility only if bilateral) and mastitis in girls, (rarely) pancreatitis and encephalitis.

Treatment
1 Rest and good nursing   2 Surgery if obstruction

Suggested nursing response

Assessment	Care
1 Pain and tenderness in the glands	Prescribed analgesia. Very gentle mouth care. Mouth washes preferred to swabbing
2 Raised metabolic rate – fever	Rest in bed if pyrexia. Glucose or milk drinks as nutrition is painful

See also care of orchitis, mastitis (2.9), pancreatitis (p 83) and encephalitis (2.5)

People with mumps are rarely nursed in strict isolation, but care needs to be exercised if vulnerable children are around (e.g. with congenital heart disease).

Cancer of the mouth

The most common site is the lip, but the tongue or mucous membrane of the mouth may be invaded.

Causes Mainly idiopathic, but higher incidences do occur in smokers (including pipe smokers), alcoholics, patients with syphilitic lesions and those with poor dental hygiene.

Effects, signs and symptoms Changes may produce:
1 Leukoplakia – a covering of white tissue over the area.
2 An obvious ulcer or sore which persists. It may be painless and some patients do not report them until serious infiltration and lymphatic spread has occurred.
3 Eventually a large fungating tumour which will make eating and speech very difficult.

Nursing notes
Early diagnosis is essential for good treatment. The nurse should be a careful observer for leukoplakia or persistent ulcers and advise. Larger lesions will need careful hygiene – hydrogen peroxide mouth washes help to clear them. Deodorants may be needed for offensive smelling tumours. The patient may be generally undernourished.

Diagnosis – investigations
1 Clinical examination and history
2 Biopsy of the lesion. Some lesions are difficult to see – a head mirror, lamp and dental mirrors may be needed as well as oral instruments.

Treatment
Lip
1 Local lesions of the lip – surgical excision
2 More extensive lesions – irradiation (external, radium needles or radium mould)
Tongue
1 Local lesions – surgical excision at the tip
2 Margins of the tongue – excision of half the tongue
3 More extensive lesions or posterior – irradiation (probably with radium needles)
Mucous membrane
1 Very small lesion – excision by diathermy
2 Larger lesions – irradiation
Lymphatic spread May need block dissection of lymph glands or irradiation

Nursing notes
Detailed nursing care of each case cannot be covered in this book. Major nursing principles for cancer of the mouth and its treatment are as follows.
1 There is a great fear of tumours in the mouth as people read of serious disfigurement (even after treatment is some cases) as well as fear of spread into the brain (rare). Severe depression may occur. Strong emphasis on early treatment and positive attitudes are needed. It is most important for a patient to be able to express his anxieties and fears.
2 There is obvious impairment of ingestion and nasogastric feeding must be adequate for full nutritional requirements. A purée of normal food is better than proprietary foods in some cases – check with dieticians.
3 Speech may well be affected both before and after treatment. Methods of communication in writing, sign language and pictures need to be employed.
4 Mouth care – dental hygiene and moistening of the mucosa is needed as frequently as two hourly in some cases. Excessive salivation and difficulty in swallowing may be dealt with by a large supply of disposable wipes. A professional dental hygienist may be needed to help and advise.

Fracture of the jaw

Usually caused by direct force, but the fracture may occur opposite the site of the force or bilateral fractures may be due to the patient falling onto the point of the jaw.

Effects, signs and symptoms Considerable pain which may lead to nausea. Difficulty in speaking. Difficulty in swallowing, possibly with increased salivation or even haemorrhage in the mouth. Dribbling of blood stained fluid from the mouth. Irregular outline of the face, pain and teeth not aligned.

Diagnosis – investigations Clinical examination and X-ray examination

Treatment
First Aid
1 Support the jaw with a pad and bandage
2 Maintain the airway
3 Beware of vomiting – place in a semi prone position and **loosen the bandage if nauseated**

Surgical
1 Approximation of the fracture edges and wiring of the jaw is performed
2 Wiring the teeth together to form a splint

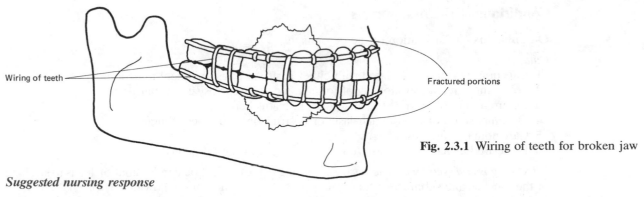

Fig. 2.3.1 Wiring of teeth for broken jaw

Suggested nursing response

Assessment	Care
1 Degree, site and nature of pain before and after treatment	Prescribed analgesia. Careful positioning in the prone or semi prone position to help drainage of fluid and avoid pressure
2 Difficulty in speaking	Arrange communication aids (call bell for help, sign language and pictures)
3 Difficulty in swallowing	Careful swabbing and aspiration of the mouth. Soft rubber tubing is used for aspirating along the side of the teeth
4 Development of oedema may continue some time after surgery. Infection and inflammation will make it become very difficult for breathing and swallowing. Obstruction could occur	Strict and regular hygiene of the mouth to prevent infection
5 Nausea and vomiting – particularly dangerous when jaws are wired	Nasogastric tube to aspirate stomach. Cut wires for the drainage of vomit

Nutrition may be started by nasogastric tube feeding but later drinking tubes can be used. Normal foods in purée form should be offered. Remember mouth hygiene after every feed.

Congenital abnormalities – cleft lip (hare lip) and cleft palate

Cause Not fully known but appears to be familial. About 1 in 1000 babies are born with varying degrees of defect.

Effects, signs and symptoms Difficulty in suckling and feeding as the tongue needs to work against the hard palate. Upper respiratory tract infections may occur because of debris entering the airway. There is an obvious cosmetic effect which distresses the parents, as well as speech defects – producing consonants is not possible.

Nursing note
Encouragement to the parents is important at the beginning, as treatment may be prolonged and it may take until adult life before cosmetic repair is complete.

Treatment Surgical repair – refashioning first the lip (2–3 months) and then the palate (may take a number of operations to complete)

Suggested nursing response
Detailed nursing care cannot be given in this book.
Principles of nursing care are:
  1 Maintaining adequate nutrition before repair is done – special teats may be used although some do better with spoon feeding.
  2 Preventing food from entering the airway. Hygiene to clean the cleft after feeding.
  3 Observations, treatment and care if infection does occur (see 2.1).
  4 Care of the child for surgery (see 2.14).
  5 Arranging speech therapy.
  6 Encouraging a normal daily living for the child with play, schooling and games.

The Oesophagus

Functions	Structures involved
1 The smooth passage of the bolus of food from the mouth to the stomach	Mucous membrane on the inside provides moist smooth passage. Blood vessels, lymphatics and mucus secreting glands are in the sub-mucous coat. Smooth (involuntary muscles) are arranged Longitudinal Outside, Circular Inside (LOCI). Outer fibrous coat
Peristalsis As the bolus enters, circular muscles relax in front and contract behind it. The longitudinal muscles push the contraction wave forward and propel the bolus to the stomach.	
2 Influence of salivation	Nerve reflexes stimulate salivary glands when food is in the oesophagus

Conditions of the oesophagus

Oesophagitis – inflammation of the oesophagus

Causes

1 Infection – possibly associated with either gastroenteritis or fungal infections
2 Following trauma – swallowing of foreign bodies or corrosive substances
3 Regurgitation of gastric contents (acid) in hiatus hernia
4 Decomposition of food in achalasia or obstruction of the oesophagus
5 Carcinoma of the oesophagus
6 Undesired effect of radiation (e.g. to carcinoma of the bronchus)

Effects, signs and symptoms These vary according to the cause. Local inflammation leads to swelling of the mucous and submucous coat. The patient has difficulty in swallowing (dysphagia) any food and may become seriously undernourished. The membrane becomes sensitive and tender. The patient complains of 'heartburn' – a deep burning pain behind the sternum.

The metabolic rate may be raised leading to pyrexia, tachycardia, tiredness and general malaise.

Diagnosis – investigations

1 Clinical history and examination
2 X-ray examination using barium – a barium swallow
3 Cold light endoscopy gives direct vision of the lesion

Treatment Depends on the cause

Suggested nursing response

Assessment	Care
1 Dysphagia – the degree of difficulty in swallowing: the nutritional state of the patient; upper arm muscles for indications of muscle wasting	Provide a full diet in liquid form if a soft normal diet cannot be tolerated. Avoid hot, spicy food, alcohol, tobacco and coffee
2 Indications of 'heartburn'	Antacids may be very helpful as prescribed
See also for individual conditions	

Foreign bodies

Usually stick in the narrowest part which is just behind the larynx. The patient feels the pain locally and removal is performed through endoscopy.

Suggested nursing response for endoscopy – oesophagoscopy
Before the procedure Nothing by mouth for 6 hours. Full explanation and assurance. Sedation may be given. Nasogastric aspiration may be requested.

Procedure Local anaesthetic spray is used. Flexible scope is passed. The patient is sitting to start with, but lying on his side for the final part.

After the procedure Withhold fluids until the swallowing reflex has returned. Observe for 24 hours for indications of bleeding and perforation.

Rupture of the oesophagus

May be due to trauma, corrosive poisoning or surgical procedures. The patient is seriously ill with indications of shock, acute respiratory distress, possibly heart failure and surgical emphysema. Urgent thoracotomy and repair would be performed and intensive care would be required.

Nursing note
Full details cannot be included in this text, but the nurse should be aware of the very serious nature of this condition. Relatives as well as the patient need a lot of support.

Treatment is aimed at surgical repair through a thoracotomy, irrigation of the thoracic cavity, antibacterial drugs and intensive support therapy (nutrition, possibly mechanical ventilation). The prognosis is guarded.

Achalasia of the cardia

A condition in which the smooth muscles in the lower part of the oesophagus fail to relax for the bolus to go through the cardiac sphincter. The cause is not known, but appears to be a failure of nerve conduction to the muscles.

Effects, signs and symptoms The oesophagus becomes enlarged above the site of the tight muscles. Food will accumulate in the large oesophagus. The patient complains of dysphagia behind the lower end of the sternum. Eventually, food cannot enter the stomach – malnutrition and weight loss will occur. At night time or if the patient lies down, food may regurgitate into the pharynx and there is danger of inhalation.

Nursing notes
The patient is advised to have very small meals and not to eat at all for two hours before retiring to bed. He should be advised to sleep with the head and shoulders raised.

Diagnosis – investigations
1 Clinical history and examination   2 Barium swallow   3 Oesophagoscopy

Treatment
1 Dilation of the narrowing by use of a water filled bag passed through the oesophagoscope.
2 Cardiomyotomy (Heller's operation) – division of the muscles at the lower end (but not penetrating the submucous and mucous coats) performed through a thoracotomy (see 2.1).

Nursing notes See oesophagoscopy and thoracotomy.
The main danger is perforation of the oesophagus.

Carcinoma of oesophagus

Causes Not known but occurs more frequently in elderly patients.

Effects, signs and symptoms Local infiltration produces inflammation, ulcerations and stenosis (narrowing). The patient complains of dysphagia which is progressive until even liquids cannot be swallowed. Severe weight loss will occur. Spread through the lymphatics and blood stream (metastases) has often occurred before the patient seeks medical advice. The tumours are usually in the lower third of the oesophagus.

Nursing notes
Careful reporting of the dysphagia and noting weight changes will help. Nurses responsible for elderly patients on long term care need to be alert.

Diagnosis – investigations
1 Clinical history   2 Barium swallow   3 Oesophagoscopy

Treatment
1 Tumours in the upper and middle third are treated by irradiation but results are not good and the radiation effects may be distressing to the elderly.
2 Tumours in the lower third, if diagnosed early enough, may be removed surgically with a section of the jejunum used to replace the removed oesophagus. A thoracotomy and laparotomy will be needed for this surgery.

Nursing notes
See *nursing care for irradiation* (2.12), *thoracotomy* (2.1) *laparotomy* and *surgery in the elderly* (2.15).
The prognosis is not very good and the patient will need terminal care eventually.
  Some surgeons will insert a tube through the tumour for the passage of food as a palliative measure for nutrition. Gastrostomy may be performed but is not tolerated well by the elderly. Neither measure seems to extend the life of these patients.

Hiatus hernia (diaphragmatic hernia)

A protusion through the diaphragm of the cardiac sphincter of the stomach, the fundus of the stomach alongside the oesophagus (para oesophageal) or (*rarely*) larger structures of the abdominal cavity through a large defect (congenital).

Causes
1 Congenital weakness – young babies are affected.
2 Possibly part of the ageing process as middle aged and elderly are affected.
3 Obesity and raised intra abdominal pressure are contributing factors.

Effects, signs and symptoms Rarely, in a large defect, abdominal contents in the baby's thoracic cavity will lead to acute respiratory distress – an emergency condition requiring specialist surgery. Some babies have regurgitation of feeds only – noted as the baby lies down after feeding.

Nursing note
Nursing the baby in a 'baby chair' usually solves the problem as the small defect will no longer allow the growing stomach to herniate.

In adults reflux of the gastric juices occurs as the cardiac sphincter fails to close. It may occur spontaneously, but it is more common when stooping, after a heavy meal, when straining on defaecation (raising intra abdominal pressure) and when lying down at night. The patient complains of the regurgitation of acid contents, sometimes into the throat and mouth. Inflammation of the mucosa in the oesophagus will cause the typical pain (heart burn). Persistent oesophagitis may lead to ulceration and bleeding. The patient develops iron deficiency anaemia and occult blood is found in the stools. Fibrosis of the inflamed oesophagus may lead to narrowing (stenosis) and obstruction. The patient then complains of difficulty in swallowing (dysphagia) and malnutrition will develop.

A para oesophageal hernia may protrude into the mediastinum and cause breathing and cardiac embarrassment. Rarely (more with a para oesophageal), strangulation can occur. An emergency thoracotomy would be needed to prevent rupture of the oesophagus.

Diagnosis – investigations
1 Clinical history and examination   2 Barium swallow X-ray examination   3 Oesophagoscopy

Treatment
1 *Postural* The patient sleeps with head and shoulders raised. Avoid stooping.
2 *Diet* Reduce weight. Avoid heavy meals. Prevent constipation.
3 *Drugs* Cimetidine reduces acidity and helps healing. Buffer agents or antacids (e.g. aluminium hydroxide) reduce the acidity.
4 *Surgery* Thoracotomy approach for repair if severe symptoms persist, or in strangulation.

Nursing notes
See the treatment above – much of it is good nursing technique. Remember to observe for the indications of iron deficiency anaemia. Iron replacements may be given, rarely a blood transfusion. Many patients are admitted for other reasons than the hiatus hernia. Most are treated at home. The care needs to be continued if they are admitted.

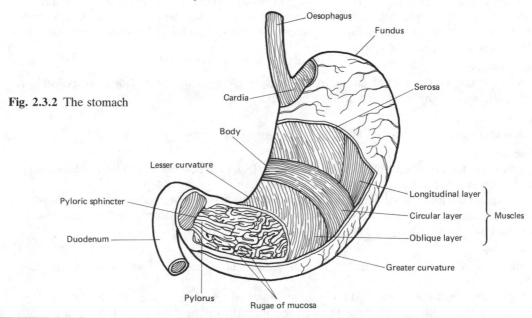

Fig. 2.3.2 The stomach

The Stomach

Functions	Structures involved
1 A reservoir for food	Whole structure and shape allow food to stay for up to about 4 hours. Emptying can be delayed e.g. after a fatty meal
2 Mechanical digestion of food	Smooth muscles churn the food with gastric juice forming chyme. Longitudinal, circular and oblique fibres
3 Chemical digestion of food: proteins are changed to peptones by pepsin; vitamin B_{12} is prepared for absorption	Glands embedded in the submucous coat are continuous with the mucous membrane and produce gastric juice comprising hydrochloric acid (mostly from near the fundus), pepsinogen (converted to pepsin by the hydrochloric acid) and intrinsic factor
4 Produces a hormone called gastrin which stimulates the gastric glands to secrete gastric juice	Glands near to the pylorus of the stomach are ductless – secretion is into the blood stream. Secretion is stimulated by the presence of food in the stomach and the action of the vagus nerve
5 Hydrochloric acid acts as a powerful antimicrobial agent	
6 Absorption of water, glucose and alcohol	Epithelial surface. Drainage is into the gastric vein, which goes via the portal vein to the liver
7 Vomiting – ejection of obstructed contents and toxic substances (peristalsis in the stomach is momentarily reversed)	Reflex action. Main stimulus for vomiting is from the vomiting centre in the medulla.

Conditions of the stomach

Gastritis – inflammation of the stomach

Causes
1 Dietary indiscretion   3 Aspirin and other drugs such as steroids
2 Alcohol consumption   4 Highly seasoned foods
5 Chronic forms may be a part of the ageing process or auto immune reactions

Effects, signs and symptoms Local inflammation may cause heartburn, epigastric pain, anorexia (loss of appetite), nausea and vomiting. Severe erosion may cause haematemesis but more commonly there will be blood loss that only appears on occult blood tests or with iron deficiency anaemia.

Many have no symptoms at all.

Treatment is symptomatic

   1 A review of the patients drug prescriptions   **2** Avoiding alcohol and highly seasoned foods

Nursing notes

This is usually a mild condition and the nurse may not be involved. It is very important to observe in patients having drugs. Occasionally the haematemesis may be severe (see p 24).

Gastroenteritis – see disorders of the intestine p 68

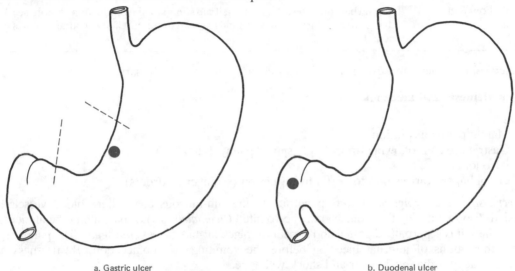

a. Gastric ulcer   b. Duodenal ulcer

Fig. 2.3.3 Position of peptic ulcers

Peptic ulcer

An ulceration either in the stomach or more commonly in the duodenum. There appears to be too much acid for the mucous membrane and of course pepsin can act on the tissues.
The exact cause is not known.

Cause factors

   1 Stress – they are more common in over anxious people and also occur after head injuries, burns, sepsis or surgery

   2 Diet – coffee drinking and cola drinks have been associated

   3 Cigarette smoking – stopping smoking may help to heal an ulcer

   4 Familial

   5 Drugs that cause erosion and gastritis

   6 Psychosomatic – psychological cause of a physical illness

Effects, signs and symptoms Erosion and crater formation in the mucous membrane. Hydrochloric acid and pepsin may extend the ulcer formation and deepen it. The patient complains of pain. The pain is localized in the epigastric region (the patient points to it) and is related to food – usually increases when the stomach is empty (typically disturbing the sleep). It is episodic – comes and goes for days (or more) at a time. Many patients describe it as a 'nagging' ache rather than severe. Classically, the pain is relieved by food or antacids. Nausea and vomiting may be related to the pain.

Ulcers near to the pyloric sphincter may cause a narrowing and obstruction may occur. This will cause a sensation of fullness and classically vomiting of large quantities in which food taken some time previously may be seen.

Nursing notes

A careful nursing assessment is necessary to help to establish a clear account of the pain. Vomitus must be measured and observed for indications of pyloric obstruction. Patients with pyloric obstruction tend to avoid eating and even if they do, absorption of nutrients is very limited. Serious malnutrition and anaemia may determine the management of the patient.

Diagnosis – investigations

   1 Clinical history and examination   **2** Barium meal X-ray   **3** Gastroscopy

Suggested nursing response – Barium meal

Preparation Nothing by mouth for at least six hours before

Procedure The patient drinks the tasteless barium sulphate. X-rays are taken. The patient may be moved into differing positions to ensure a clear view. (Remember to ensure that your patient is fit to tolerate this.)

Digestive conditions

Treatment

1 Rest – bed rest is usually prescribed either at home or in hospital. Reduce anxiety
2 Drugs – antacid drugs between meals. Cimetidine or carbenoxolone will act as antacids and promote healing
3 Discourage cigarette smoking, alcohol and any foods that cause pain

Suggested nursing response

Assessment	Care
1 Evidence of anxiety and acceptance of bed rest	Diversional therapy may be needed. Discuss anxieties with the patient and his family
2 Tolerance of diet limitations and avoidance of smoking	Diet can be more interesting but smell can stimulate the production of more acid! Giving up smoking may be very difficult – a lot of support and encouragement is needed

If medical treatment and care is not successful, then surgery is necessary.

Haematemesis and melaena

Causes

1 Mainly peptic ulceration
2 Gastric erosion following drugs (e.g. aspirin, phenyl butazone)
3 Alcoholic
4 Oesophageal varices due to portal hypertension (see liver disorders)

Effects, signs and symptoms Ulcers penetrate to the sub-mucous coat where blood vessels are eroded. Blood entering the stomach may be vomited (*haematemesis*) or pass along the alimentary tract where it is is partially digested and appears as black tar-like faeces (*melaena*). The patient may show indications of internal bleeding before the vomiting and defaecation. Restlessness and anxiety, tachycardia, air hunger and shock will appear.

Nursing note

These early observations are very important – watch particularly for the restlessness and anxious look.

This is a medical emergency and efficient teamwork is important.

Treatment

1 Replace blood loss with transfusion.
2 Protect the airway during vomiting.
3 Surgery if control not obtained.

Suggested nursing response

Assessment	Care
1 Indications of internal bleeding and shock: restlessness, anxiety; tachycardia; hypotension; gasping for air (air hunger); oliguria	Intravenous infusion – plasma or dextran first, followed by whole blood. Position the patient with feet raised, but in recovery position (semi prone)
2 Evidence of bleeding – vomitus and stools observed	
3 Protection of the airway if vomiting continues	Some physicians like a nasogastric tube passed to keep the gastric contents reduced
4 Note evidence of prolonged fear and anxiety	Sedation may be prescribed by the doctor. Some use morphine with an antiemetic drug. Give careful assurance

Notes: Melaena is offensive smelling and deodorants may be used for the patient's and relatives benefit, but they could mask a new incident if too strong. Visual observations should continue. Some physicians will only allow ice to be sucked, others prefer to give a soft diet as an empty stomach is more active.

Perforation of peptic ulcer

The ulcer erodes through the muscle coat and eventually ruptures through into the peritoneal cavity, allowing the gastric juice to cause acute peritonitis. Only in a few cases would a blood vessel be involved and at operation there is rarely evidence of bleeding. Indeed, perforations may be difficult to find because they can be so small. This is a surgical emergency and urgent preparation of the operating theatre team is necessary. Some patients do not reach hospital.

The patient will have acute abdominal pain, with rigid 'guarding' of the abdominal muscles (muscles held very tight). They will be suffering from shock which will be neurogenic due to the severity of the pain. If a blood vessel ruptures, hypovolaemic shock will occur (prognosis – not good). Patients will be very frightened. They may vomit suddenly, possibly as a result of the pain.

Suggested nursing response

Assessment	Care
1 Degree of shock – blood pressure	Position according to the patients comfort, but protect the airway if vomiting
2 Severity of pain – the patient often lies very still	Analgesia may be part of pre-medication
3 Degree of fear and anxiety (including fear of surgery)	Careful assurance – speed and efficiency as well as words of comfort
See surgery of the stomach	

If there is delay, severe dehydration and electrolyte imbalance will occur. Intravenous therapy and nasogastric aspiration, with correction of electrolyte imbalance may be needed before surgery.

Carcinoma of the stomach

Cause Unknown

Factors thought to influence the development are still not clear. There are geographical incidences. It tends to occur in older people, mainly men and patients with chronic gastritis and gastric ulcer seem to be more susceptible. 5–7% of gastric ulcers become malignant, but not duodenal ulcers.

Effects, signs and symptoms Local infiltration occurs most commonly on the greater curvature of the stomach (ulcers more frequently on the lesser). Ulceration around the tumour is clearly defined on gastroscopy. The patient may have few symptoms or those of a peptic ulcer: loss of appetite, vomiting, loss of weight and anaemia. Haematemesis and melaena may occur.

Polypoid sizes vary from small polyps with no symptoms to large palpable masses. Extensive spread through the stomach wall may cause obstruction around the pylorus, hardening and rigidity of the stomach and *linitis plastica* (leather bottle stomach). The spread may also involve other organs (colon, pancreas) and 'seed' tumours through the peritoneum. Late symptoms – see pancreatic tumours and colon tumours.

Lymphatic spread is to the para aortic chain of nodes. Haemorrhagic spread is through the gastric vein and portal vein to the liver (see hepatic tumours). Very late spread to lungs and brain.

Sadly, the patient has usually become very weak and ill by this time with extensive weight loss, sallow complexion and possibly jaundice. Prognosis is very poor at this stage.

Diagnosis – investigations
1 Clinical history and examination (for a palpable mass particularly)
2 Barium meal and gastroscopy
3 Liver function tests and scanning (possibly liver biopsy)

Treatment

Surgery Very tiny tumours have been removed with very little gastric tissue disturbance. Usually resection of part or the whole of the stomach is needed.

Extensive tumours and those with liver metastases are inoperable but palliative surgery may be done to prevent obstruction if possible.

Suggested nursing response

Assessment	Care
1 Indications of weight loss, anorexia, vomiting	Attempt to provide light nutrient diets. Give prescribed antiemetic drugs. Appetisers such as sherry may be helpful if no erosive haemorrhage. Care of the emaciated skin. Mouth care for dryness and faetor
2 Indications of metastases *1* liver – jaundice, ascites, indigestion, haemorrhoids *2* lungs – respiratory infections (see 2.1) *3* brain – behavioural changes (see 2.5)	Careful positioning for comfort. Possibly paracentesis if ascites embarrasses the breathing. Antacids for indigestion. Care with elimination (for haemorrhoids)

Psychologically, the patient is usually very low and needs great understanding and support from nursing staff and the family. See also surgery of the stomach.

Surgery of the stomach

Pre operative assessment and preparation

Nutritional state and hydration may be poor and should be corrected with diet and fluids orally when possible, or intravenously if necessary.

Respiratory condition The operation site is near to the diaphragm and all patients with upper abdominal incisions are in danger of respiratory complications. Chest X-ray should be performed. Pre operative physiotherapy for breathing needs to be encouraged by nursing staff too.

Evidence of anaemia Blood will be taken for haemoglobin and total blood cell count. Blood transfusion may be needed before surgery.

State of the mouth and teeth Dental caries or mouth infections may lead to complications at the operation site and in the post operative period when oral intake is controlled.

Skin conditions for hygiene Shaving is usually from the neck to the knees, but is at the surgeon's discretion. Bathing may not be possible if perforation of an ulcer means urgency.

Fasting Is for six hours and some surgeons ask for a nasogastric tube to be passed before surgery.

Remember many patients (especially with ulcers) are, by nature, very anxious. They will need assessment of their fear and careful reassurance and sedation before the pre medication.

Surgery

Incision Usually upper para-median incision

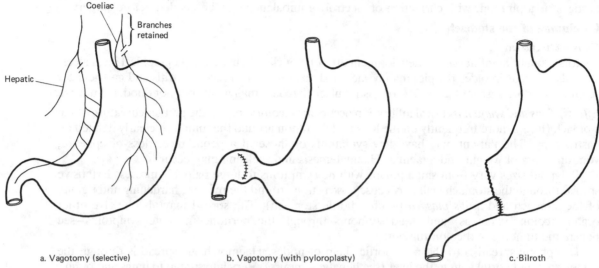

Fig. 2.3.4 Surgery of the stomach and duodenum

Vagotomy (selective) Reduces the secretion of hydrochloric acid in the stomach

Vagotomy (with pyloroplasty) Some surgeons ensure better drainage from the stomach by refashioning the pylorus to empty more easily

Bilroth Resection of diseased part of stomach with anastamosis to duodenum or jejunum, leaving the duodenal stump for the digestive enzymes to enter

Post operative care and assessment

Assessment	Care
1 Condition of the airway, breathing and coughing	Protect the airway with artificial tube, suction. Position carefully. Use analgesia of post operative drugs to encourage deep breathing and coughing while supporting the abdominal wound
2 Evidence of haemorrhage: blood pressure; pulse; observe wound and drain for bleeding and inflammation	If stable blood pressure, early sitting up will help breathing. Aseptic dressings to the wound. Drain removed on surgeons orders. Sutures may be soluble or removed after 7–10 days
3 Hydration and early nutrition	Care of intravenous infusion
4 Evidence of gastric filling, nausea, vomiting and, later, evidence of emptying	Protect by suction (aspiration) of nasogastric tube. Controlled small amounts of fluid orally (e.g. 15 mls hourly) according to surgeon's orders, gradually increasing until normal diet in a few days

Nasogastric tube is removed when emptying is efficient and bowel sounds are heard through a stethoscope. Early movements and ambulation are as for all surgery. Post operative prognosis is good.

Specific post operative complications

1 *Nutrition* With extensive gastric resection, some food may not be digested properly and cannot be absorbed leading to weight loss.

More commonly, relief of symptoms tends to cause the patients to overeat for the size of their remaining stomach. The nurse can ensure that they only have small portions to begin with.

Rarely, vitamin B_{12} absorption will be affected and pernicious anaemia occurs (total gastrectomy).

2 *Dumping syndrome* After partial gastrectomy, possibly related to a sudden dilation of the jejunum, the patient may suddenly feel epigastric fullness, sweating, giddiness, extreme weakness and fatigue whilst eating a meal. Dry food, avoiding hot fluids and resting after the meal will ease the symptoms. Careful explanation may ease the anxiety.

Congenital pyloric stenosis

Cause Not known but seems to be genetic. The incidence in boys is quite high – up to 1 in 150 (girls 1 in 60).

Effects, signs and symptoms There is an overgrowth (hypertrophy) of the smooth muscle around the pyloric sphincter, causing a narrowing of the lumen which eventually becomes obstructed. The stomach becomes dilated and gastritis may be caused by stagnant food.

The baby may appear normal for a few weeks, but then starts vomiting – small amounts initially, but later large volumes and as the dilated stomach contracts, projectile vomiting may occur – mainly the whole feed with mucus but may contain 'coffee ground' particles – indicating gastritis with bleeding. There may be visible peristalsis after a feed. The baby becomes dehydrated and malnourished. The skin appears wizened and loose with 'sunken eyes' and fontanelles. Weight may be below birth weight.

Diagnosis – investigations
1 Clinical history (including family history)
2 Clinical examination
3 Milk test for visible peristalsis (some use air through a nasogastric tube)

Treatment Surgery to refashion the pyloric sphincter – Ramstedt's operation

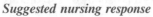

Fig. 2.3.5 Ramstedt's operation

Suggested nursing response
Pre operative assessment and preparation
Observations of the degree of dehydration and nutritional state. Intravenous therapy may be commenced and surgery is delayed until fluid, electrolyte and acid/base balance are restored. Note indications of gastritis and prevention of further vomiting. Examine all vomitus. A nasogastric tube will be passed to aspirate and wash out the stomach.

Surgery General anaesthetic. See Fig. 2.3.5 for incision and effect.

Post operative assessment and care
1 Clear airway.
2 Evidence of haemorrhage and infection – apply aseptic dressings.
3 Return to feeding. Some surgeons allow the baby to resume normal full strength feeding unless gastritis is present. It is more usual to follow a graduated regime e.g. sterile glucose solution 2 hourly; after 6 hours – half strength milk feeds; 48 hours – full strength milk feeds. (Ideally, breast milk of course.)
See also *aspects of baby surgery* 2.14.

The small intestine

Functions	Structures related
1 Continual passage of chyme from the stomach to the colon at a controlled rate	Smooth muscles continue peristalsis and produce segmentation. They are mainly controlled by the action of the parasympathetic nervous system through branches of the vagus nerve
2 Mechanical digestion of food by movement	
3 Emulsification of fats by the action of bile (breaks molecules up from each other – similar to a detergent)	Bile is secreted from the liver and gall bladder through the common bile duct
4 Changing the acid chyme to alkaline	Hydroxide ions in pancreatic and intestinal juice
5 Chemical digestion of food *1 Pancreatic juice* **Proteins** Trypsin changes peptones to polypeptides **Carbohydrates** Amylase changes starches to maltose **Fats** Lipase changes emulsified fats to lipids (fatty acids and glycerol)	Pancreatic juice from the pancreatic duct. Common bile duct and pancreatic duct enter through the Ampulla of Vater and the sphincter of Oddi
2 Intestinal juice (Succus entericus) **Proteins** Erepsin changes polypeptides to amino acids **Carbohydrates** Maltase changes maltose to glucose. Lactase changes lactose to glucose and galactose. Sucrase changes sucrose to glucose **Fats** Lipase continues to convert fats to lipids	The glands secreting intestinal juice were thought to be in crypts between the villi. Some now think that it is secreted by cells on the villi themselves. The flow of juice seems to be influenced by mechanical stimulation of food in the lumen of the intestine
6 Absorption of digested foods: amino acids, monosaccharides (e.g. glucose), lipids, water, salts and vitamins. Absorption may be by simple diffusion or through transfer agents	Micro villi on the surface of the columnar cells, the villi and the folds within the intestine give the large surface area for absorption. All but the lipids are carried through the blood vessels in the villi to the mesenteric veins and through the portal vein to the liver. The lipids are carried through the lymphatics (lacteals)

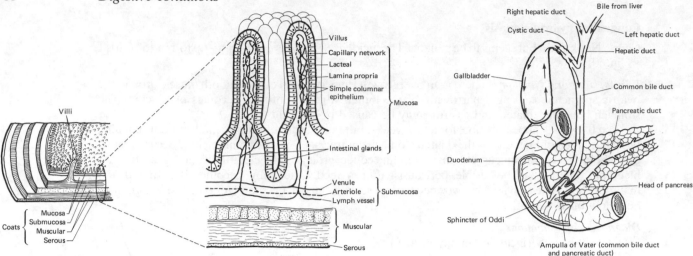

Fig. 2.3.6 Small intestine villi   **Fig. 2.3.7** Ampulla of Vater and sphincter of Oddi

Conditions of the small intestine

Enteritis – inflammation of the small intestine

Gastroenteritis is more common with the stomach involved too. In adults it is usually due to dietary or alcoholic indiscretion, but may be due to infection.

Gastroenteritis in children

Causes
1 Sometimes idiopathic or may be due to feeding problems
2 Organisms causing infection are viruses and coliform bacteria from an outside source

Effects, signs and symptoms Inflammation of the stomach and intestinal mucosa. Vomiting and diarrhoea will occur, and will in turn lead to severe dehydration and electrolyte imbalance. Organisms continue to survive in faeces and the condition is highly infectious unless strict hygiene is observed. The metabolic rate is increased. The child may present with a fever, tachycardia and be very irritable. Some are exhausted and listless.

Diagnosis – investigations
1 Clinical history and examination
2 Stool specimens to identify organisms
3 Serum electrolyte levels to determine needs

Treatment
1 Isolation to prevent spread.
2 Restore fluid and electrolyte balance with intravenous infusion.
3 Antibacterial agents are rarely used.

Suggested nursing response
Nurse in cubicle

Assessment	Care
1 Amount of vomit and its characteristics	Care of the mouth. Provide vomit bowls and support the head
2 Stools are usually very runny, green and offensive smelling	Disinfection of faeces before disposal
3 Degree of dehydration and electrolyte imbalance: sunken eyes and fontanelles; dry, loose skin; wizened appearance	Maintain intravenous infusion (scalp vein may be used). Prevent child from playing with infusion site. Check fluids carefully, using 'metroset' and intravenous regulator
4 Evidence of raised metabolic rate: rectal temperature; tachycardia; irritability or ominous quietness	Glucose may be given intravenously and orally as vomiting stops. Nutrition gradually restored as baby improves

Notes: Dehydration can be severe enough to cause haemolysis with danger of renal failure. Parents will be alarmed as the baby appears (and is) very ill, but recovery is sometimes remarkably quick.

Enteric fever – typhoid and paratyphoid

Cause Salmonella organisms – salmonella typhoid and paratyphoid A and B

Effects, signs and symptoms Infection of the intestine follows a period of septicaemia with bacilli in the blood. The metabolic rate increases with a rising pyrexia and severe malaise. As inflammation occurs in the intestine, severe diarrhoea with frequent green, watery stools is the main symptom. Ulceration of the mucosa may occur – Peyer's patches are involved. Bleeding may be slight, but there is a danger of fatal haemorrhage or bowel perforation. A typical rash – 'rose spots' – may appear on the abdominal wall.

Diagnosis – investigations
1 Clinical history and examination   2 Examination of faeces for bacilli
3 Blood for haemoglobin and electrolyte balance

Treatment
1 Isolate   2 Replace fluids by intravenous infusion   3 Give chloramphenicol

Suggested nursing response

Assessment	Care
1 Degree of fever and malaise – may be very ill indeed	Strict isolation. Bed rest. Cooling fans. Encouragement. Glucose intravenously
2 Degree of dehydration	Intravenous infusion
3 Dangers of haemorrhage perforation, heart failure	Urgent medical help needed

Prevention
1 Strict food hygiene must be stressed. The health education role of the nurse is important here.
2 Isolation of cases and carriers. Carriers may not have evidence of the disease. (Organisms are often carried in their gall bladder)
3 Immunization programmes need to be encouraged – monovalent typhoid vaccine is more commonly used than TAB and causes far fewer reactions.

Food poisoning

Generally causes gastroenteritis and should be considered here.

Causes
1 Intestinal allergies
2 Poisonous foods e.g. eating toadstools instead of mushrooms
3 Chemicals e.g. arsenic
4 Bacterial – salmonella is usually transmitted through poor food handling, infected foods (duck eggs, for example, should be well cooked!) and reheated meat dishes. Staphylococci is usually transmitted through infected lesions on the hands of food handlers and *clostridium welchii* through uncleaned foods. (Botulism is a rare food poisoning in which *clostridium botulinum* produces a toxin that paralyses the patient. Transmission is in poor canning and preserving. The prognosis is very poor.)

Effects, signs and symptoms
For diagnosis, treatment and nursing response – see gastroenteritis.
Staphylococcal food poisoning is more dangerous as a toxin is released into the blood stream which may cause a severe toxaemia with *shock* within 2–6 hours of ingestion.

Nursing note
Urgent and intensive care may be needed but recovery is usually very good. Dangerous in young children and the elderly though. See notes on prevention.

Crohn's disease – regional enteritis or ileitis

Cause Unknown. May be auto immune – an abnormal immune response to an unknown stimulus (antigen)

Effects, signs and symptoms Inflammation may occur anywhere along the alimentary tract but the most common site is the latter part of the ileum, near to the ileo caecal valve. All the coats of the intestine may be inflamed including the outer coat of the peritoneum. Abscesses may form and as loops of intestine adhere, fistulas may occur.

The patient's usual complaint is pain. It may be similar to that in acute appendicitis. It may be colicky (severe spasmodic pain). There may be tenderness and guarding over the site. Diarrhoea is common, the stools may be loose or formed. If the colon is involved, mucus and pus may be seen. Malabsorption leads to weight loss and with the chronic inflammation, anaemia. Metabolic rate is increased with a recurrent low pyrexia, tachycardia and progressive weakness.

Diagnosis – investigations
1 Clinical history and examination – sometimes a mass may be felt in the area inflamed (right lower quadrant of the abdomen)
2 Barium meal and follow through   3 Barium enema to assess if the colon is involved

Treatment
1 *Medical* Anti-inflammatory and immunosuppressive drugs may be used – oral corticosteroids, corticotrophin (ACTH) or tetracosactrin. Azathioprine is an immune suppressive agent which may help some cases. Antibacterial drugs can be used if abscess develops
2 *Surgical* Resection of the inflamed areas, but may need extensive resection which causes malabsorption problems

Suggested nursing response

Assessment	Care
1 Degree and type of pain	Careful positioning. Prescribed analgesia
2 Degree of diarrhoea – observe stools and frequency	Position near the toilet or provide commode. Prescribed anti inflammatory agents should reduce frequency
3 Dehydration and malnutrition; note the nature of skin, sunken eyes, measure muscle dimensions (upper arm circumference)	May need intravenous infusion, electrolytes and parenteral nutrition. High protein, high carbohydrate diet given as tolerated. Vitamin and iron supplements may be needed
4 Raised metabolic rate; pyrexia, tachycardia, weakness	Nurse at rest in bed if temperature elevated. Light clothing and a gentle fan may help control temperature. Glucose drinks will help restore energy

Major complication is *intestinal obstruction* – see below
Surgery – see resection of gut
Crohn's disease is a chronic disorder and the patient will have a long history of ill health with miserable signs and symptoms. Some remain remarkably cheerful but some need a great deal of psychological support to cope.

Intestinal obstruction – mechanical

Causes

1 Within the lumen – foreign body, gall stones (in the colon – impacted faeces).
2 Lesions in the wall of the intestine – Crohn's disease, tumours.
3 Lesions outside the wall of the intestine – adhesions (fibrous bands from previous peritonitis or surgery) or strangulation of a hernia sac.
4 Lesions due to abnormal movement of the intestine – intussusception (when one piece of intestine becomes trapped within another) and volvulus (due to a twisting action of the intestine).

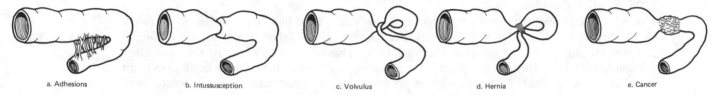

a. Adhesions   b. Intussusception   c. Volvulus   d. Hernia   e. Cancer

Fig. 2.3.8 Examples of intestinal obstruction (mechanical)

Effects, signs and symptoms

Obviously, peristalsis cannot move chyme beyond the obstruction. The degree of effect depends to some extent on the site but the consequences can be dangerous wherever it occurs. Approximately 8 litres of fluid are secreted by the gastric, pancreatic and intestinal juices and bile in addition to any food. This fluid cannot be absorbed, will accumulate in the intestine above the obstruction and cause distension before eventually being vomited. Serious dehydration and electrolyte loss will occur.

Higher obstruction Pain is frequent and felt in the upper abdomen. Vomiting is copious and early. Dehydration will be rapid and may cause shock due to hypovolaemia. Bowel action early, but then no flatus or faeces.

Lower obstruction Pain is more vague over the lower abdomen. Vomiting may be delayed. If very low, faecal colour and smell may be noted. Distension obvious and constipation.

Strangulation Colicky pain may be felt. Bacterial toxins may cause toxaemia and increase the degree of shock.

Intussusception Classically in infancy. The pain is severe with the baby crying with knees bent up. Usually passes a stool which is blood stained – 'cherry red' stool.

Diagnosis – investigations

1 Clinical history and examination
2 Abdominal X-rays will show distensions, trapped flatus and fluid levels

Nursing note

The patient will need supine and erect X-rays taken. Check with the medical staff when the patient, who may be shocked and very ill, is fit to go to X-ray department.

Treatment

1 Laparotomy to confirm the cause and relieve the obstruction.
2 Foreign bodies are removed. Adhesions can be dissected out.
3 If the piece of intestine will no longer function then resection of gut, including its mesentery will be performed.
4 For obstruction in the colon, a temporary colostomy may be performed to relieve the obstruction first. More extensive surgery will then be performed later. The patient would be at serious risk in these operations unless care before surgery was carried out. The aims are to:

1 empty the stomach and prevent vomiting.

2 rehydrate and correct electrolyte imbalance – especially in the shocked patient.

3 prevent toxaemia if strangulation has occurred.

Suggested nursing response

Assessment	Care
1 Degree of vomiting, type and frequency – record on fluid balance chart	Provide vomit bowl. Pass nasogastric tube and aspirate frequently
2 Degree and nature of pain – the patient is often restless and uncomfortable most of the time	Careful positioning. Give prescribed analgesia early
3 Degree of dehydration, electrolyte imbalance and shock. Observe: urine output; skin; behaviour; pulse and blood pressure; central venous pressure	Intravenous infusion may be quite rapid. Plasma or electrolyte solutions are given. Position according to the blood pressure. Feet may be raised but do not put the trunk down – pressure on the diaphragm may embarrass breathing (Danger of vomit being inhaled goes if nasogastric tube is in place)
4 Evidence of toxaemia (raised metabolic rate) – pyrexia; tachycardia	Prescribed antibacterial drugs may be given intravenously – check carefully. Light clothing and a fan. Glucose intravenously
5 Evidence of anxiety as the possibility of extensive surgery is high – note facial expression (anxiety of relatives too!)	Careful assurance. Sensitive listening to the patient's fears. Explain the reasons for tubes and procedures carefully
See also – *care before creation of a stoma*	

Intestinal obstruction – paralytic ileus The cessation of peristalsis in the intestine

Causes

1 Peritonitis – generalized inflammation of the peritoneum.

2 Inexpert or extensive handling of the intestine in surgery of the abdominal cavity.

Effects, signs and symptoms Are as for intestinal obstruction, including the toxaemia.

Treatment

1 Rest the intestine until inflammation has resolved.

2 Give parenteral nutrition, fluid and electrolytes.

Suggested nursing response

1 Nasogastric aspiration is continued.

2 Nothing is given by mouth – therefore oral hygiene must be intensive.

3 Intravenous infusion will be continued for some time – giving sets should be changed every 24 hours usually (see manufacturer's instructions).

4 Antibacterial agents are given either intravenously or intramuscularly – care with checking and handling of the solutions.

5 Two difficult problems for the nurse in many patients

  1 boredom and irritation especially at meal times,

  2 anxiety as to when they will be able to eat again.

6 Return to oral fluids and eventual nutrition depends on listening for peristalsis restarting – bowel sounds – may be heard through a stethoscope. A nurse may hear them but a doctor should confirm.

The large intestine (the colon), rectum and anus

Functions	Structures involved
1 The movement of undigested materials (mainly cellulose) and fluids from the ileocaecal valve at the end of the small intestine to the rectum prior to elimination through the anus	Peristalsis is continued into the rectum. Efficiency of peristalsis is influenced by the bulk of the contents – depends on the fibre content of the diet and the presence of bile salts.
2 Absorption of water and some vitamins	Columnar cells on the inner lining (mucous membrane)
3 Synthesis of some B vitamins and vitamin K	Commensal bacteria (coliform organisms) in the lumen of the colon (also prevent fungal infections)
4 Storage of faeces before elimination	The rectum will distend
5 Elimination of faeces, water, bile pigments – defaecation	Nerve receptors in the wall of the rectum. Sphincters in anus. Motor nerves of the autonomic and central nervous system
6 Deoderization (reducing the unpleasant smell)	Bile salts in the faeces

The functions of the appendix are still not firmly established in humans. It seems to be concerned with cellulose metabolism in other animals. The lymph nodules suggest that it should be considered as part of the lymphatic system – as a defence mechanism against micro-organisms.

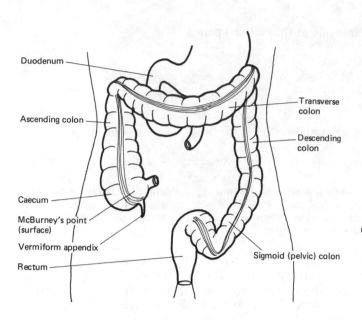

Fig. 2.3.9 Large intestine

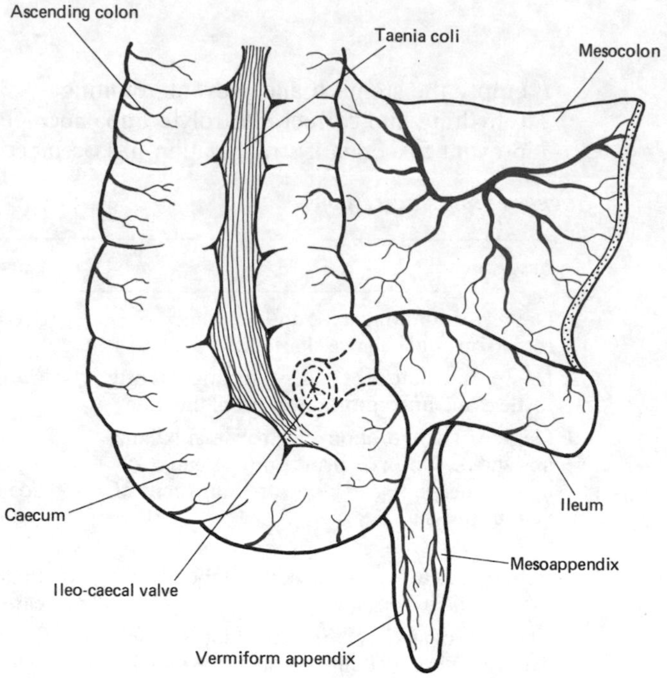

Fig. 2.3.10 Vermiform appendix

Conditions of the large intestine

Note that many conditions have effects through the alimentary tract. As seen previously, conditions like gastroenteritis and regional enteritis (Crohn's disease) will affect the colon. Diarrhoea, particularly, is a feature of disturbance in either the small intestine, large intestine or more commonly both.

Appendicitis – inflammation of the vermiform appendix

Causes

1 Infection by coliform organisms. This follows damage to the mucous membrane which would normally be able to withstand the presence of coliforms. Obstruction of the lumen of the appendix by a faecolith (stone-hard faecal lump) is common.
2 Lack of cellulose in the diet may be a contributing factor.

Effects, signs and symptoms Inflammation of the appendix locally causes a piece of the greater omentum (of the peritoneum) to enfold the organ. The patient feels unwell due to the raised metabolic rate and may complain of anorexia and nausea. The mouth may be dry, coated and halitosis (smelly breath) may be present. They are usually constipated. Pyrexia and tachycardia may be rising. Palpation of the site will cause tenderness and guarding. Pain is referred to the umbilical region and colicky pain may cause vomiting.

The classical site is McBurney's point, but note also that the appendix may lie over the bladder producing symptoms of cystitis or it may lie in the pelvis and cause diarrhoea.

Blockage and further inflammation may lead to the occlusion of the appendicular artery, causing gangrene (necrosis of tissue). As the pressure inside rises, the damaged wall will perforate. Locally, following perforation, an abscess may form in the right iliac fossa (appendix abscess) or in the pelvis (pelvic abscess). The pain is more localized to the right lower quadrant of the abdominal cavity. The abscess mass is extremely tender.

The main problem following perforation is general peritonitis. This may be very diffuse and produce a severe toxaemia. The high temperature may fall (although the core temperature is still high). Severe tachycardia and low blood pressure will give indications of toxic shock. Paralytic ileus will also occur with the peritonitis (see p 71).

Nursing notes

Nursing observations, particularly in children, need to be continual and recordings made frequently of temperature, pulse, blood pressure, vomiting, the changing characteristics of the pain and other signs of the inflammation.

Appendicitis is still a life threatening condition.

Diagnosis – investigations

1 Clinical history and examination – especially rectal examination.   2 Careful observations.
3 Blood – shows increased polymorphonuclear white cells.
4 Abdominal X-ray for gas and fluid levels.

Nursing note

It is a notoriously difficult diagnosis, especially in children. A careful nursing assessment and again meticulous observations are essential.

Treatment
1 *Appendicectomy* Usually for inflamed appendix and most perforations now with strong antibacterial drug cover.
2 *Drainage of abscess* first, followed by removal later.
3 *Conservative treatment* Treat as for paralytic ileus and give antibacterial drugs. Most would still have removal later.

Suggested nursing response
Pre operative

Assessment	Care
1 Condition of the skin over the incision site	Wash and shave to reduce danger of infection
2 Site and nature of pain	Analgesia is difficult until diagnosis is confirmed – can then be given with pre-medication
3 Evidence of nausea, vomiting	Nasogastric tube should be passed and aspirated regularly. Mouth care should start before surgery if possible. No drinks or food
4 Evidence of dehydration	Intravenous infusion will be set up giving saline and glucose
5 Raised metabolic rate pyrexia, tachycardia	Rest in bed. Cooling by light clothing
6 Degree of fear, including parents of children, although many may not be aware of the dangers	Assurance and listening to fears. Careful explanation. Sensitive communication with parents

Antibacterial drugs will usually be given intravenously.

Surgery Usually grid iron incision (McBurney's) in the right iliac fossa. Some surgeons may do a right lower paramedian incision if they anticipate difficulty locating the appendix or extensive toilet of the abdominal cavity is needed. Drainage from the bed of the appendix.

Post operative – specific

Assessment	Care
1 Wound for haemorrhage or infection, including the drain	Aseptic dressings. Nurse as upright as possible for drainage. Drain removed on surgeon's orders as drainage diminishes
2 Pain – may inhibit breathing if peritonitis	Prescribed analgesia followed by breathing and leg exercises
3 Metabolic rate remains high for some time after surgery	Bed rest, but passive exercise. Mobilize as pyrexia and tachycardia settle down (usually 24–48 hours – but watch). Glucose needed
4 Rehydration	Intravenous infusion and later, oral fluids
5 Protection from vomiting until peristalsis is restored – note bowel sounds	Aspirate the nasogastric tube. Fluids and nutrition orally are introduced as surgeon indicates

Antibacterial drugs are continued until course is completed (5–7 days).

Complications are usually sequels to infection
1 Local abscess formation
2 Sub phrenic abscess or pelvic abscess following peritonitis. A sub phrenic abscess is dangerous, it may 'track' into the thoracic cavity and lead to lung abscess. The patient will be very ill and surgical drainage is necessary.
3 Burst abdomen – follows more extensive incision with gross wound inflammation. Very frightening for the patient.

Action Cover the viscera with wet sterile towels and resuturing in theatre.
Antibacterial drugs will usually prevent, but some patients' resistance to infection is often very low.

Ulcerative colitis

Cause Not known, but thought to be an abnormality of the immune system (auto-immune disease). Although psychological factors appear to be involved, proof that they cause the disease is not established. The fastidious, hypersensitive characteristics of the patient may be a result of the disease.

Effects, signs and symptoms Inflammation with ulcer formation occurs in the mucous and submucous coat of the colon. It may be localized in the rectum (proctitis), the ascending colon or it may involve the whole length of the colon. Attacks may be caused by infection elsewhere and antibacterial drugs.

The patient complains of diarrhoea. Loose stools with streaks of mucous, blood and pus. In severe forms, the stools are extremely watery and defaecation may be necessary up to twenty times in a day. There is abdominal discomfort and painful straining during defaecation (tenesmus).

The raised metabolic rate will give rise to a pyrexia, tachycardia, energy loss and malaise. Weight loss is increased in the acute phase. The recurrent diarrhoea (often offensive smelling) causes acute embarrassment to patients and a serious loss of self esteem. Relapses often occur during a time of stress. Behaviour varies considerably, but often there is a deep concern about personal hygiene and appearance.

Suggested nursing response

Assessment	Care
1 Frequency and nature of diarrhoea – record stool quantity; consistency and presence of blood; mucus and pus	Nurse near to the toilet. A bedside commode is reassuring, but should be discreet
2 Psychological state and nature of the patient	Listen to fears and anxieties. Respect fastidiousness. Provide deodorants and scented toiletries

In severe colitis, dehydration may be severe and the patient will show evidence by thirst, dry hot skin, sunken eyes and headache. Haemorrhage may be steady over a long period and the patient will show indications of anaemia. Acute haemorrhage may lead to shock.

Danger arises mostly from:
   1 acute dilation of the bowel with toxaemia and possible perforation with faecal peritonitis.
   2 stricture may cause intestinal obstruction.
   3 carcinoma of the colon often develops in patients with long standing ulcerative colitis.

Diagnosis – investigations
   1 Clinical history and examination   **2** Rectal examination is needed
   3 Barium enema (not in acute colitis though)   **4** Sigmoidoscopy and proctoscopy.

Suggested nursing response for sigmoidoscopy
Before procedure
   1 Assure the patient carefully and explain the test   *2* Light breakfast may be given
   3 Some surgeons require light enema to clear the rectum, but great care is needed if inflammation is present

Procedure
   1 The patient is usually in a left lateral position
   2 Air may be introduced which may cause pain (some patients feel faint)
   3 Biopsy may be taken

After procedure – observe for indications of bleeding or infection at the biopsy site

Colonoscopy is performed with a fibre optic tube. More extensive bowel preparation is needed and possibly a general anaesthetic. Great care is needed over inflamed tissues.

Treatment
Medical
   1 Anti-inflammatory agents – corticosteroid drugs – (usually prednisolone retention enema twice daily and systemic prednisolone)
   2 Poorly absorbed sulphonamide – sulphasalazine in acute phases and for long term care.
   3 Increase the bulk of the stool to reduce fluid loss by use of a high fibre diet or methyl cellulose additives.
   4 Correct dehydration and anaemia.

Surgical if medical treatment fails, perforation or fear of cancer occurs
   1 *Colectomy* – most surgeons include the rectum (*proctocolectomy*)
   2 An *ileostomy* will be performed also. Some surgeons may later try to anastomose the ileum with the rectum left behind at a later operation.

Suggested nursing response

Assessment	Care
1 Progress of inflammation should be controlled by treatment: reduce metabolic rate; decrease diarrhoea. The patient feels much better (steroids do make them euphoric and increase the appetite)	Give prescribed drugs. Prednisolone enemas should be given slowly with the patient inclined for retention. Give extra fluids with sulphasalazine. Encourage all signs of improvement
2 Increased bulk of stool initially may cause some abdominal discomfort	High fibre diets contain cellulose and bran. The patient needs a lot of encouragement to continue
3 Correction of hydration	Initially intravenous infusion, but mixed oral fluids are better as soon as possible
4 Correction of anaemia – note colour, pulse	Initially blood transfusion, later high protein diet and iron supplements

Surgery – see p 41 for bowel surgery

Ileostomy

The fashioning of a spout of the ileum (small intestine) onto the abdominal skin surface.

Nursing notes

1 *Before ileostomy* Careful assessment and preparation is needed. The patient must have a clear understanding of what is to be done and that he will be able to cope well enough to lead a normal life. A talk with a member of the Ileostomy Association before surgery is advisable – not all patients can bear the sight of a recently formed ileostomy.

2 *After ileostomy* Learning to master the appliances. Careful guidance by a stoma therapist is helpful. Ileostomy contents are fluid and caustic to the skin. Ask your surgeon to give a long enough spout for fitting the appliances. Waterproof adhesives are used.

Many patients become very depressed following surgery and on discharge home. The nurse should be aware and warn of this explaining what to do – contact his Primary Health Care team, the Stoma Clinic perhaps or a fellow member of the Ileostomy Association.

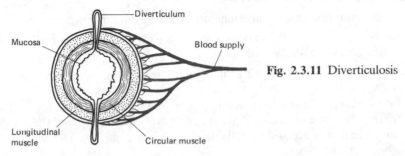

Fig. 2.3.11 Diverticulosis

Diverticulosis

The presence of diverticula – pouches of the submucous and mucous coat of the intestine bulging out through the muscle coat.

Causes Increased pressure within the colon due to a lack of bulk in the faeces. A common disease of the elderly in Western civilizations.

Diverticula themselves may be symptomless. If found before serious disease has developed, they may be controlled simply by introducing a high fibre diet.

Diverticulitis

Effects, signs and symptoms The diverticula become inflamed due to impacted faeces and infection. The patient will complain of recurring bouts of acute lower abdominal pain. They are usually constipated but they may alternate between constipation and diarrhoea. There are associated bouts of fever with pyrexia, tachycardia, malaise and progressive weakness.

Fistula In an acute phase, the inflamed colon and peritoneum may adhere to other structures. The eroding infection may then cause a fistula – sometimes into the bladder or the vagina – allowing faecal contents to enter them. The patient will have indications of cystitis or vaginitis. An alarming feature is the passing of flatus through the urethra or vagina.

Peritonitis Abscesses may form around the colon and give rise to local and general peritonitis. Acute tenderness and guarding over the site will be followed by severe board like rigidity over the whole abdomen, with toxaemia and possibly collapse due to shock.

Perforation of a diverticulum will likewise produce acute peritonitis.

Intestinal obstruction Progressive inflammation and fibrosis may narrow the lumen and stricture may cause intestinal obstruction.

Haemorrhage Severe bleeding with collapse is possible.

Nursing note

It can be seen how the nurse's advice to patients about nutrition and increasing fibre intake could prevent much misery and potential hazards for patients – especially the elderly who are at risk.

Diagnosis – investigation

1 Clinical history and examination   **2** Barium enema examination

Nursing notes

Bowel preparations vary widely in different centres for barium enema and no regime is given here. The aim is to try to get the colon as clear of faeces as possible. Patients will be tipped to different angles in X-ray department. Do warn if the elderly patient has other conditions.

Treatment

Diverticulosis

1 High fibre diet   **2** Education for good bowel habit restoration

Diverticulosis complications

1 Surgical treatment

2 May need a temporary colostomy first and more extensive surgery when fit

Suggested nursing response

The majority of patients with minimal disease may be nursed at home, but may need hospital admission in the acute phase.

Assessment	Care
1 Raised metabolic rate: pyrexia; tachycardia; weakness	Rest in bed. Regulate the temperature. Give glucose drinks. Prescribed antibacterial drugs
2 Degree and characteristics of pain: look for peritonitis; guarding; increasing severity	Prescribed analgesia, but great care not to miss worsening condition
3 Nature of faeces: observe for bowel pattern. Some patients may bleed	A fluid diet initially. Cellulose may be given in artificial form. Inform the doctor if bleeding

Carcinoma of the colon and rectum

The most common malignant condition of the alimentary tract in Great Britain.

Cause Not known, but it has been associated with a lack of fibre (cellulose) in the diet, ulcerative colitis and (rare) a familial disease called polyposis.

Effects, signs and symptoms These depend on the type and site of the tumour, and whether spread has occurred.

In the ascending colon and the caecum, the tumour grows out from the wall like a polyp (polypoid). There may be some ulceration, inflammation and bleeding around the tumour. Obstruction is rare because the faeces are still very fluid. The patient complains of weakness (due to anaemia) and possibly melaena.

They are sometimes found during laparotomy for appendicitis.

In the sigmoid colon and rectum, they grow around the colon, leading to a ring-like stricture (annular). Ulceration, inflammation and bleeding can occur again. The patient presents with an altered bowel pattern, passing blood and mucus in his faeces.

Obstruction is more likely and will present as a low intestinal obstruction with faecal vomiting eventually. Perforation is possible, leading to peritonitis. In the rectum, the tumour often presents as an ulcer first, with bleeding and inflammation. The patient passes blood and mucus in the faeces.

Nursing note

It is very important to advise patients who pass blood per rectum to seek medical opinion. Most will be benign lesions or haemorrhoids, but all need to be examined.

Metastases

Lymph nodes in the mesentery may be enlarged but do not always present symptoms. The most serious problem is fairly rapid spread through the mesenteric veins to the portal vein and the liver – prognosis is poor when the liver is involved.

Diagnosis – investigations

1 Clinical history and examination
2 Rectal examination
3 Barium enema
4 Sigmoidoscopy or colonoscopy

Treatment Surgical removal

Suggested nursing response for surgery of the colon and rectum

Pre operative management should take a few days and not be hurried.

Physical

1 Skin cleansing and shaving should be thorough and include particularly the perineum.
2 Any anaemia may need to be corrected by blood transfusion before surgery.
3 Nutrition is given in the form of a no or low residue regime – depends on the surgeon's preference.
4 The bowel is emptied of faeces – some surgeons like colonic washouts. Broad spectrum antibacterial drugs and metronadiozole are given to reduce the bacterial content of the colon.
5 The day of the operation – a nasogastric tube is passed to prevent vomiting.
6 Urinary catheter is passed to keep the bladder drained and free from the operation site.

Psychological

1 Careful explanation by the surgeon and support by nurses to assure the patient.
2 If stoma is to be performed, introduce to the Colostomy Welfare Association who will provide a member of the same age and sex if possible to give assurance. Use a stoma therapist if available. Treat all patients individually here and listen to their fears and anxieties.

Surgery

It is not possible to cover all the operation in this text, but note that:

1 The pelvic region is highly sensitive and neurogenic shock is possible.
2 In abdomino-perineal excision of the rectum there are two extensive incisions to consider in addition to the colostomy

Specific post operative management Assessment and care for:
  1 Shock and haemorrhage – observations, intravenous infusion
  2 Little or no peristalsis initially – listen for bowel sounds
  3 Preventing infection – aseptic technique (difficult) and antibacterial agents.

Suggested nursing response for colostomy
  1 Observe frequently for its retained position.
  2 First action may be very loose and profuse and a well fitting appliance is essential at all times. Always measure *before* changing the appliance.
  3 Gentle introduction of the patient to self care on an individual basis. Persistent encouragement may be needed and congratulations do help.

Haemorrhoids (piles)

Are really prolapses of the submucous and mucous coat of the anal canal. The plexus of veins within the coat prolapses with the membrane. The cause is not fully known.

Cause factors
  1 Chronic constipation, pregnancy, pelvic tumours
  2 Part of portal hypertension with cirrhosis of the liver

Effects, signs and symptoms These depend on the degree of prolapse. There are three degrees.
1st degree Slight prolapse, but may be torn by the passing of hard faeces and will bleed (usually stops after defaecation). The patient complains of a splattering of blood in the lavatory after defaecation. They may be painless.

2nd degree Prolapse on defaecation which may return or may be replaced by a gloved finger.
If the sphincter grips the prolapse, the blood in the veins becomes congested and may clot. The patient may then have acute pain and the pile may need to be incised and the clot evacuated.
If the arteries are occluded, a strangulated pile will cause great pain. The patient may need morphine and cold compresses to relieve it. Bed rest is required.

3rd degree Complete prolapse which persists – strangulation can occur. Pruritis – irritation of the skin – is common around the anus. The patient may be quite anaemic after repeated haemorrhages.

Diagnosis – investigations
  1 Clinical history – bowel habits   **2** Examination – direct view, rectal palpation
  3 Proctoscopy or sigmoidoscopy to exclude carcinoma of sigmoid colon or rectum

Treatment
  1 Application of local anaesthetic creams or suppositories
  2 Injection of 5% phenol in almond oil into the piles. (Obliterates the plexus of veins)
  3 Haemorrhoidectomy

Suggested nursing response for strangulation
  1 Rest in bed, but difficult to find a comfortable position   **2** Give prescribed analgesia
  3 Continue application of cold compresses

Suggested nursing response for haemorrhoidectomy
Post operative management
  1 Observe carefully for reactionary *haemorrhage* and if a ligature slips (blood can accumulate in the rectum). Later there is danger of secondary haemorrhage if infection occurs.
  2 Prevent infection by regular bathing, drying carefully and dressings.
  3 Difficulty in passing the first stool. Varying techniques may be used: liquid paraffin or gentle aperients may be started, or an olive oil enema may be given. Ideally, a well formed stool may prevent stricture. Stricture is treated by anal dilation (the patient may do it himself).
Some surgeons are using wide anal dilation under a general anaesthetic instead of haemorrhoidectomy.

2 The liver and gall bladder

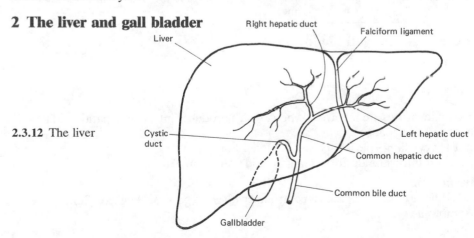

2.3.12 The liver

The liver

Functions	Structures involved
1 The metabolism of carbohydrates, proteins and fats **Carbohydrate** – glucose in excess of immediate needs is stored as *glycogen* and released for use by the action of *glucagon* **Protein** – amino acids are used in the manufacture of the plasma proteins albumin, globulin, fibrinogen and prothrombin. Excess are changed by deamination to *urea* for excretion **Fats** – lipids are distributed for storage and reactivated for release of energy	Liver cells receive blood from the hepatic artery and portal vein. The cell products enter the blood stream, leaving the liver by the hepatic vein
2 Detoxication of substances (including drugs)	All liver cells
3 Changing fat soluble bilirubin (from red cell breakdown) into water soluble bilirubin. Manufacture of *bile* – approximately 500 ml daily	Bile is secreted, through tiny 'capillaries' known as bile canaliculi, drains through hepatic ducts, is stored in the gall bladder and released for the digestion of fats through the common bile duct
5 Foetal erythropoiesis	
6 Generation of heat	High rate of metabolism in cells and huge blood supply

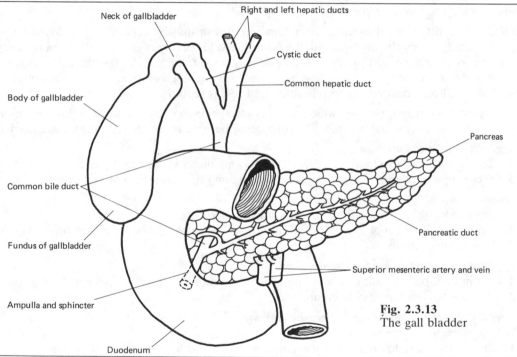

Fig. 2.3.13
The gall bladder

The gall bladder

Functions	Structures involved
1 Storage of bile	Delivered from the liver through the hepatic duct and the cystic duct
2 Concentration of bile	Absorption of water through the mucous membrane
3 Release of bile into the cystic duct and common bile duct in response to the presence of fat in the intestine	Smooth muscles contract after being stimulated by the hormone cholecystokinin (enters blood stream from cells in the intestine)

Conditions of the liver and gall bladder

Hepatitis is inflammation of the liver

Acute hepatitis

Causes

1 Infection Two main viruses are involved: type A which produces infective hepatitis and type B which produces serum hepatitis
2 Drugs The list is very long – please see the National Formulary
3 Poisons e.g. carbon tetrachloride (dry cleaning fluid), fungi and alcohol

Type A – Infective hepatitis
Incubation period is about 1 month. Spread is controlled with good personal hygiene. Some patients only have mild symptoms

Type B – Serum hepatitis

Incubation period is 3 months or more. Transmitted through infected serum – danger to hospital staff handling equipment containing blood – even syringes and needles. Often occurs in drug dependent patients. Also transmitted by close sexual contact

Effects, signs and symptoms Prodromal illness (before specific signs and symptoms). The patient has a raised metabolic rate with fever, malaise and weakness. Abdominal discomfort, nausea and vomiting occur. Because of liver enlargement pain may be felt in the upper abdomen and the liver is tender on palpation. Eventually, swelling in the liver impedes the secretion of bile through the canaliculi.

Jaundice causes yellowing of the sclera first and then of the skin, which becomes irritable. The urine is dark in colour (bilirubin is present) and the stools become pale and offensive smelling.

A few patients (mainly type B) will have an overwhelming inflammation (fulminating) leading to liver failure (see below). Many patients become very depressed with hepatitis.

Diagnosis – investigations

1 Clinical history and examination.
2 Blood – presence of viruses; serum transaminases are raised; serum bilirubin is raised
3 Urine – bilirubin present; urobilinogen is present early on, absent when jaundice present and reappears as jaundice recedes

Urobilinogen is made in the liver by acting on bile that has been absorbed from the intestine. It cannot be made if there is obstruction to the flow of bile.

Treatment There is no specific treatment

Suggested nursing response

Assessment	Care
1 Raised metabolic rate: pyrexia; malaise (sometimes bradycardia due to the action of bile salts)	Rest in bed. Glucose drinks for energy and fluid replacement. High protein diet for tissue repair (but see liver failure)
2 Effects of jaundice and liver damage:	
1 skin irritation	Apply soothing lotion (e.g. Calamine)
2 intolerance to fat	Reduced fat diet
3 intolerance to alcohol	Avoid alcoholic drinks
4 depression	Assurance and tolerance of 'black' moods – needs sensitive handling

All patients should be isolated. Major care with disposal of excreta.

Cirrhosis of the liver

Is a chronic fibrosis of the liver

Causes

1 Sometimes follows acute hepatitis
2 May be due to obstruction of the common bile duct of long standing
3 Many cases – no known cause
4 Strongest association is with alcoholism

Effects, signs and symptoms May be summarized in two ways but they are related.

1 *Damage to the liver* (hepatocellular effects)
   1 Failure to manufacture plasma proteins
   2 Low albumin reduces osmotic pressure in the blood capillaries – oedema and ascites will occur.
   3 Low globulin reduces resistance to infection. There is often a low grade fever present.
   4 Low prothrombin and fibrinogen impairs blood clotting. Bruising and bleeding can take place.
   5 Spider naevi may be present. (Spider naevi consist of a red raised spot on the skin, with radiating red lines from it. They go white when pressed.)
   6 Failure to make bile may lead to constipation, sometimes the passing of fatty, pale, offensive stools.
   7 Patients cannot tolerate fatty foods very well.
   8 Jaundice occurs at the *late* stage of cirrhosis.

Although many patients have a low grade pyrexia, they usually complain of an intolerance to cold.

2 *Portal hypertension* (as the liver becomes more shrunken and hardened)
   1 Dilation of veins in the oesophagus (oesophageal varices). These may rupture and bleed profusely.
   2 The stomach – the patient complains of indigestion (may have alcoholic gastritis too).
   3 The mesentery – ascites will develop and gross abdominal distension occurs.
   4 The spleen – becomes enlarged (splenomegaly) and tender.
   5 The rectum – haemorrhoids may occur. Again these may bleed easily.

Some patients only have very mild symptoms of abdominal discomfort. Some have no symptoms at all and it is found in surgery for something else or at post mortem.

Diagnosis – investigations
1 Clinical history and examination
2 Blood – serum bilirubin and serum transaminases may both be raised.
3 Liver biopsy – using a large needle

Nursing notes – liver biopsy
The liver capsule usually closes over the small hole and little discomfort occurs. It may be torn or blood clotting is delayed and haemorrhage may persist for a long time. Observations should continue for evidence of internal haemorrhage for 24 hours after the procedure.

Treatment There is no specific cure for the cirrhosis. Surgical bypass of the portal vein into the inferior vena cava is done to relieve severe portal hypertension. Patients who give up alcohol may survive for many years.

Suggested nursing response

Assessment	Care
1 Metabolic rate – low grade fever and weakness	Rest in bed if pyrexia persists. High caloric fluids for energy
2 Intolerance to cold	Keep the patient warm
3 Degree of ascites and oedema – note the girth measurements – discomfort increasing	Low sodium diet Prescribed diuretics usually work very well. Rare now – drainage of the ascites – paracentesis abdominus. Careful positioning and lifting for care of pressure areas
4 Intolerance to fat – fatty stools	Low fat diet. Deodorant if conscious of smell
5 Note any tendency to bleed 1 bruising 2 haematemesis 3 rectal bleeding	Urgent action – treat for shock, intravenous infusion, prepare for surgery
6 If alcoholic, note any withdrawal symptoms	Great care and encouragement may be needed. Possibly psychiatric help

Cancer of the liver

Primary tumours of the liver are in fact rare. Metastases from other tumours are common and the prognosis is very poor.

The effects vary in the early stages, but eventually those similar to cirrhosis will occur but with gross weight loss. Liver failure and coma will eventually lead to death, but many die of an overwhelming infection first.

Liver failure – hepatic coma

The effects as for cirrhosis will occur. Eventually, the most serious problem that occurs in the liver is the failure to convert the ammonia from protein catabolism into urea. Serum ammonia rises and will eventually cause hepatic coma.

The patient may have a flapping tremor of his hands before this. There is a characteristic smell of the breath called faetor hepaticus – described as a sweet smell of a decomposing corpse!

Treatment and care
These are aimed at keeping the patient alive and awaiting recovery of liver cells.
1 High calories are given – oral strong glucose drinks or intravenous infusions to prevent protein catabolism being used to give energy.
2 Low protein diet is given to reduce ammonia levels.
3 Coliform organisms produce ammonia – the contents of the bowel are washed out and an antibacterial drug, usually neomycin, is given.

Nursing note
This is another situation that demands a total nursing care plan – apply one of the nursing models in Section 1, remembering the range of problems already given above.

Rupture of the liver

This is a dangerous consequence of violent injury such as steering wheel injuries in road traffic accidents or as a result of kicking or stabbing in fights.

Effects, signs and symptoms May be a slow leak of blood from a torn liver capsule. The patient will have pain and gradually rising pulse, falling blood pressure and increasing restlessness and anxiety. There may be profound injury with massive blood loss, severe pain and fear. The patient is in danger of dying from shock (hypovolaemic and neurogenic).

Treatment
1 Laparotomy and suturing of the liver capsule
2 Some liver tissue may be resected
Suturing of tissues and the capsule is not easy

Suggested nursing response
In accident centre
1 Quick assessment and treatment for shock
2 Blood transfusion, analgesia and assurance
3 Prepare for admission for observation or immediate surgery

In the ward Observe: pulse, blood pressure (¼ hourly recordings); behaviour; pain and response to analgesia; girth measurements

Following surgery Needs intensive nursing care for laparotomy, sometimes thoracotomy, peritonitis, ileus and liver damage. Large volumes of blood are required and it is usually warmed for rapid infusion.

Cholelithiasis – gall stones

Cause The cause is not known but appears to be related to fat metabolism in Western civilization. The stones may contain bilirubin, cholesterol (or both) with calcium salts. The contents vary in different patients. Cholesterol is found in 75% of gall stones.

Effects, signs and symptoms Many gall stones produce no symptoms or functional disorders at all. They may produce however:

1 *Cholecystitis* Inflammation of the gall bladder which may become infected with coliform bacteria. The inflammation may be mild or lead to gross distension with ulceration of the gall bladder wall. Rarely, perforation may allow bile into the peritoneum (biliary peritonitis).

The main symptoms are upper abdominal pain and tenderness with referred pain in the shoulder, a history of indigestion and an aversion to fatty meals. More acute disease may cause biliary colic, but that is more due to obstruction.

2 *Biliary tract obstruction* may cause severe spasmodic contractions of the smooth muscles – known as *biliary colic*. The pain is intense and the patient may appear shocked, restless and anxious.

Nursing note
There is an urgent need for prescribed analgesia – usually pethidine is given with an antispasmodic drug such as morphine may cause spasm of the sphincter of Oddi.

3 *Jaundice* occurs with yellowing of the sclera and skin with pruritis, the production of dark urine with bilirubin present and pale, offensive smelling, fatty stools.
Blood clotting is affected because fat soluble vitamins (especially vitamin K) cannot be absorbed and prothrombin production is reduced.

Diagnosis – investigations
1 Clinical history and examination
2 Abdominal X-rays
3 Cholecystogram and cholangiogram
4 Blood for serum bilirubin
5 Urine for bilirubin (urobilinogen not present)
6 Stools for fat content
7 Ultrasound

Treatment
Medical Acute cholecystitis
1 Rest in bed, analgesia and antibacterial drugs are given.
2 A fat free diet is given until cholecystectomy is performed at a later admission.
3 Gall stones (predominantly cholesterol) have been treated medically, by use of chenoxycholic acid oral capsules – dissolving cholesterol stones over a period.
4 Some patients may still need surgery.

Surgical Cholecystectomy (removal of gall bladder)
Cholangiogram will help to decide if exploration of the common bile duct is done also.

Suggested nursing response for acute cholecystitis
Assessment and care of a febrile patient, noting the characteristics of the pain, evidence of biliary colic, biliary obstruction and perforation.

Suggested nursing response for cholecystectomy
Pre operative management
1 Assessment and care if jaundice is present or if liver damage has occurred. Prothrombin estimation is important. Vitamin K may be given prior to operation.
2 Prepare for an upper abdominal incision (many patients are obese). Breathing and coughing exercises before surgery. (Sputum to exclude chest infection.)
3 Prepare for a period of nasogastric aspiration after surgery. Pass the nasogastric tube before surgery.

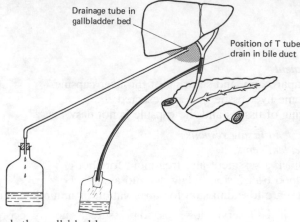

Fig. 2.3.14
Drains following
cholecystectomy

Surgery

1 Deep retraction is necessary to reach the gall bladder.
2 The gall bladder is adherent to the liver capsule and capillary bleeding may persist after removal (note blood clotting factors). Drain to the bed of gall bladder needed.
3 Exploration of the common bile duct causes oedema and possible obstruction. A T tube is inserted to ensure free flow of bile through the common bile duct and drainage of excess into an outside bag.

Post operative management

1 *Breathing* – care of the airway immediately; sit up as soon as possible; use post operative analgesia to encourage deep breathing and coughing exercises while supporting the wound – as soon as possible.
2 *Drains* Observe and measure blood from the gall bladder bed. Remove after a few days – depends on cessation of drainage and surgeon's instructions.
T tube After about 48 hours, clamp the tube for short periods and observe the patient for indications of obstruction (pain). If no reaction, clamp for longer periods – continue to observe (note urine and stools too). 7–10 days after operation, cholangiogram is performed and T tube removed if the duct is patent. Give strong analgesia before removing the tube.
3 *Diet* Fluids in sips only unless bowel sounds are heard, then gradually increased. Normal diet may be introduced gradually but many still prefer a reduced fat intake – will need advice to try out for himself.

3 The pancreas

Functions	Structures involved
1 Manufacture and secretion of pancreatic digestive juice containing the enzymes amylase, trypsinogen (becomes trypsin in the duodenum) and lipase. Sodium bicarbonate neutralizes the hydrochloric acid in chyme leaving the stomach	Exocrine glands and ducts in the pancreas. The ducts unite to form the pancreatic duct, which joins the common bile duct in the Ampulla of Vater before releasing secretions through the sphincter of Oddi in the wall of the duodenum
	Secretion is controlled by vagus nerve activity and by hormone action – secretin and pancreozymin are released from the intestinal mucosa when food is present.
2 Manufacture and release into the blood stream of the two hormones:	
1 insulin – main function is thought to be in the cell membranes to allow glucose to enter for energy release	Beta cells of the islets of Langerhans – crops of endocrine glandular tissue throughout the gland
2 glucagon – releases glucose into the circulation by conversion of glycogen to glucose in the liver	Alpha cells of the islets of Langerhans

Conditions of the pancreas

Pancreatitis is inflammation of the pancreas.

Acute pancreatitis

Cause

1 Not known in many cases
2 Related to gall bladder disease
3 Associated with alcoholism
4 A complication of mumps (rarely)

Effects, signs and symptoms

Apart from inflammation, the digestive enzymes may start digesting the tissues of the gland itself.

Mild cases – swelling and oedema of the tissues cause severe pain in the abdomen following alcohol or a large meal.
Severe cases – gross tissue destruction with haemorrhage. The patient may collapse in shock – blood pressure very low, severe tachycardia. Often confused with perforated peptic ulcer if peritonitis occurs.

Diagnosis – investigations

1 Careful clinical history and examination
2 Blood for serum amylase in the early stages
3 Ultrasound shows enlarged pancreas
4 Laparotomy

Treatment
1 Treat for shock   2 Nasogastric aspiration
3 Intravenous fluids, electrolytes and nutrition
4 Pain relief – methadone or pethidine with an antispasmodic drug (morphine causes spasm of the sphincter of Oddi)
5 If haemorrhage, a blood transfusion is needed
6 Antibacterial drugs to prevent secondary infection

Surgery
1 Laparotomy may be needed to confirm diagnosis
2 Relief of obstruction of the ducts may help
3 Rarely, pancreatectomy is done, but the patient would need insulin and pancreatic enzymes with meals for life afterwards

Suggested nursing response

Assessment	Care
1 Degree of shock – blood pressure and pulse recorded every 15 minutes in early stages	Rest in bed. Position for comfort
2 Degree and type of pain – a 'pain chart' may help	Giving prescribed analgesia but observe carefully. Strong narcotics are used and if continued for some time, physical dependence may occur
3 Position and patency of the nasogastric tube – test and aspirate frequently	Position and aspiration. Nothing given by mouth apart from sips of water
Without food in the intestine, the hormones that stimulate pancreatic enzyme production reduce their activity.	
4 Patency and continuing intravenous infusion, possibly using blood, plasma or electrolyte fluids. Central venous pressure may be needed in severe cases	Check the bag, the giving set, the site of injection and the patient's reaction
5 Psychological effects – possibly withdrawal from alcohol (see physical drug dependence too)	Understanding assurance and listening to the fears. Medical and psychiatric help for severe symptoms
Antibacterial drugs are used to prevent infection – but see undesired effects in National Formulary.	

Chronic pancreatitis

1 Usually associated with alcoholism
2 Defective production of pancreatic enzymes leads to malabsorption syndrome – loss of weight, anaemia, possibly a pale bulky stool if bile duct affected too
3 Treatment is by giving pancreatic enzymes with meals and avoiding alcohol

Nursing note
The nurse's role as a health educationalist may lead her to advising on alcohol consumption. Physical effects such as cirrhosis of the liver and pancreatitis with the misery they can cause are often missed out.

Cystic fibrosis

This is the commonest genetic condition of consequence in Britain in which all exocrine glands are affected as well as the pancreas. Pancreatic enzymes are deficient in infancy and need to be replaced (malabsorption otherwise). The main problems are in the airway where bronchiectasis may cause repeated chest infections.
More patients now survive to adulthood and genetic counselling is needed. An interesting diagnostic test is the 'sweat test' – there is an increase in the sodium content.

4 The abdominal wall – hernias

A **hernia** is a protrusion of an organ or part of an organ outside its normal cavity.

Causes
1 Congenital weakness of the muscles
2 Excessive physical strain (often when lifting)
3 Coughing excessively
4 Poor wound healing

Effects, signs and symptoms There is swelling at the site which
1 may be obvious and enlarge on coughing.
2 may be reduced as the protrusion is gently replaced (reducible).
3 may not return to the natural state by pressure (irreducible).
Many patients are unaware of a hernia until it strangulates. There may be local discomfort rather than pain which the patient is made aware of by coughing and straining at stool.

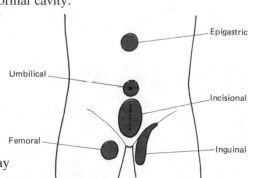

Fig. 2.3.15 Types of hernia

Strangulation The pressure of the muscles on the sac may occlude the venous return first, and later the arterial supply to the section of the organ (usually a loop of small intestine). The loop becomes inflamed and ultimately will become necrosed. Intestinal obstruction will occur and toxins from bacteria in the intestine entering the blood stream cause severe toxaemia. The patient is in severe pain, has nausea and vomiting; abdominal distension occurs and toxic shock will follow.

Diagnosis Is by clinical examination

Treatment
Surgery Repair of the hernia–*herniorrhaphy*. If strangulation has occurred re-establishment of fluid and electrolyte balance and treatment for shock are carried out before urgent surgery. Herniorrhaphy may need to be accompanied by resection of necrosed intestine.

Suggested nursing response
Patients may ask advice about swellings from the trained nurse. *Always* refer them for a medical opinion, even if they are painless. Trusses may still be supplied (rarely). Advice on cleaning and maintenance of them should be given.

Pre operative management
1 Herniorrhaphy–note whether the patient smokes or has a chest infection
2 Strangulation–see intestinal obstruction (p 70) and care before surgery

Post operative problems
1 Reduce the effects of coughing and straining by supporting the wound.
2 Note for internal haemorrhage–inguinal hernia–look for haematoma in the scrotum which can be quite tender (as well as embarrassing). A scrotal bridge or suspensory bandage may help.
3 Strangulation–the patient will still be very ill after surgery. Ileus may persist for some time. Toxaemia may continue–antibacterial drugs needed.

Psycho-social effects Many patients with hernias are physically fit, active people who will be anxious about their work and exercise tolerance following repair. Advice and assurance about returning to normal activity should be given.

2.4 Renal conditions

The renal system

This system will be considered as follows.

1 **The kidney**   2 **The urinary tract**–ureters, bladder and urethra

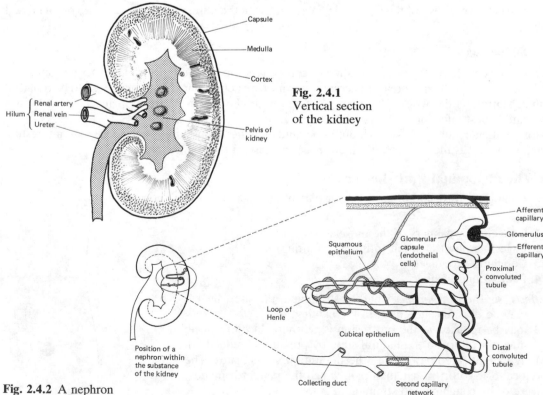

Fig. 2.4.1
Vertical section
of the kidney

Fig. 2.4.2 A nephron

1 The kidney

Functions	Structures involved
1 Formation and secretion of urine by:	
1 Filtration of blood (170 litres per day 120 ml per minute)	Glomerulus and Bowman's capsule. Filtration is governed by: (a) the arterial blood pressure exerting enough force through the afferent blood vessels (70–80 mm Hg systolic needed) (b) the lumen of the arterioles which are controlled by the sympathetic nervous system
2 Selective reabsorption of water (168.5 litres per day)	Tubules of the kidney. 65% reabsorbed in proximal tubule but continues throughout. Final control is by antidiuretic hormone (ADH.)
3 Selective reabsorption of glucose, amino acids and lipids	All reabsorbed in proximal tubules normally
4 Selective reabsorption of electrolytes (salts) e.g. sodium, potassium, calcium and chloride ions (maintains electrolyte balance) and hydrogen ions (maintains the pH of blood at 7.4). Urine is normally acidic – high number of hydrogen ions but lower pH (4–6)	Throughout the tubule including the Loop of Henle and distal tubules. Final control is in the distal and collecting tubules by the action of the hormone aldosterone
5 Secretion of some electrolytes (potassium, ammonium and hydrogen) and secretion of toxins, drugs and urinary pigments	Distal tubules mainly
2 The production of erythropoietin – the hormone that influences red cell production in the bone marrow	Renal tissue
3 Controlling blood pressure by the release of renin which changes angiotensinogen to angiotensin. Angiotensin causes constriction of peripheral arterioles and increases blood pressure	Renal tissue near the glomerules. There is increased secretion of renin when the kidney is damaged or if the blood flow to it is diminished for any reason

Conditions of the kidney

Nephritis – inflammation of the kidney
Three conditions will be considered: glomerulonephritis, pyelonephritis and nephrotic syndrome.

Glomerulonephritis

Cause Antibody/antigen reaction. The antigens are most commonly the immune complexes formed after an infection by beta haemolytic streptococci but others may be responsible. There is usually a period of 1–3 weeks following infection.

Effects, signs and symptoms Raised metabolic rate. The degree of fever may vary considerably, but in some people the temperature may be very high and rigors can occur. Tachycardia may be marked and the patient appears very tired and feels miserable and ill.

Inflammation of the glomerulus may cause leakage of plasma proteins through the filter. Some patients only have proteinuria. There may, however, be leakage of red cells and some may enter the urine. The urine appears cloudy and may appear grey in colour (described as 'smoky'). If tested, blood and protein will be found. More frank haematuria may occur in severe cases.

Poor filtration of the blood will lead to fluid retention (sodium is retained too) and low urine output (oliguria). This causes oedema which is first noticed under the eyes, then the face becomes 'puffy' and ankle swelling may be seen. There may be pulmonary congestion with breathlessness and possible pleural effusion. Blood pressure will rise and (rarely) hypertensive encephalopathy may produce fits and brain damage.

A few patients may go into acute renal failure with severe oliguria or even anuria. They are then in danger from the retention of potassium in the blood (hyperkalaemia) and hydrogen ions which will cause acidosis.

The majority of patients make a spontaneous recovery with a diuresis (as the filter functions again). Proteinuria may last a few days, but some patients go on to develop nephrotic syndrome (see p 87) and some may develop chronic renal failure (see p 90).

Diagnosis – investigations
1 Clinical history and examination
2 Urine – visible description is important and the volume and proteinuria are checked daily
3 Blood for antistreptolysin titre, electrolytes and urea levels
4 Throat swab for haemolytic streptococci (but often negative at this stage)

Treatment
1 Rest in bed until fever settles
2 Penicillin may be prescribed
3 Fluid control (see nursing)
4 Diet – low sodium, low protein and high carbohydrates for energy

Suggested nursing response

Assessment	Care

1 Metabolic rate
  1 observe temperature 4 hourly and pulse frequently (but record at least 4 hourly).
  2 observe for rigors or convulsions in children.
  3 vomiting is common in children too
	Rest in bed. Cooling with light clothing and a fan. Glucose to drink (but fluid restrictions)
	
	Assurance and support (including parents)
	Vomit bowl. Mouth care

2 Urine output and fluid balance
  1 measure accurately!
  2 urinalysis (test for protein)
  3 report increase in obvious haematuria
	Fluids are restricted to 500 ml plus the equivalent volume of the previous days output. Care of the mouth is vital
	Note carefully: when diuresis occurs, patient could be dehydrated

3 Acceptance of diet restrictions
  1 low sodium
  2 low protein
	Needs a lot of encouragement
	Salt free butter, no chocolate
	Reduced meat intake

4 Evidence of increasing fluid retention
  1 oedema – face
  2 hypertension – headaches, fits
  3 pulmonary congestion – breathlessness
	Report quickly to doctors
	Skin care for oedema
	Position for breathlessness and oxygen therapy. May need pleural aspiration if effusion

For evidence of acute renal failure see p 89.

Pyelonephritis

Is inflammation of the pelvis of the kidney and the kidney tissue – mainly the renal tubules.

Cause
  1 Ascending infection through the urinary tract
  2 Micro-organisms – coliform bacteria (*Escherichia coli, Pseudomonas, Proteus, Streptococcus faecalis*) and staphylococcus epidermidis
  3 Factors influencing urinary tract infection
    1 poor genital hygiene and nappy care in infants
    2 incontinence
    3 sexual intercourse
    4 congenital disorders of the tract
    5 tumours and stones in the tract
    6 catheterization – poor technique or hygiene (incidence increases when catheters are left in for more than five days)

Effects, signs and symptoms Metabolic rate may be severely raised with high pyrexia, tachycardia and malaise. Rigors may occur. Nausea and vomiting are common.

Inflammation of the renal pelvis causes distention and the patient complains of pain and tenderness in the loin.

Inflammation of the tubules interferes with tubular reabsorption and the patient may pass large volumes of urine which has a low specific gravity. Micro abscesses may form in the tubules. The urine may have streaks of pus in it. The classic 'fishy' smell is due to the action of escherichia coli. There may even be a faecal smell.

Many children do not get specific urinary symptoms and the condition may be missed if careful observation of urine is inadequate. Some patients with pyelonephritis progress to severe renal damage and chronic renal failure (see p 89). Chronic pyelonephritis is one of the most common causes of chronic renal failure.

It should be remembered that the effects of cystitis and urethritis, described later, will very likely be present in an ascending infection.

Nursing note
Prevention of urinary tract infection is one of the nurse's important functions in health education and preventive medicine. Learn the factors and note the misery and serious consequences for a whole family when, typically, a mother may have chronic pyelonephritis.

Diagnosis – investigations
  1 Clinical history and examination
  2 Mid stream specimens or catheter specimens of urine for culture of micro-organisms
  3 Renal function tests if severe damage suspected

Treatment
  1 Rest
  2 Increase fluid intake
  3 Antimicrobial agents e.g. co-trimoxazole, sulphonamides, gentamicin or ampicillin according to culture of organisms. Usually given for *2 weeks*, followed by a further *2 weeks* following a second culture test.

Suggested nursing response

Assessment	Care
1 Raised metabolic rate: pyrexia; tachycardia; weakness, malaise; sweating; nausea and vomiting	Rest in bed. Cool with fans (rarely now – tepid sponging). Glucose drinks needed. Skin care. Vomit bowl. Mouth care
2 Evidence of dehydration: skin may be hot and dry; headaches; irritable and restless	Give at least 3 litres of fluid in 24 hours (better – ensure at least 250 ml hourly while awake)
3 Note the colour, consistency, smell and volume of urine	Frequent urinals or bed pans needed. Careful hygiene of genitalia with soap and water and drying
4 Self consciousness if smell	Deodorants may help
5 Pain and tenderness in loin	Prescribed analgesia. Patients find comfort in local warmth
6 Acceptance of prescribed therapy	Important to impress on patients the need to complete long courses of antibacterial drugs
7 Undesired effects of drugs – see details in the National Formulary	

Note especially: Broad spectrum antibacterial drugs may cause moniliasis in a long course. Oral 'thrush', diarrhoea and vaginitis may occur. Sulphonamides (including co-trimoxazole) may cause crystalluria if inadequate fluid intake. Rarely, they cause bone marrow damage

Nephrotic syndrome – proteinuria and oedema

Proteinuria – plasma proteins leak into the urine
Oedema is widespread
In addition, there is usually a low resistance to infection.

Causes
1 May be an auto immune condition or due to unknown allergens
2 May be a sequel to glomerulonephritis
3 Due to diabetes mellitus – diabetic nephropathy
4 A consequence of mercury poisoning
5 Due to amyloid disease or lupus erythematosus

Effects, signs and symptoms
Loss of plasma proteins through changes in the glomerulus.

Loss of albumin will lower the osmotic pressure in the blood capillaries, reduce tissue fluid return and causes the oedema. Classically, there is oedema of the face (under the eyes), ascites may develop and dependent oedema may endanger skin on the sacral areas, ankles and heels.

Loss of globulin (immunoglobulins) leads to a loss of antibodies and lowers the resistance to infection. The patient may present with a fever due to infection elsewhere. (Note the special dangers for the diabetic patient with this condition.)

Some patients make spontaneous recovery. Some progress to chronic renal failure. Continual loss of protein will lead to loss for muscles and muscle wasting and weakness will be present. There is usually an abnormality of fat metabolism too, with increased cholesterol in the serum. They are more prone to thrombosis development.

Diagnosis – investigations
1 Clinical history and examination
2 Urine test for proteinuria. 3–50 gram per day may be lost
3 Mid stream specimen to exclude infection
4 Blood shows low serum albumin; high serum cholesterol
5 Renal function tests
6 Renal biopsy will be performed in adults and older children, but great caution in infants

Suggested nursing response for renal biopsy
Before the procedure
1 Clear explanation to the patient and consent
2 X-rays to locate kidney – usually intravenous urogram
3 Skin marked
4 Blood cross matched

During the procedure
1 Local anaesthetic used through a long needle (there are pain receptors in the kidney)
2 Usually done by X-ray guidance

After the procedure
1 Rest quietly for 24 hours
2 Observe for haemorrhage – restlessness; pulse and blood pressure; all urine for haematuria
3 Observe for pain and give prescribed analgesia
4 Observe for infection – pyrexia, tachycardia. (*Note:* Secondary haemorrhage could follow infection.)

Treatment
1 High protein diet 80–100 gram per day (unless renal failure)
2 Low sodium intake
3 Diuretics may be useful to reduce the oedema
4 Some patients benefit from corticosteroid drugs (but note dangers)

Suggested nursing response
Nephrotic syndrome may present with a considerable number of nursing problems.

Assessment	Care
1 Condition of the patient's skin: oedema; ascites; striae	Very careful: lifting of the patient; care of pressure areas; washing and drying of the skin as danger of infected lesions
2 Circulation: danger of thrombosis; possible hypotension if gross loss of osmotic pressure; possible hypertension if renal failure	Passive exercises but muscles are weak and wasted. Position carefully
3 Respiration: danger of chest infections	Breathing exercises. See care of chest infections (2.1)
4 Digestion and nutrition: acceptance of the high protein diet with no added salt	Sick patients find a high protein diet very difficult to digest, apart from the loss of taste (salt substitute should be used)
Note: with renal failure there is a change to a *low* protein diet. This may confuse ward staff	
5 Renal system *1* danger of urinary tract infection *2* effects of diuretic drugs *3* daily weighing	Hygiene and high fluid intake
6 Psychological state *1* changed body image with gross oedema *2* fear and danger of renal failure	Care with appearances and reactions Listen to fears and anxieties. Assurance of recovery and care available

Obviously, individuals will present different problems but it is a very demanding condition for the nursing team. Even worse is to add on the problems of the diabetic patient (see 2.8). In diabetes, amyloid disease and lupus erythematosus, the prognosis is very poor.

Tumours of the kidney

Renal carcinoma (previously hypernephroma)

Cause Unknown

Effects, signs and symptoms The tumour may erode a blood vessel causing haematuria with blood clots that may cause renal colic. Low grade inflammation may lead to tenderness, abdominal pain and fever.

Unfortunately, metastases to the lungs, liver and bones present symptoms before renal effects. Prognosis is very bad then.

Treatment Surgical removal
See *nursing for surgery of the kidney* – p 93.

Wilms' tumour (nephroblastoma)

Involves the pelvis of the kidney as well as renal tissue.
Occurs in childhood.
Needs early diagnosis, surgical removal and radiotherapy.

See *nursing for surgery, radiotherapy* and *care of children*.

Congenital defects of the kidney

A number of abnormalities do occur and present specialist surgical problems e.g. abnormal position, such as pelvic, or structures, such as horseshoe. These cannot be covered in this text but principles are as for renal surgery.

The most important hereditary defect though is polycystic kidney.

Polycystic kidney

Cause It is an autosomal dominant trait

Effects, signs and symptoms The kidneys are grossly enlarged with large cysts throughout the renal tissue. As renal tissue may continue to function in spite of the conditions, symptoms rarely appear until adult life (30–40 years old). There may be haematuria if renal damage occurs or renal pain and tenderness but often the symptoms of hypertension may be the first indicators (headaches, breathlessness). Renal failure is inevitable. Care is symptomatic and as for chronic renal failure (p 90).

Rupture of the kidney

Causes
1 A blow to the loin area (sometimes surprisingly minor blows) as in accidents or violence (kicking, thumping)
2 Puncture wounds due to stabbing or gun shot wounds

Suggested nursing response – first aid
1 Treat for shock – severe pain and haemorrhage
2 Strict observations and care for internal haemorrhage
3 Apply dressings to external wounds
4 Nil by mouth and early transfer for hospital assessment
5 Observe any urine for blood staining

Management
Only if severe haemorrhage would surgery be indicated. Emergency intravenous urogram is performed.
More commonly: blood transfusion to replace blood loss; analgesia to relieve pain; rest in bed (usually for about 2 weeks) and antibiotics to prevent infection.
Secondary haemorrhage following infection would possibly indicate the need for nephrectomy.

Suggested nursing response

Assessment	Care
1 Indications of severe haemorrhage (profound shock) or continuing bleeding into the abdominal cavity (girth measurements) or ureters (blood in urine)	Blood transfusion care. (Prepare for emergency surgery possibly.) Assurance while observations continue as anxiety continues
All urine specimens saved for assessment of when bleeding has stopped.	
2 Degree of pain – may interfere with ventilation too; tenderness if abscesses form	Prescribed analgesia and breathing exercises encouraged
3 Indications of infection (raised metabolic rate – pyrexia, tachycardia)	Prescribed antimicrobial drugs. Rest in bed. Cooling. Fluids with glucose added

Acute renal failure

Causes Usually related to failure of the glomerular filter
  1 *Hypotension – low blood pressure*
    1 Shock   *2* Haemorrhage
    Inadequate pressure for filtration and perfusion of kidney tissue. Lack of oxygen to the tissues.
  2 *Glomerular damage*
    1 Acute glomerulonephritis   *2* Septicaemia
  3 *Impairment of filter*
    1 Agglutinated red cells (incompatible blood transfusion)
    2 Free circulating haemoglobin (haemolysis)
    3 Metabolites from crush injuries when released or as tourniquets are released (crush syndrome)
    4 Pigments (e.g. bilirubin)

Effects, signs and symptoms
Suppression of urine. As the filter does not function, there is a marked failure of urine output (oliguria) and even complete cessation (anuria).

Nursing note
Observations of urine output following trauma or surgery and during blood transfusions are much more concerned with the production of urine, rather than retention. It may be necessary to calculate in volumes less than 20 ml hourly and the nurse should learn to palpate the bladder.

Accumulation of electrolytes The most serious are:
  1 Retention of potassium ions (hyperkalaemia) which may cause severe muscle spasm with pain in the legs. Much more dangerous are cardiac arrhythmias including cardiac arrest.
  2 Retention of hydrogen ions (acidosis) which will lead to over breathing (hyperventilating) to try and overcome the effect. Serious disturbances can occur leading to coma and death.

Raised blood urea which again can eventually have toxic effects on the brain leading to coma and death.
A glance at the causes and effects of acute renal failure should indicate how dangerously ill patients are in this condition. They are prone to infection also, and it can be seen why the mortality rate is still quite high.

Diagnosis – investigations
  1 Clinical history and examination – nurse's observations are critical
  2 Blood for serum electrolytes, pH, urea and creatinine levels

Treatment

1 Strict fluid balance control
2 Restricting sodium and potassium intake. Serum potassium can be lowered with the use of an exchange resin (Resonium) given orally or rectally. Some physicians prescribe insulin and glucose which transfers the potassium ions from the serum into the cells
3 Control of urea by reducing the protein intake – usually to about 30 gram (normal is about 70 gram)
4 Calcium gluconate is sometimes used to prevent cardiac arrhythmias
5 Prevent and treat infections. Isolation is needed and antimicrobial agents may be prescribed
6 Peritoneal or haemodialysis would be used as early as possible

Suggested nursing response
– in addition to nursing management of the cause of the renal failure, using Model of nursing A (1.3)

Assessment	Care
1 Safe environment	
1 need for isolation and barrier nursing	Sympathetic explanation of need for barrier nursing
2 dangers of bed rest	Care of the skin, pressure areas
2 Communicating	Explaining all procedures carefully
1 need for understanding of the problems	
2 anxiety of relatives	Listen to fears and assure
3 Breathing	
1 note for indications of chest infection	Care for chest infections – special care of sputum
2 breathlessness due to arrhythmias – needs ECG monitor	Prescribed drugs (often intravenous). Possible defibrillation
3 hyperventilating if acidotic	Give bicarbonate solutions
4 danger of cardiac arrest	Immediate resuscitation
Note: cramp-like muscular pain indicating raised serum potassium	
4 Eating and drinking: acceptance of fluid and food restrictions (fluid balance chart)	Explanations. Give 500 ml of fluid per day plus the equivalent volume of previous 24 hours. Give low protein diet. Low sodium and potassium. (*Note*: many salt substitutes contain potassium.) Give regular mouth care
5 Eliminating	
1 danger of constipation	High fibre in the diet
2 acceptance of rectal resonium	Difficult enema to give
6 Personal cleansing and dressing	Light clothing in bed
7 Controlling body temperature – metabolic rate may rise if infection (pyrexia, tachycardia)	Keep cool with light clothing and fans. Extra glucose – 'Hycal'
Note: 1 A shocked patient would have a low temperature and feel cold but should not be over heated. 2 Over a long period, protein may be metabolized to provide energy, increasing urea levels and hence increasing the need for even more glucose – but difficulty in giving exists, as fluids are restricted.	
8 Mobilizing – likely to be immobile for some time	Passive exercises of all limbs
9 Anxieties about work and prospects after serious illness – financial difficulties	Involve work welfare/personnel services. Social workers needed
10 Difficulty in sleeping	Good nursing care needed for sleep as there is limitation on drug therapy when renal damage is serious
11 Dying: death may be sudden or may follow long periods of treatment and care	Resuscitation attempts. Handling relatives in shock. Sensitive care of staff may be needed

Patients who survive usually go on after the *oliguric* phase to a *diuretic* phase when the glomeruli suddenly allow filtration to occur. The nurse needs to observe for this to prevent dehydration due to fluid restriction.

Chronic renal failure (uraemia)

Usually gross distortion and damage to all kidney tissue

Causes

1 Chronic glomerulonephritis   2 Chronic pyelonephritis   3 Polycystic kidney
4 Hypertension – structural damage due to the high pressure. Note also though, damaged renal tissue increases the release of renin which leads to raised blood pressure.
5 More rarely – diabetic nephropathy; drugs and poisons; gout; amyloid disease; connective tissue diseases; obstruction (bilateral)

Effects, signs and symptoms   The effects are a raised blood pressure (occasionally malignant), failure to regulate electrolyte and fluid balance, failure to excrete urea and failure to produce erythropoietin. There is also interference with vitamin D metabolism. These effects are so widespread that it is common to consider them by body systems, but we should also note the psychological and social effects. Applying Model B (1.4), it is possible to devise a nursing care plan also.

System	Effects
Skin	May become pigmented (brown). Irritation (pruritis) occurs in areas where sweating occurs (due to urea crystals). In terminal stages 'uraemic frost' may appear around the lips
Circulation	Heart failure due to hypertension. Anaemia due to loss of erythropoietin. Pericarditis due to urea deposits
Respiration	Danger of chest infections. Smell of breath – uraemic or ammonia
Digestion	Hiccoughs due to urea effect on the diaphragm. Nausea and vomiting. Constipation or diarrhoea
Nervous	Peripheral neuropathy due to urea. May be confused or have convulsions. Headaches and visual disturbances due to hypertension
Renal	May pass large volumes of urine but cannot concentrate it. Urine may be infected.
Locomotor	Arthritis due to urea and altered calcium metabolism. Bone changes may lead to pain and occasionally pathological fractures. Muscular cramps
Reproductive	Loss of gonad functioning – impotence and loss of libido
Psychological	Self image may be seriously affected. Serious anxieties about the future. Depression and anxiety states may be serious enough to need psychiatric intervention. Need to learn much about their condition
Social	Serious effects on married life. Work prospects may be poor

Diagnosis – investigations
  1 Clinical history and examination including nursing observations
  2 Creatinine clearance test – a major indicator of the glomerular filtration rate
  3 Blood for urea, electrolyte, pH and creatinine   4 Intravenous urography   5 Renal biopsy

Treatment
  1 Control urea levels by restricting protein intake – sometimes 30 grams, but may be much less.
  2 High carbohydrate amounts are given to prevent protein breakdown for energy purposes
  3 Electrolytes are controlled according to serum levels
  4 Blood transfusion is needed for anaemia   5 Haemodialysis is indicated – but is expensive
  6 Renal transplant is the ideal treatment if possible

Dialysis will correct all the effects apart from anaemia. Renal transplant, if successful, can give the individual normal daily living. If severely damaged kidneys are continuing to cause a rising blood pressure, then bilateral nephrectomy is indicated (followed, of course, by dialysis).

Suggested nursing response
Question Mr Joseph Walker is a vagrant, age 68 years, and has been admitted to your medical ward from Accident Centre. He attended there with a painful toe but the Consultant has diagnosed that he has the terminal stages of chronic renal failure.

Describe a nursing care plan for Mr Walker for the first 48 hours in your ward.   100%

Analysis This is asking for a description and, therefore, a reason for your care will be needed.

It is logical to use a problem solving approach and here it may be helpful to use Model B.

Plan This should include nursing observations and care of Mr Walker's:
  1 *Skin* Pigmentation may be marked. Pruritis could be complicated by infestation
  2 *Circulation* Pericarditis may cause soreness. Anaemia will make him very tired and weak. Blood pressure may be raised
  3 *Respiration* Breath may smell of urine
  4 *Digestion* May have nausea and vomiting. Hiccups may be troublesome

You are invited to complete this plan now using the model of patient needs.

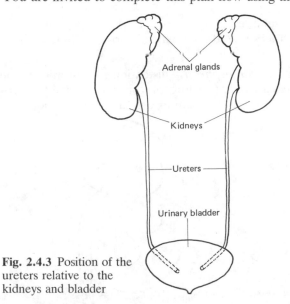

Fig. 2.4.3 Position of the ureters relative to the kidneys and bladder

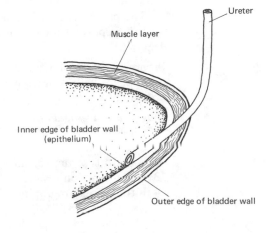

Fig. 2.4.4 Position of the ureter relative to the bladder wall

2 The urinary tract

Function	Structures involved
1 Conducting of urine from the collecting tubules of the nephrons to the urinary bladder. Movement is assisted by peristaltic movements	The pelvis of the kidney is considered to be a dilated part of the ureter Smooth muscle coat
2 Self protection of the tissues from the effects of acid (and occasionally alkaline) urine	Transitional epithelial tissue is resistant to acids and alkalis and is able to stretch to accommodate dilation when urine flows
3 Prevention of reflux of urine back into the kidney tissue	The critical angle at which the ureters enter the base of the bladder prevents reflux by closing the ureter when the bladder is distended

Conditions of the ureters

Pyelitis

Inflammation of the renal pelvis. It is rarely considered alone now as the renal tissue is nearly always inflamed. Therefore, see pyelonephritis (p 86).

Renal calculi (stones)

Commonly form in the pelvis of the kidney and damage the ureter if they try to pass through (small ones)

Cause factors
1 Inadequate fluid intake
2 Excessive fluid loss by perspiration
3 Urinary tract infections
4 Excessive calcium in the urine which may be due to hyperparathyroidism or may be due to long term bed rest (calcium mobilised from bone tissue)
5 Increased uric acid excretion (e.g. gout)
6 Congenital abnormalities
7 Possibly dietary factors

Effects, signs and symptoms Stones are made up of combinations of substances such as calcium, ammonium, magnesium, phosphate and oxalate ions or trace elements and metabolites (products of metabolism). They may be very small, like grit, or as old men call it, gravel. They may be the size and shape of the renal pelvis when they are known as staghorn calculus.

Many patients have few signs and symptoms, some have dull pain and tenderness, haematuria, or get recurrent pyelonephritis. Some patients develop renal colic.

Renal colic

A small stone obstructs the ureter. Severe spasm of the smooth muscle attempts to overcome the obstruction. Reflux into the renal tissue causes excruciating loin pain, the patient writhes in agony and may be shocked. Vomiting often occurs. Later the patient may pass the stone in the urine and quite often pass blood in the urine too (haematuria).

Nursing notes

This is an acute emergency and a doctor is required urgently to prescribe strong analgesia (often pethidine) and an antispasmodic drug.

The patient is very frightened and needs assurance.

It is important for the nurse to retain all stones passed – the patient's urine is filtered before disposal.

Progressive development of obstruction may cause *hydronephrosis* – distension and distortion of the renal pelvis with progressive damage to the renal tissue. (Hydronephrosis may be due to unco-ordinated peristalsis and obstruction of the ureter from other causes e.g. abdominal tumours.)

Diagnosis – investigations
1 Clinical history and examination (nursing observations of urine for stones and haematuria)
2 Blood for serum calcium
3 Renal function tests
4 Intravenous urography

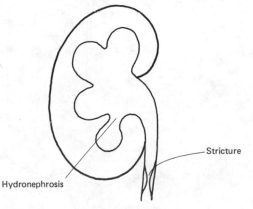

Fig. 2.4.5 Hydronephrosis

Hydronephrosis

Stricture

Suggested nursing response for intravenous urogram (intravenous pyelogram)

Before the procedure

1 Assess for any known allergies
2 Explain the procedure to the patient
3 Light diet the previous day
4 Aperient the evening before
5 Food and fluids withheld for 6–8 hours

During the procedure Assess for any allergic reaction–rash, wheezing, shock.

After the X-ray Return to normal eating and drinking.

Treatment

1 Surgery to remove the stone
2 Refashioning of the pelvis in hydronephrosis (pyeloplasty).

Suggested nursing response for surgery of the kidney and ureters

Pre operative management

1 Ensure that results of all renal function tests are available.
2 Assess and prepare the skin over the operation site–depends on surgeon's preference for either abdominal route or lumbar approach. The surgeon will mark the side–the nurse should check that this is done correctly.
3 Assess and prepare the patient's breathing. Chest infection must be excluded. Breathing exercise should be taught and practised before surgery.
4 Assess and help to prepare the patient's circulatory system. Many patients need blood transfusion for anaemia before surgery as well as afterwards.
5 Most surgeons prefer the bowel evacuated before surgery by use of enemas or suppositories. Catheterization is *not* always performed for surgery in the upper part of the urinary tract.

Operations Most surgeons attempt to avoid nephrectomy if possible

Nephrectomy The kidney is removed and a drain inserted into the site through separate stab wound

Pyeloplasty The pelvis of the kidney is refashioned and a nephrostomy tube sometimes inserted, draining into a closed bag system

Post operative management

1 *Breathing* Ensure a clear airway initially. As soon as possible, with the help of analgesia, the patient is sat up and deep breathing encouraged.
2 *Wounds and drains* Strict aseptic technique is vital. Observe for haemorrhage and haematuria. Nephrostomy tubes are managed strictly according to surgeon's instructions. Nursing towards the affected side assists drainage.
3 *Digestion* 'Paralytic' ileus often occurs. Some surgeons would use a nasogastric tube for all patients as vomiting is always possible. Intravenous fluids and nutrition is needed. Observe for bowel sounds and introduce drinks and diet as soon as possible.
4 *Mobilization* Passive movements initially, but active mobilization should be as for other abdominal operations.

Complications

1 Haemorrhage is the main hazard
2 Infection would be very dangerous–hence strict asepsis
3 Chest infections

Congenital defects of ureters There are various abnormalities which occur due to malformation of the foetus. They require specialist surgical care and details are not given in this text book. The general nurse should realize though that they do predispose to urinary tract infection and renal calculus formation.

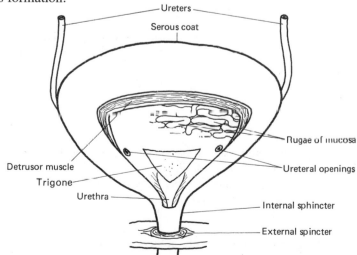

Fig. 2.4.6 Urinary bladder

Urinary bladder (*see Fig. 2.4.6*)

Functions	Structures involved
1 Reservoir for urine – a normal adult bladder holds approximately 300 ml	Inner lining of transitional epithelium allows for expansion and protection of submucous folds from urine (usually acid). Expansion causes distension in front of the peritoneum
2 Control of micturition *1* initially a reflex action	The trigone at the base of the bladder is sensitive to pressure as the bladder fills. Sensory nerves synapse in the spinal cord with intermediate nerves which synapse with motor nerves of the parasympathetic nervous system. The motor nerves cause the detrusor muscle in the bladder wall to contract and the internal sphincter to relax, thus emptying the bladder
2 later develops as a controlled function	Voluntary nerves control the external sphincter in the urethra – constricting it to prevent emptying until socially acceptable

Conditions of the bladder

Cystitis – inflammation of the bladder

Causes
   Usually infection
   1 Coliform organisms – Escherichia coli, Pseudomonas, Proteus, Streptococcus faecalis
   2 Skin commensal organisms – Staphylococcus epidermidis
   3 Some are non specific

See *pyelonephritis* for other predisposing factors.
   Inflammation may result from a stone irritating the epithelium or invasion by a tumour.

Effects, signs and symptoms Inflammation of the bladder increases the sensitivity of the trigone to even small amounts of urine in the bladder. The patient complains of frequency of micturition, passing small volumes (as little as 50 ml). There is usually urethritis too and a burning sensation is felt when the urine is passed. The bladder may be sore and uncomfortable.
   The metabolic rate may rise and the patient may have a pyrexia, tachycardia and feel tired and ill.

Diagnosis – investigations
   1 Clinical examination and history
   2 Mid stream specimen of urine for bacteriology
   3 Cystoscopy later if stones or tumour are suspected

Treatment Rest, fluids and antibacterial drugs if organisms isolated.

Suggested nursing response

Assessment	Care
1 Raised metabolic rate: pyrexia; tachycardia; behaviour	Rest in a chair (frequency makes bed rest difficult). Cool. Glucose drinks
2 Frequency of micturition. Colour and smell of urine. Test for nitrites (products of bacterial action)	Increase fluid intake to at least 3 litres per day. Care of the genitalia. Give prescribed antibacterial agents
3 Soreness and burning of micturition	Mild analgesia as prescribed

Cystitis should not be treated lightly. Observations for the development of pyelonephritis should also be followed (see p 86).

Bladder stones (calculi)

Calculi may form in the bladder if there is a node of inflammation or a foreign body in the bladder (e.g. a catheter tip). They also tend to occur in patients on long term rest as do ureteric calculi.
   The effects are to produce recurrent cystitis with strangury (frequent desire to micturate, but passing only small amounts with pain and difficulty), scalding and haematuria. Occasionally they cause obstruction leading to retention of urine, reflux and hydronephrosis.

Treatment Surgical removal by the transurethral route or by suprapubic lithotomy.

Suggested nursing response
   1 Prevention by ensuring adequate fluid intake for all patients and advising. Regular turning of patients on long term bed rest allows deposits to drain.
   2 Observations for recurrent cystitis, any difficulty or pain on micturition and for haematuria.
   3 Care is as for bladder and prostate surgery (p 98).

Tumours of the bladder

All new growths in the bladder are now considered to be malignant.

Cancer of the bladder

Cause factors

1 Cigarette smoking
2 Calculi
3 Chronic inflammation
4 Chemicals in certain industrial proccsses, although many have now been withdrawn from use

Effects, signs and symptoms The tumours usually start as papillomas on the epithelium and in the early stages produce no signs or symptoms.

The first indication is usually when the tumour erodes a blood vessel and *haematuria* occurs but is usually painless. The urine is usually bright red in colour, but may have some clots formed – the patient complains of clot retention (acute, painful retention of urine). Local infiltration into the bladder wall is quite rapid and early diagnosis is essential. Surrounding tissues will also be invaded – sacral nerve invasion causes severe pain.

Metastases are most common in bones and the lungs, but could be the liver as the peritoneum is infiltrated. Early symptoms could be due to the metastases e.g. pain in bones, chest infection in the lungs.

Diagnosis – investigations

1 Clinical history and examination. Painless haematuria is especially important.
2 Cystoscopy and biopsy
3 Intravenous urography
4 Micturating cystogram

Treatment

Early stages Cauterization by diathermy through an endoscopy

Later stages (unless metastases have occurred): radiotherapy; total cystectomy and formation of an ileal loop conduit; cytotoxic drugs by installation into the bladder e.g. thiotepa, Ethoglucid.

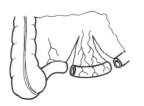 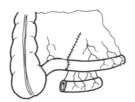 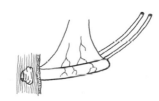

a. Ileal segment is isolated   b. Parent mesentrey is closed   c. A stoma is formed and the ureters are embedded in the ileal segment either individually or joined together

Fig. 2.4.7 Ileal loop conduit

Suggested nursing responses

Radiotherapy

1 Some patients develop diarrhoea and cramp-like pain in the bowel following radiotherapy in the pelvic cavity.
2 A low residue diet may be indicated.

Total cystectomy and ileal loop conduit

1 Many patients have considerable degrees of 'surgical' shock following surgery.
2 Pain relief is very important.
3 Ileal loop conduit is virtually handled as an ileostomy, but obviously urine is collected in the bag, which must be well fitting.
4 There is usually a period of paralytic ileus following surgery as in bowel surgery.

Cytotoxic therapy

1 Strict asepsis needed for catheter instillation.
2 Careful handling of cytotoxic drugs by the staff involved (some recommend gown, gloves, mask and eye shields when mixing the drugs).
3 Reverse barrier nursing if reduction of leucocytes.

Rupture of the bladder Is usually caused by a severe blow to the lower abdominal region, stab wounds or gun shot wounds. It is often a complication of fractured pelvis. It used to be a result of incompetent abortionists' work.

The effects may be delayed, but haematuria and developing hypovolaemia will occur and abnormal tenderness or urine leaks into the peritoneal cavity.

Treatment is by temporary suprapubic cystostomy and antibacterial drugs to prevent and treat infection. They should be catheterized on the ward as further damage may occur.

The Urethra

Functions	Structures involved
1 The passage of urine from the urinary bladder to the external meatus	Tube of transitional epithelial tissue, submucous tissues embedded in various structures: 20 cm in a man and curved; 4 cm in a woman and straight.
2 Voluntary restraint on micturition until socially acceptable	External sphincter is controlled by voluntary nerve fibres from the pudendal nerve
3 In the male, passage of semen on ejaculation	Semen enters through the ejaculatory duct which joins the urethra within the prostate gland

It is more relevant to consider the functions of the prostate gland in the reproductive system (2.9) but conditions within it cause most problems in their effects on the urinary system and will be included in this section.

Conditions of the urethra

Urethritis – inflammation of the urethra

Causes
  1 Infection by coliform organisms and skin organisms (see *cystitis* and *pyelonephritis*).
  2 Gonorrhoea in men causes urethritis about 7–14 days after sexual contact.
  3 Non specific urethritis is also a sexually transmitted condition.
  4 It may follow the passage of calculi.
  5 Sometimes occurs around an indwelling catheter.

Effects, signs and symptoms Inflammatory changes in the transitional epithelium cause loss of resistance to the effects of urine being passed. It is made worse by the action of proteus organisms acting on the urea to produce ammonia which is strongly alkaline.

The patient complains of a burning or scalding sensation on passing urine. The man with gonorrhoea will also have a white or yellow creamy discharge from the meatus. Metabolic rate may be raised but only minimally, usually.

Diagnosis – investigations
  1 Clinical history and examination
  2 Mid stream urine specimen for bacteriology
  3 Swab – of discharge

Treatment
  1 Extra fluids to dilute the urine usually reduces the scalding
  2 Antibacterial agents according to culture

Nursing notes
  1 A lot of encouragement is needed to reach good fluid intake levels – about 3 litres per day are needed.
  2 Analgesics may be needed to relieve scalding but have limited effect.
  3 The main concern is the danger of ascending infection again – see *pyelonephritis*.

Rupture of the urethra

Is caused by a direct blow in the perineum which tears the urethra directly or as a complication of fractured pelvis. Blood will be seen at the meatus and bruising of the penis or pubic area may be observed directly.

Catheterization is dangerous and the patient is usually examined in theatre. A suprapubic cystostomy will be performed. Repair of the urethra with a 'catheter split' may be performed at the same time or be delayed for a few weeks.

Stricture of the urethra

With eventual retention of urine is a common complication of urethritis (especially gonococcal) and rupture.

It is treated by intermittent passing of bougies of increasing size to dilate the urethra.

Nursing notes
  1 Observation of blood at the urethral meatus is an important indication of ruptured urethra.
  2 Strict concern to prevent introduction of infection is critical.
  3 There is considerable embarrassment and anxiety about conditions affecting the urethra. A professional, sensitive approach is most important.

Congenital defects of the urethra

The main problem is that of *hypospadias* – the abnormal positioning of the external meatus of the urethra.

It requires specialist refashioning by a genito urology surgeon and details are not included.

Nursing notes

The problem in the infant is excoriation and soreness of the scrotal and perineal area and danger of urinary tract infection. Immaculate nappy care is essential.

A boy with hypospadias should not be circumcised – the prepuce (foreskin) may be used in the refashioning operation.

Disorders of the prostate gland

Prostatitis (inflammation of the prostate). This may be associated with cystitis in men (see p 94) or may be a sequel to gonorrhea. The patient has deep perineal pain and (rarely) develops retention of urine.

It usually develops into a chronic form with fibrosis and retention of urine.

Benign hypertrophy (enlargement) of the prostate gland is a phenomenon of ageing in men. It does not always cause symptoms, but it is the most common cause of retention of urine. An enlarged prostate gland will press onto the trigone, especially when the patient is in bed and frequency of micturition may occur before retention.

Carcinoma of the prostate gland

Cause Not known, but it is much more common in elderly than younger men.

Effects, signs and symptoms
Local infiltration very often is slow and the patient may have few symptoms. Gradually, enlargement will cause retention in a similar way to hypertrophy. There may be difficulty passing urine (dysuria) prior to retention of urine.

Metastases are most commonly found in bones and the patient complains of 'bone pain' and may be anaemic. Some are prone to bleed easily. Metastases in the lungs would produce chest infections which in the elderly would of course be very dangerous.

Diagnosis – investigations
  1 Clinical history and examination
  2 May be discovered on cystoscopy or transurethral resection
  3 Skeletal X-rays for bone metastases   4 Chest X-ray
  5 Blood – raised serum acid phosphatase

Treatment
  1 Transurethral resection when retention of urine has occurred.
  2 Stilboestrol – preparation of female hormones – oestrogen reduces the size and development of the primary tumour and metastases.

Nursing notes
See Retention of urine and Surgery of the prostate and bladder neck.
Stilboestrol tends to produce feminizing effects such as breast enlargement, nipple tenderness and pigmentation. It may also cause nausea, fluid retention with ankle swelling and occasionally cardiac embarrassment.

The nurse may need to explain carefully to the patient and drug therapy may need adjustment. The patient should also be encouraged though, as prognosis for their latter years can be optimistic.

Retention of urine is usually described as either *acute* or *chronic*.

Acute retention of urine

Due to acute obstruction of the urinary flow. The bladder does not always distend greatly and may be palpated just above the pubis in some patients. The volume can be surprisingly small (may be less than 1 litre).

The patient is in severe distress with acute lower abdominal pain. Analgesia has limited effect. Aseptic catheterization is urgent to relieve the retention. Some surgeons would leave a fine catheter in position, some may remove it after relief is obtained.

Chronic retention of urine

Again due to obstruction, but it may have been gradual as partial bladder emptying may have occurred. The bladder is much more enlarged but the patient may not be aware of its size. The volume can be gross when the patient is eventually catheterized. The problem is that there may have been back pressure through the ureters and kidneys causing distension (hydro-ureter and hydronephrosis) and renal damage. Some patients get an 'overflow' of urine through the urethra as if they were incontinent (described as retention with overflow). Palpation of the bladder is performed for all incontinent patients.

Aseptic catheterization is performed and continual closed circuit drainage is commenced. Strict catheter care to prevent infection is even more vital if renal damage is already present. Some surgeons prefer to stop the drainage for a period after the first litre has drained (some patients went into acute renal failure following sudden drainage): others prefer to continue the drainage.

Suggested nursing care for surgery of the prostate and bladder neck

Pre operative management

Assessment and care of breathing Many patients are elderly with increased anaesthetic risk – should be free from chest infection and be able to breathe deeply before surgery. Chest X-ray will be taken.

Assessment and care of the urinary tract Renal function tests will have been performed and results should be available. Immaculate catheter care before surgery and possibly prophylactic antibacterial drugs may be given.

Assessment and care of the circulation Pulse, blood pressure and electrocardiograms will assist the doctor in his estimation of fitness. Active and passive leg exercises will be taught before surgery. Blood may be needed to correct anaemia.

Assessment and care of the skin The skin over the pubic region, scrotum and perineum should be inspected for infected lesions, washed thoroughly, dried and shaved before surgery.

Surgery

Anaesthetic Many elderly patients are given epidural anaesthetics. The nurse should note that they may cause headache after surgery and hypotension (due to peripheral vasolidation in the legs).

Operations most commonly used are transurethral resection and retropubic approach, involving a wound.

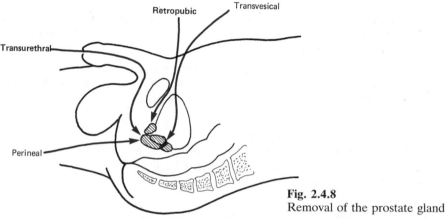

Fig. 2.4.8
Removal of the prostate gland

All patients may bleed following surgery. The surgery itself is specialist. Aseptic catheterization is used – most surgeons use a bladder irrigation system now.

Post operative management

Haemorrhage Observations of the wound and urinary drainage. Continue irrigation. If there is clot retention the patient is in severe pain and drainage stops. Bladder irrigation and analgesia are necessary and possible return to operating theatre if intractible. Some surgeons use a thrombolytic agent such as aminocaproic acid to prevent this.

Breathing The patient should be sat up as soon as possible, but this depends on the blood pressure. Deep breathing and coughing are encouraged.

Catheter care Closed circuit drainage is used and irrigation continues. There is strict hygiene around the catheter. Observations of urine for amount, colour and for blood. Catheter removal is very individual according to surgeons' preferences. Some still clamp periodically to restore bladder 'tone' before eventual removal. Most agree that removal should be as early as possible.

Hydration Intravenous fluids initially followed by plenty of oral fluids (at least 3 litres per day)

Mobilization as soon as possible for elderly patients.

Psychological care It is easy for nurses working on a genito-urinary ward to become so familiar with catheter care that they forget the deep embarrassment for some old men. A professional and sensitive approach is most important.

Sexually active men will need assurance that total impotence is rare following prostatectomy but sexual hygiene is necessary to avoid infection.

Dialysis

Full details cannot be covered in this text but the general nurse is required to understand the principles of dialysis and be able to care for a patient having peritoneal dialysis.

Principles

1 Blood is brought to one side of a semi-permeable membrane.
2 A *dialysate* (fluid prepared and adjusted in different concentrations) is placed on the other.
3 Substances of higher concentration in the blood will normally cross into the weaker solution of the dialysate. Hence, high concentrations of urea, electrolytes and toxins may be removed.

Practice

Haemodialysis Blood is taken from a shunt or fistula in the patient and directed through a kidney dialyser. The dialysate is directed from a mixing device.

Peritoneal dialysis The dialysate fluid is introduced into the peritoneal cavity. The peritoneum acts as the semi permeable membrane.

Suggested nursing response for peritoneal dialysis

Before procedure
1 Careful explanation to the patient
2 Strict cleansing of the skin
3 Strict aseptic technique for introducing the catheter through a trochar. (The bladder should be empty to avoid perforation)

During procedure
1 Careful measurement of fluid in and fluid out. Changes of position will help to drain all fluid
2 Fluid (up to 2 litres) is introduced and left in for ½–2 hours
3 Weigh the patient regularly throughout to detect fluid retention
4 Check blood pressure at least hourly
5 Careful observations for evidence of infection are continued and antibacterial drugs would be given as prescribed

The patient may of course be dangerously ill from renal failure or acute poisoning – see nursing care for those conditions too.

2.5 Nervous conditions

The nervous system

This system will be considered as follows.
1 **Nerve tissues** – neurones and neuroglia
2 **Nervous system as a whole**
3 **The supporting and protective structures** – meninges, skull and spinal column

Notes on eye and ear conditions will be at the end of this unit

1 Nerve tissues

Functions	Structures involved

1 The transmission of impulses
  1 from the brain to functioning parts (motor activity).
  2 from nerve endings to the brain (sensory activity).
  3 from one nerve to another through synapses.
	Dendrites and nerve endings receive impulses. Axons transmit them along the neurones. Nerve bodies contain nucleus and granular markings in cytoplasm (Nissl granules) – give the grey appearance. Axons are grey or white according to the thickness of the myelin sheath. Nodes of Ranvier help the impulse to travel quickly through long nerves. Synapses contain chemical transmitters (main ones are acetyl choline, noradrenaline and adrenaline) which are activated by impulses but then deactivated by enzymes.

Neurones are particularly sensitive to oxygen and glucose levels in the blood	
2 Providing support and nutrition for the neurones	Individual neurones – the myelin sheath is maintained by the Schwann cells. Collections of neurones – brain and spinal cord. The neurones are supported by a special connective tissue known as the neuroglia

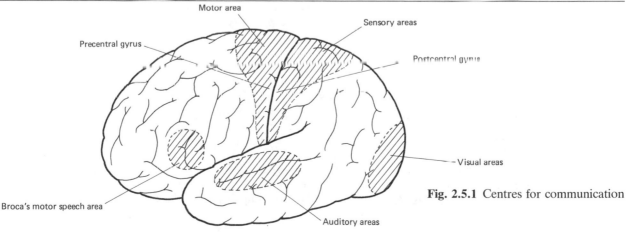

Fig. 2.5.1 Centres for communication

2 The nervous system as a whole

Functions	Structures involved
1 Consciousness – self awareness of the individual	All parts of the system are involved but centres in the cerebrum are: sensory cortex, occipital lobe for vision, temporal lobe for hearing and frontal lobe for awareness and personality. Brain stem and the reticular formation control conscious state
2 Centres for communication: speech; reading; eye contact	Cerebral centres identified on Fig. 2.5.1. Speech centre is known as Broca's area
3 Sensitivity to the environment and changes in it	Sensory nerve endings in the skin (touch, cold, pressure and pain), eye (vision), ear (hearing), nose (smell) and tongue (taste). Sensory nerves synapse in the thalamus
4 Controlled and co-ordinated movements (voluntary)	The motor cortex of the cerebrum. Pyramidal tracts with cross over fibres in the medulla. Lower motor neurones to muscle groups. Nerves from the cerebellum synapse in basal ganglia: the fibres follow the extra pyramidal tract and enable controlled, co-ordinated muscle activity. Nerves of the reticular formation control inhibition and excitation
5 Autonomic control of body functions – glandular secretions and smooth muscle activity	All centres have not yet been identified but some important ones are: the hypothalamus for body temperature and appetite and the medulla oblongata for the cardiac centre, respiratory centre, vaso motor (blood pressure) centre and vomiting centre
6 Protection by reflex activities	
1 coughing, swallowing, sneezing	Centres in the medulla
2 withdrawal reflexes	Intermediate nerves in the spinal cord and the brain
7 Ensuring sleep and rest	Partially through awareness but also the working of the reticular formation systems

The over active brain can prevent the inhibiting effect of the reticular formation and disturb sleep patterns. Important point for your study sessions!

3 The supporting and protective structures – meninges, skull and spinal column

Functions	Structures involved
1 Providing a soft support for the brain and spinal cord with nutrition for the organs	*The meninges* Pia mater – next to the brain and spinal cord. Arachnoid mater – fine (spiders web) honeycomb containing cerebro spinal fluid which is formed in the choroid plexus in the lateral ventricles and drains through the third and fourth ventricles into the arachnoid space. Dura mater – tough, fibrous double layer which is adherent to the periosteum of the skull and the vertebrae, and the inner layer following contours of the brain. Two supporting folds are present: the Falx cerebri between cerebral hemispheres and the Tentorium cerebri – 'tent' covering between the occipital lobe and the cerebellum
2 Providing a hard protection for the brain and spinal cord	The bones of the skull – especially the cranium and the vertebral column (down to the lumbar vertebrae where the cord divides)

Blood supply to the brain is through the circle of Willis. Try to make him more friendly.

Motor and sensory pathways If you have difficulty remembering which cortex is in front and which fibres are in the front of the cord, try this mnemonic
Anterior – Motor, Posterior – Sensory **AMPS**

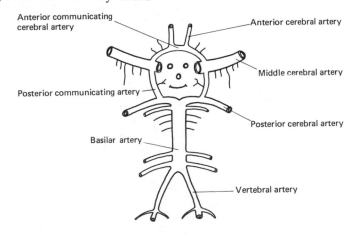

Fig. 2.5.2 Arteries at the base of the brain and the circle of Willis

Conditions of the nervous system

Inflammations affecting the nervous system

Meningitis is inflammation of the meninges

Cause

1 Micro-organisms: viruses, pyogenic (pus forming) bacteria e.g. meningococci and pneumono-cocci (occasionally coliform bacteria); haemophilus influenzae; mycobacterium tuberculosis.

2 Infection may be secondary to other infections e.g. otitis media, a complication of compound fractures or due to congenital defects e.g. meningocele.

Note: Blood in the meninges gives similar effects of meningitis

Effects, signs and symptoms There may be a short history of a 'flu like illness before, but sometimes events are very dramatic. The first problem is that the amount of cerebrospinal fluid and its pressure is increased and causes the patient to complain of a headache.

Cerebral irritation will occur and causes stiffness of the neck–possibly leading to rigidity and resistance to any stretching of the spinal cord. This is detected by *Kernig's sign* (flexion of the hip followed by resistance to knee extension is a positive sign). Some children develop opisthotonos–a backward arching of the neck and spinal column.

The patient has increased painful sensitivity to light (photophobia) and sound. Some patients have a typical high pitched cry (meningeal cry).

Rising intracranial pressure will cause vomiting to occur, increase the severity of the headache and may slow the pulse and cause the blood pressure to rise. The rate, rhythm and volume of breathing may alter and the patient will eventually become unconscious.

The metabolic rate will be very high with a high pyrexia (39–41°C or even higher). Febrile convulsions may occur in infants. Tachycardia may be evident but rising intracranial pressure may slow the pulse.

Meningococcal meningitis often causes a purpuric rash (used to be called 'Spotted fever'). It is a highly infectious form and is notifiable. All patients with meningitis are regarded as infectious.

Diagnosis – investigations

1 Clinical history and examination, including nursing observations

2 Lumbar puncture cerebro spinal fluid for culture and sensitivity. Pressure is high and the fluid usually appears cloudy

Suggested nursing response for lumbar puncture

Before the procedure

1 Explain carefully to the patient and assure them that it is painless but that headache may follow.

2 Report any indications of rising intracranial pressure (lumbar puncture is dangerous in this condition). Pressure inside the cranium may force the brain stem (shaped like a cone and containing the vital centres in the medulla) down into the foramen magnum at the base of the skull (known as *coning*).

3 Prepare the trolley and equipment.

4 Place the patient in a lateral position with knees drawn up (a child may need to be firmly held).

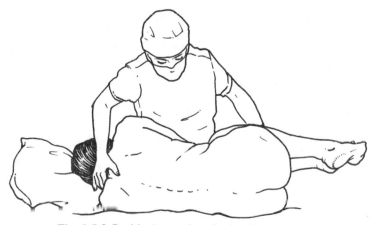

Fig. 2.5.3 Positioning patient for lumbar puncture

During the procedure

1 Observe the patient for any anxiety

2 Assist the doctor by checking anaesthesia; noting the pressure, colour and consistency of fluid; collecting samples in bottles or culture medium and checking the dressing. Queckenstedt's test is not always done (pressure is applied to the jugular vein and should normally cause a rise in cerebro spinal fluid pressure).

After the procedure
1 Observe the patient for any anxiety and assure that coning has not occurred.
2 Position carefully – headache can be prevented by lying down for a few hours. In meningitis, they would be in a semi prone position already.
3 Check the dressing.

Treatment
1 Rest in safe position
2 Give antibacterial agent e.g. benzylpenicillin for meningococcal and pneumococcal and chloramphenicol for haemophilus influenzae. Intrathecal penicillin is not usually given now
3 Care of the unconscious patient
4 Occasionally, steroids may be used for a very ill patient

Suggested nursing response

Assessment	Care
1 Infectious disease	Isolation is indicated
2 Indications of cerebral irritation: stiffness of the neck; opisthotonos; photophobia and sound hypersensitivity	Careful positioning and avoid unnecessary moving. Sedation may be prescribed. A darkened quiet room. Care of the eyes
3 Indications of a rising intracranial pressure	
1 severe headache	Prescribed analgesia but care is needed with observing conscious levels
2 vomiting	Provide a vomit bowl. Mouth care
3 levels of consciousness (see *head injuries* p. 108)	Care of the unconscious patient
4 Raised metabolic rate: pyrexia; exhaustion; dehydration (constipation later)	Control temperature by use of a fan, tepid sponging. Intravenous fluids and glucose. Mouth care. Bowel care. Drugs may be given intravenously
5 Nutritional state	Nasogastric feeding may be used later if the patient remains unconscious. Not to be used if vomiting is occurring
6 Anxiety state of relatives and parents	Assurance about the progress of the patient. Prognosis is good if treatment is started early
7 Possible deafness is a complication	Referred for ENT guidance

Encephalitis – inflammation of the brain

Cause
1 Infection by viruses or pyrogenic bacteria
2 Bacterial infection is secondary to infection in the nasal sinuses or ears
3 May be due to haemorrhagic spread from chest infections

Effects, signs and symptoms Oedema leads to swelling of the brain with raised intracranial pressure. The patient has a severe headache, may vomit, become confused, drowsy and ultimately unconscious. Epileptiform fits may occur. Localization of infected material leads to cerebral abscess.

In addition to the above symptoms and signs, limb paralysis may occur. Metabolic rate is raised with pyrexia, tachycardia (unless intracranial pressure is raised)

The prognosis is guarded both for survival and return to normal daily living.

Diagnosis – investigations
1 Clinical history and examination
2 Lumbar puncture
3 Brain scan for abscess

Treatment
1 As for meningitis
2 Steroids are used for viral disease
3 Surgical drainage of abscess through a burr hole in the skull

Suggested nursing response
Is as for meningitis but observation for fits and paralysis is important. Prognosis is much worse and mental impairment is much more likely on recovery.

Poliomyelitis

An acute viral infection which affects the anterior horn cells of the spinal cord and the brain stem. The virus enters, through the nasopharynx and the intestine, into the blood stream. It is infectious through faecal contamination of food, water and poorly cleaned swimming areas.

The meninges are affected first and a mild, flu like illness with neck stiffness may be the only signs and symptoms. The paralytic stage is reached when the anterior cells are affected. Muscle groups are paralysed. Bulbar paralysis is when the brain stem is affected. Breathing muscles, swallowing muscles, eye muscles may become paralysed.

Treatment and nursing care are the care of the paralysed patient with possibly intermittent positive pressure ventilation.

Nursing notes The disease is now rare in this country because of a very good immunization programme. The nurse as a health educationalist needs to reinforce the need for vaccination and good hygiene.

The oral, live, attenuated vaccine contains all three virus strains that cause the disease. Three doses are required – the timing of these varies in different Health Authorities – make sure you know the one for yours.

Polyneuritis – inflammation of many nerves

Cause Not always known but uraemia may cause it, as well as some viruses (e.g. causing glandular fever).

Effects, signs and symptoms Usually, mixed motor and sensory nerves are affected. The patient complains of symptoms starting in the hands and feet and spreading upwards until in some cases all muscles may be paralysed.

The early effects are numbness – often described as a 'burning' numbness and pins and needles. There is a weakness and wasting of the muscles served by motor nerves. Total anaesthesia of hands and feet may occur (glove anaesthesia) and is dangerous if the patient gets near to sharp or very hot implements. Reflexes are absent in affected limbs.

An acute infective type follows a pyrexial illness and is known as '*Guillain-Barré*' syndrome.

Recovery depends on the cause. The acute infective type may produce severe paralysis (including facial) but patients usually make a complete recovery.

Diagnosis – investigations
1 Clinical history and examination, including nursing observations
2 Lumbar puncture shows high levels of protein in the cerebro spinal fluid

Treatment and nursing Are based on protecting the patient and care of paralysis until recovery takes place.

Neuro-syphilis

Cause
1 Infection by Treponema pallidum – the spirochaete transmitted sexually

Neurosyphilis is part of the tertiary syphilis and may occur many years after the primary untreated disease.

Effects, signs and symptoms Inflammation of the meninges may give the effect of meningitis and thickening of the cerebral arteries may cause thrombus formation, with paralysis of a cranial nerve or limb.

Sensory nerve root damage in the posterior part of the spinal cord – known as *tabes dorsalis* – causes the patient to have 'lightning' pains in the limbs and, sometimes, constricting pains of the trunk. They lose the sense of where limbs are in space (loss of proprioception) and develop a typical gait. They put toes down first, then stamp the heels – as if testing water. The feet are wide apart. Loss of bladder sensations leads to retention of urine with overflow.

Gross changes in the joints occur as in arthritis (Charcot's joints). The eyes may be affected – small irregular pupils that do not react to light (Argyll Robertson pupils).

Changes in brain cells may produce general paralysis of the insane with marked mental deterioration and unpredictable behaviour changes needing psychiatric care.

Diagnosis – investigations
1 Clinical history and examination including a search for other effects of tertiary syphilis
2 Lumbar puncture and blood tests for the Wasserman reaction

Treatment Procaine penicillin 1.2 grammes daily for 10–12 days with repeated courses until activity ceases (only moderate results with tabes dorsalis).

Nursing notes
The incidence of primary syphilis has continued to rise since the Second World War. There are often unrecorded cases in excess of those notified.
The nurse needs to follow three roles in the care of syphilis:
1 To educate for prevention of sexually transmitted disease.
2 To encourage anxious patients to seek early treatment to avoid further infection and tertiary disease.
3 To give confidential treatment in all stages of the disease.

Herpes zoster – shingles

An inflammatory condition of the ganglia on the posterior roots of spinal nerves and occasionally the trigeminal nerve.

Cause Viruses are thought to be the cause – often associated with chicken pox virus

Effects, signs and symptoms Inflammation initially causes severe pain in the nerve affected. Red patches and later vesicles (fluid filled swellings like blisters) will appear along the nerve pathway – typically on the trunk.

Nursing note
Some elderly patients think that if the red patches appear on both sides and meet, then death is inevitable, (this is an *old wives' tale* but does increase anxiety).

It sometimes affects the eyes (ophthalmicus). The facial nerve may be involved and lead to facial palsy.

Many patients become very depressed with shingles due to the prolonged pain.

Treatment and nursing
  1 Strong analgesia   2 Application of idoxuridine may help. Cover any vesicles

Multiple sclerosis

Is the formation of hardened scar tissue in the myelin sheath of nerves of the central nervous system (the brain and spinal cord).

Cause factors These are mainly unknown but possible factors are
  1 Long acting virus
  2 Dietary factors as yet unidentified
  3 Hereditary factors
It usually affects women between 20 and 40 years.

Effects, signs and symptoms Initially, patches of inflammation are found in the myelin sheath. Later they form hardened fibrous plaques and total loss of nerve function is seen.

In the early stages, there may be transient episodes such as vision loss, unexplained falls due to limb paralysis or dropping of objects without reason. Many patients find themselves tiring easily.

There may be long intervals between attacks but these become progressively shorter and symptoms become worse.

System	Effects
Eyes	There may be a blurring of vision or double vision. Total loss of vision in one eye or both may be temporary or permanent. Rhythmic uncontrolled movements of the eyeball (nystagmus).
Speech	May be slurred.
Upper limbs	Numbness and loss of sensation of the limb in space leads to clumsiness. Muscle groups are weakened and intention tremors will make feeding difficult. Fine skills such as sewing may be lost.
Lower limbs	Numbness and loss of sensation in space. Involuntary movements (ataxia) and weakness lead to unsteadiness of gait and falls. Eventually paraplegia may occur.
Urinary tract	Initially there may be urgency and frequency of micturition. Paraplegia will lead to incontinence. Urinary tract infection is common and dangerous.
Bowel	There may eventually be faecal incontinence
Psychology	These patients often display swings of mood from euphoria to deep depression. Self perception (body image) is affected.
Social	The disease often has serious effects on marriage and family life.

Paraplegia will eventually lead to a vulnerability to pressure sores which are painless due to loss of sensation.
Respiratory tract infections are common in the later stages.

Diagnosis – investigations
  1 Clinical history and examination
  2 Nursing history may help to identify episodes previous to diagnosis

Treatment No specific treatment. ACTH (adrenocorticotrophic hormone) is given with good results in acute phases but does not halt the progress of the disease.

Physiotherapy and occupational therapy are important to help maintain daily living for as long as possible.

Suggested nursing response
It will be necessary here to include care required at home and in hospital for the terminal stages of the disease. The role of physiotherapists and occupational therapists will be included in the assessment and care plans.

Assessment	Care
1 Effects on the eyes: any difficulty of vision should be noted; nystagmus should be reported	Care of the partially sighted or even blind patient: careful positioning of articles for use; good orientation and clear speech when approaching; provide large print books
2 Slurring of the speech	Patient listening. Use of writing pads or sign cards. Speech therapy may help
3 Upper limbs	
1 physiotherapists would assess the state of the muscle groups and degree of paralysis	A planned programme of stretch and tension exercises initially to avoid wasting. Later, when paralysed, a full range of passive movements
2 occupational therapist would assess the problems of daily living activities e.g. cooking, dressing, bathing	Adaptions and re-teaching to use implements. Feeding is helped by making food that can be held in fingers
3 nurses would need to help with the assessments above but also need to assess those activities that she would do herself – hair dressing, finger nail care, make up, hygiene	Washing and nail care, hair dressing, applying make up – the nurse may need to do this in latter stages. Families do it at home
4 Lower limbs	
1 physiotherapists would assess walking abilities	Planned exercises and assistance with sticks may be needed. The wheel chair is the last resort
2 occupational therapists would assess problems of mobility around the home	Modifications of the house may be needed (arranged by Social Services department)
3 the nurse would assess the feet for nail growth and hygiene; problems with shoes and stockings; danger of pressure sores on heels	Careful hygiene of the feet and nail trimming. (If loss of sensation, great care is needed.) Application of sheepskin bootees to prevent friction sores
5 Urinary tract for indications of infection: fever; check urine for smell and presence of pus; the degree of incontinence	Care of urinary tract infection. Frequent changing and drying but ultimately, an indwelling catheter may be needed permanently
6 Bowel for degree of faecal incontinence	Establish regular bowel clearance (glycerine suppositories help)
7 Psychology: mood and behaviour changes	Patient and careful relationships are needed. May need psychiatric help
8 Effects of strained family relationships	May need professional guidance

Paralysis If totally immobile and justified, a mobility allowance is paid towards the cost of specially adapted transport.

The paralysed patient needs special care of the skin with regular change of position to prevent pressure sores, a well balanced diet to preserve tissues and good hygiene.

Progressive immobility will cause hypostatic pneumonia – the nurse needs to observe cough and sputum. Prescribed antibacterial agent will be given. The nurse may be the one to encourage patients to join the Multiple Sclerosis Society where patients and families can share experiences and help in this distressing disease.

Cerebral vascular accident (stroke)

Cause
1 Cerebral thrombosis. A sequel to atherosclerosis due to hypertension, high lipids in diet and cigarette smoking.
2 Cerebral embolism. May be a thrombus formed in the heart in atrial fibrillation or a mural thrombus in myocardial infarction which breaks through into the cerebral circulation via the carotid arteries.
3 Cerebral haemorrhage. Cerebral arteries weakened by arteriosclerosis which are then subject to hypertension (especially sudden rises) may rupture and bleed into brain tissue.

Effects, signs and symptoms There is usually a sudden loss of consciousness. This may be a transient 'black out' or the patient may be deeply unconscious for some time. Some authorities say that prognosis is very poor if unconsciousness lasts for more than 48 hours. Cerebral haemorrhage is most hazardous and mortality is very high.

Occlusion of blood will cause necrosis of brain tissue with inflammatory reaction around it. Haemorrhage may flood the tissues of the brain leading to widespread reaction. The effects will depend on the part of the cerebral cortex damaged. The most common is the middle cerebral artery with damage to the *motor cortex*. There will be either slight paralysis (paresis) or total paralysis of the limb or limbs supplied. As damage is above the medullary cross over fibres, the limbs on the opposite side to the lesion will be affected. One sided paralysis is hemiplegia. Initially the muscles are loose (flaccid) due to cerebral shock. As this wears off and 'tone' returns the muscles become tight (spastic) and contraction deformities will occur.

If Broca's (speech) area is involved, the patient has difficulty verbalizing although his mental state is not impaired. Most are usually associated with right hemiplegia. Other areas may produce symptoms associated with function. A lesion in the posterior cerebral artery may produce visual disturbance. Optic nerve fibres may be affected too. Hemianopia is defective vision of one half of the visual field and can be disturbing to the patient.

A rare lesion affects the frontal lobe of the brain and personality changes have occurred.

Blood pressure usually falls after a stroke and oxygen supply to the brain may be wholly depleted. There is often confusion and emotional disturbance for some time after the stroke.

Diagnosis – investigations
1 Clinical history and examination – the doctor may need help if the patient is still unconscious
2 Lumbar puncture
3 Brain scan

Treatment No specific treatment but neuro surgery is possible in certain cases and long term physiotherapy and occupational therapy are needed.

Suggested nursing response
Initially the care of the unconscious patient (see p 110) and maintaining life.

It is an area of team work between nurses, physiotherapists and occupational therapists to aim at rehabilitation, starting as soon as the patient is admitted.

Early nursing care to prevent pressure sores, urinary tract infection (catheter should be the last resort) and respiratory tract infections will make rehabilitation much more likely. The patient will need positive encouragement enough without complications.

Aims for rehabilitation
1 *Prevent deformities*
  1 Careful positioning of the patient as a whole, including limbs, hands and feet, starts in the unconscious phase
  2 Use passive exercises when attending to the patient, then involve the family and teach the patient to use good limbs to move paralysed limbs
2 *Training in activities involving affected limbs* Learning to balance
  1 Learning to use one leg to move the other paralysed one for turning and moving
  2 Learning to stand and walk
  Appliances are kept to the minimum but the nurse should ensure that they are used correctly
3 *Training in speech*
  This is difficult and early assurance is important. A speech therapist will help. The nurse needs to encourage
4 *Retraining in daily living activities*
  1 The team needs to assess individual capabilities, home circumstances and possible work facilities
  2 A planned programme of learning, e.g. cooking, dressing, bathing, craftwork
  3 Supervising and encouragement from all the team

Psychology
1 Loss of body image and frustrations in coping with retraining and communication may lead to depression and despair
2 Listening carefully and establishing communication should start early – talking to the unconscious patient even
3 Positive encouragement with feeding, personal hygiene and control of micturition are necessary
4 The family need to be involved from the start in restoring the patient's dignity and integrity as well as his physical rehabilitation

Sub arachnoid haemorrhage
Causes
1 Ruptured aneurysm – usually near the circle of Willis
  An aneurysm is a thin walled sac formed by the dilation of an artery as a result of congenital weakness, arteriosclerosis or trauma of the vessel.
2 Head injury
3 Brain tumours
4 Rupture of an angioma (congenital abnormal collection of blood vessels)

It may be a complication of leukaemia or aplastic anaemia, or associated with hypertension.

Effects, signs and symptoms
Blood pouring into the cerebrospinal fluid in the arachnoid spaces leads to:
1 Sudden intense headache – patients describe it as 'pain in the head'
2 Cerebral irritation similar to meningitis (meningism) – stiff neck, positive Kernig's sign, photophobia and convulsions
3 Rising intracranial pressure – vomiting (sometimes preceded by nausea), loss of consciousness and changes of pulse, blood pressure and respiration
4 Hemiplegia may occur as motor fibres are affected. If the optic chiasma is involved (near to the circle of Willis) there may be loss of vision, double vision or drooping of the eye lid (ptosis)

Diagnosis – investigations
1 Clinical history and examination
2 Lumbar puncture for blood in the cerebrospinal fluid
3 Cerebral angiography

Suggested nursing response for cerebral (carotid) angiography
Before the procedure
1 Careful explanation to the patient
2 Warning of the need to lie still during procedure; 'burning' sensations in the head, face and behind the eyes will only last a few seconds
3 Some patients are given a prescribed sedative
4 Withhold food before test according to local instructions

After the procedure
1 Neurological observations – conscious response levels; speech defects; motor or sensory changes (e.g. hemiparesis); pulse or blood pressure changes
2 Injection site – observe for haematoma; aseptic dressing
3 Emboli to other arteries – note changes in hands or feet; check all pulse sites

Treatment
Medical
1 Strict bed rest for 4–6 weeks
2 Antihypertensive drugs if needed
3 Antifibrinolytic drugs may be given
4 Corticosteroids (e.g. betamethasone or dexamethasone) may be used to reduce inflammatory effects and reduce cerebral oedema

Surgical
1 Craniotomy and clipping of the aneurysm. There are different techniques according to the nature of the deformity
2 Occasionally, a carotid artery in the neck may be ligated to reduce pressure in the circle of Willis and the aneurysm, to prevent rupture
Transfer for neuro surgery cannot be done for 2–3 days after haemorrhage and is a hazardous undertaking.

Suggested nursing response

Medical
1 Strict bed rest for 4–6 weeks in a darkened, quiet room
2 Continue careful observations as further haemorrhage is common
3 Avoid straining – bowel care; use commode rather than bedpan
4 Avoid stress that may increase blood pressure – involve relatives in the importance of this
5 Give prescribed drugs but look for undesired effects

Surgical – Craniotomy
Pre operative management
1 Assist with neurological tests
2 Careful record of pre operative neurological observations for comparison
3 Maintain care of the patient – continue prescribed drugs (e.g. steroids)
4 Wash hair and warn that the head may be shaved
5 The patient is usually catheterized
6 Careful assurance and guidance about the operation itself

Post operative management
1 Maintain respirations to avoid hypoxia and carbon dioxide retention (which increase cerebral oedema)
2 Careful neurological observations for motor responses, reflexes and conscious levels
3 Maintain body temperatures (heat regulation may be disturbed) – cooling fans or sponging
4 Assess for signs of rising intracranial pressure – pulse, blood pressure, respirations, vomiting, conscious levels
5 Relief of pain – analgesia that does not affect neurological responses (aspirin)
6 Steroids may be continued to reduce cerebral oedema
7 Observe for leak of cerebrospinal fluid and meningitis
8 Observe for fits and care of patient in them

Specific observations for hemiplegia should follow surgery on the blood vessels. They may undergo periods of spasm during which poor blood supply (ischaemia) to brain tissue may give signs of a cerebro vascular accident.
Prognosis following surgery for sub arachnoid haemorrhage is good though and assurance can be given.

Head injuries

Causes

1 Accidental injury   **2** Violence   **3** Self inflicted injury

Effects, signs and symptoms Any severe blow to the head may cause distortion of the brain stem, disturb the reticular formation that controls consciousness and lead to loss of consciousness (concussion). This may be momentary black prolonged periods (years in a few cases).

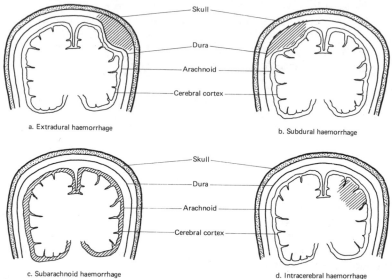

Fig. 2.5.4 Types of intracranial haemorrhage

Haemorrhage may occur with or without fracture of the skull. Three types are described.

Extra dural haemorrhage Bleeding between the dura mater and the skull causes a separation of the two. After a period of apparent recovery, the bleeding increases the pressure inside the cranial cavity (raised intracranial pressure), compresses the brain tissue (cerebral compression) and, most dangerously, the brain stem and medulla are coned towards the foramen magnum of the skull.

Raised intracranial pressure will cause a progressive loss of consciousness, vomiting (sometimes without previous nausea), rising blood pressure, slowing pulse rate and slowing, shallow respirations (occasionally, abnormal rhythm as in Cheyne-Stokes breathing). Rising pressure may also cause a portion of the temporal lobe of the cerebrum, known as the uncus, to protrude through the fold of dura mater known as the tentorium. This protusion presses onto the occulomotor nerve pathway on the injured side. The result is a fixed, dilated pupil that does not react to light.

Sub dural haemorrhage Bleeding between the dura mater and the arachnoid. It is more usually associated with a fracture, may be very acute and is often fatal. The patient remains unconscious, cerebral compression and raised intracranial pressure are rapidly progressive. However, there is a more chronic type in which there is a slow blood loss and symptoms and signs do not show for days or even weeks.

The patient usually complains of headache, drowsiness and, in some cases, hemiplegia. Relatives may notice behaviour changes. Typically, they will be alert one minute, drowsy and uncommunicating the next (but easily roused). Occasionally fits (convulsions) may be reported.

Sub arachnoid and intracerebral haemorrhage Severe bleeding will again lead to raised intracranial pressure. Otherwise the effects are similar to sub arachnoid haemorrhage with cerebral irritation causing headache, neck stiffness, photophobia and irritability with a meningeal cry. Other signs and symptoms will depend on the area of the cerebrum that is damaged. Amnesia (loss of memory) is quite common. Epilepsy may occur early or later.

A contrecoup injury occurs when the brain movement causes damage on the opposite side to the blow – bleeding could occur from both sites.

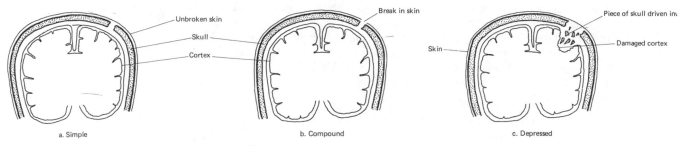

Fig. 2.5.5 Fractures of the skull

Fractures of the skull (see Fig. 2.5.5)

Rhinorrhoea A frontal bone fracture allows cerebrospinal fluid into the frontal sinuses to appear in the nose. (Test for sugar – positive for CSF)

Otorrhoea A temporal bone fracture involving the petrous portion allows cerebrospinal fluid into the external ear.

In all compound fractures or if cerebrospinal fluid leaks, meningitis may be a serious complication. Damage involving the hypothalamus may lead to a loss of control of body temperature. High pyrexia could lead to even further cerebral damage.

Diagnosis – investigations
1 Clinical examination and history
2 Results of neurological observations
3 Skull X-ray
4 Echo encephalogram. Angiography
5 Lumbar puncture (but dangerous if intracranial pressure is high)

Treatment
1 Care of the unconscious patient

2 Surgery
  1 Drainage of haematomas or release of intracranial pressure through burr holes
  2 Resection of tissues
  3 Repair, elevation or plating of fractures

3 Reduce cerebral oedema
  1 Dexamethasone, a steroid, reduces oedema by reducing inflammatory response
  2 Osmotic diuresis – using mannitol. Osmotic diuretics produce a strong solution in the renal tubules which counteracts the reabsorption of fluid. Catheterization is necessary to cope with the large urine output
  3 Prevent hypoxia and carbon dioxide retention which can increase cerebral oedema

Suggested nursing response – first aid
1 Treat all patients who are 'knocked out' or cannot remember as head injuries
2 Place in semiprone position and maintain the airway. Remove dentures, debris, mucus or vomit. Give expired air resuscitation if necessary
3 Give nothing by mouth
4 Send a record of neurological state to Accident Centre. Conscious state, bizarre behaviour, pulse rate changes and vomiting must be reported
5 Cerebrospinal fluid and wounds – apply a light pad but do not plug orifices
6 Stay with the patient and ensure their safety

Suggested nursing response – hospital care

Assessment	Care
1 Respirations	Needs constant care
1 Ensure a clear airway and adequate ventilation. Observe for loss of cough and swallow reflexes; secretions, vomit or blood in the mouth and nose; jaw tends to fall backwards	Maintain airway. Semiprone position, changing sides at least 2 hourly for ventilation of both lungs. Aspirate the mouth and airway to avoid obstruction. Jaw is held forward (remove dentures)
2 Depression of rate rhythm and volume of breathing	May need endotracheal tube (tracheostomy after 48 hours) and positive pressure ventilation
3 Cyanosis may be first indication of severe hypoxia	Oxygen therapy is wise before cyanosis appears

continued overleaf

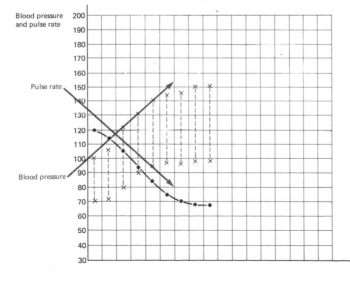

Fig. 2.5.6 'Cross of danger' in rising intracranial pressure

continued from previous page

Assessment	Care
2 Indications of rising intracranial pressure – conscious response levels; falling pulse rate and rising blood pressure; vomiting; depressed breathing; pupil sizes and reactions to light	Report changes immediately – Be ready to prepare for surgery
3 Indications of damage to the hypothalamus – rising body temperature (using an oesophageal probe for core temperature – above 40°C is dangerous)	Patient unclothed covered by a light sheet. Apply fan cooling. Tepid sponging or cool wet blankets may be needed. Occasionally, ice packs are applied. Prescribed chlorpromazine will help to reduce the shivering
4 Indications of cerebral irritation and oedema – headache or pain; neck stiffness; photophobia; meningeal cry	Nurse in a subdued light (but enough to observe the patient). Eyes may be lightly covered
5 Loss of reflexes	
1 staring eyes	Insert oily drops. Gently cover
2 unco-ordinated violent movements of limbs	Padding of cot sides. Do not restrain
3 no cough or swallow	See care of the airway. Nasogastric aspiration
6 Prescribed underhydration and therapy to reduce cerebral oedema. Fluid balance chart	Intravenous fluids given. Catheterization – fine bore catheter with strict asepsis should not introduce infection. Give prescribed dexamethasone and mannitol intravenously
7 Confusion and amnesia on recovering consciousness is normal	Give assurance of where the patient is, who you are and what is happening even when they are unconscious

For *epileptic fits* – see p 110
For *hemiplegia* – see patient with *cerebral vascular accident* (p 105)
Relatives of patients with head injuries need a lot of assurance and support, especially if unconsciousness is prolonged

Care of the unconscious patient
Using Model B of our nursing models in Section 1.3 in brief note form. Try other models of care too.

Assessment		Care
1 **Skin**	*1* hygiene	Regular washing and drying
	2 pressure areas	Relieve pressure. Turn 2 hourly. Give nutrition
	3 wounds and lesions	Aseptic dressings
2 **Circulation**	*1* pulse, blood pressure	Careful positioning
	2 danger of thrombosis	Passive exercises
	3 danger of hyperthermia	Cooling methods
	4 if haemorrhage	Blood replacement
3 **Respiration** (see in *Head injuries care*)		
4 **Digestion**	*1* nutrition	Intravenous or nasogastric nutrition as soon as possible, using pureed normal diet
	2 vomiting	Aspirate nasogastric tube. Change feeding regime
	3 elimination	Glycerin suppositories. Enemas. Manual evacuation as last resort
5 **Excretion**	*1* renal	Catheter care
	2 urine output	
	3 urinalysis	Report
	4 if diabetes mellitus	Stabilization needed
6 Nervous control (see *care of head injuries*)		
7 Locomotion – paralysis, spasticity		Passive exercises. Careful positioning
8 Communication – patients can often hear while unconscious		Encourage relatives and nurses to talk to the patient. Play favourite music or voices

Epilepsy

Caused when brain cells suddenly produce a burst of large bio-electrical waves.

Cause
1 Idiopathic There is some evidence of inherited trait but not conclusive
2 Brain damage or disease – following head injury; due to inflammation; due to cerebral tumour
3 Factors known to bring on a fit include: hypoglycaemia (see diabetes mellitus); strong excitement or fear; flashing lights – from television screens (special danger from 'strobe' lights at discos); infection; alcohol

Effects, signs and symptoms
Petit mal Usually affects children. Brief lapses of consciousness described as 'absences'. This type of fit is reported by parents or school teachers as the child may be unaware of what happened.
Focal epilepsy There is a local brain lesion producing specific effects. E.g. temporal lobe gives a sense of taste or smell before the fit.

Jacksonian fit Starts with twitching of fingers, toes or mouth, spreading to other areas on the same side before loss of consciousness.

Grand mal Tonic–clonic seizures
1 The aura, or warning may be a form of hallucination (e.g. hearing sounds)
2 The tonic phase–acute contraction of all muscles. Air forced out of lungs causes a cry. Clenching of the teeth may bite the tongue or cheek. Cyanosis usually occurs.
3 The clonic phase–all muscles relax and contract intermittently. Mucus may gather in the mouth. Incontinence may occur.
4 The coma–all muscles relax. Respirations become noisy. The face is usually flushed. The patient may drift from coma into normal sleep or go through a period of disorientation

Post epileptic automation or fugue Some patients have a period of bizarre behaviour following grand mal and have been known to commit murder, suicide, or more harmless anti-social activities!

Status epilepticus The patient does not recover consciousness but immediately goes into one fit after the other. This is a dangerous medical emergency as there is danger of death or severe brain damage due to the hypoxia resulting from the breathing problems during attacks.

There is no evidence that epilepsy affects intellectual development. There are some patients who display personality traits but these are now thought to be due to the brain damage that caused the epilepsy or possibly prolonged use of drugs.

There is still a stigma attached to epilepsy and the patients complain of other people's superstitions about them (it used to be thought of as being possessed by the devil!).

Diagnosis – investigations
1 Clinical history and examination
2 Nursing observations of the fit in detail is important
3 Electro encephalogram will usually detect abnormal waves, but not always

Treatment
1 Long term usually a single antiepileptic drug is given, either phenytoin or carbamazepine for grand mal and sodium valproate for petit mal
2 Status epilepticus–intravenous diazepam is usually given (occasionally may be given rectally)

Suggested nursing response – first aid
A calm confident approach is essential
1 Protect the patient

1 Clear the surroundings	*3* Do not put anything in the mouth
2 Undo tight clothing remove dentures if possible	*4* Semiprone position when in coma

2 Check if the patient carries a card
3 Advise about taking medication

Transfer to hospital is not always necessary, but send a written account of the fit with the patient if it is done.

Grand mal

Aura Write down any hallucinations described by the patient. Note the time of day of any precipitating factors

Tonic phase Ensure safety of the patient by clearing surroundings, loosening clothing, moving from danger

Clonic phase Do not attempt to forcibly restrain limbs, but prevent them striking lockers, bed frames or cot sides

Coma Place in semiprone position (see care of unconscious patient). Change if incontinence has occurred

Automatism Observe the patient carefully for some time after the fit

Status epilepticus
1 Treat as an unconscious patient
2 Give prescribed drugs intravenously
3 Careful observation of all stages of fits is important
4 In rare cases, if cyanosis is persisting, anaesthesia and positive pressure ventilation may be needed

Psychological and social care
1 Assurance that a normal life is possible *if medication is maintained*
2 Driving is allowed but only if the patient has been free of day time fits for two years. It is better to discourage driving
3 Certain occupations are not possible and dangerous sports should not be undertaken. Re-employment may be necessary (and difficult)
4 Exercise and normal activity should be encouraged
5 Alcohol and smoking are discouraged

6 Contact with the British Epilepsy Association is advised
7 The patient's family need a lot of guidance to avoid over protection on one hand but having to help through difficult social crises occasionally
8 There is no reason why marriage and parenthood should not be considered

Tumours of the nervous system

Malignant changes in nerve cells (neurones) are quite rare. The supporting cells and tissues may be affected by new growths, some of which are benign, others are malignant.

Meningioma

Usually a benign tumour in the dura mater which is well localized and may be removed surgically.

Neuromas

May originate in specific nerves – sometimes the cranial nerves. They are usually benign but symptoms may be quite distressing. For example, acoustic neuroma on the vestibulo cochlear nerve will affect hearing, but may enlarge to press on the cerebellum and brain stem, leading to a bulbar paralysis which could be fatal.

Metastases

Secondary tumours in the brain may be sequels to carcinoma elsewhere – most commonly the bronchus and breast. They are usually multiple and grow rapidly. No treatment is available.

Brain tumours are referred to as *gliomas*.
Gliomas include tumours of different types of glial cells – the most common is the *astrocytoma*.

Astrocytomas

May be benign but are usually malignant. The malignancy varies too – some develop slowly, some very rapidly (known as glioblastomas).

Cause Not known

Effects, signs and symptoms
Infiltration of the tumour gradually produces a 'space occupying lesion' causing a rise in intracranial pressure. Local infiltration in specific parts of the cerebrum will produce individual effects.

Raised intracranial pressure The patient complains of a headache and vomiting. Papilloedema may be seen in the eye (swollen optic disc and distended retinal veins)

Local effects of tumours – examples
1 Frontal lobe – personality changes; memory loss; euphoria and amoral behaviour; focal epilepsy; hemiparesis on the opposite side
2 Parietal lobe – loss of sensations; Jacksonian epileptic fits
3 Occipital lobe – visual impairment or hallucinations

Tumours in the cerebellum would alter co-ordination and equilibrium. Tumours in the brain stem would affect the cranial nerve functions e.g. swallowing, speaking. There is usually a rapidly progressive deterioration in health as nutrition will have been poor, leading to cachexia – general wasting of body tissues with muscle weakness, unhealthy skin and prone to infection.

Diagnosis – investigations
1 Clinical history and examination including the nurse's neurological observations
2 Skull X-rays
3 Brain scanning
4 Angiography

Treatment
1 Dexamethasone may be prescribed
2 Surgical resection or partial resection to reduce intracranial pressure
3 Shunt of cerebrospinal fluid into the blood stream to reduce pressure
4 Radiotherapy
5 Cytotoxic chemotherapy

Suggested nursing response

Assessment	Care
1 Rising intracranial pressure	
1 increasing headache, especially on bending down or straining	Prescribed analgesia. Careful positioning. Bowel care to avoid straining
2 vomiting	Prescribed antiemetic drug. Mouth care
3 loss of consciousness with changes of blood pressure, pulse and respirations as the brain stem is compressed	Care of the unconscious patient (p 110)

continued next page

continued from previous page

2 Local tumour effects	
1 epileptic fits	Care of epilepsy
2 hemiparesis	Careful positioning and protection of limbs
3 visual impairment e.g. blindness, drooping eye lid	Care of the blind patient. Covering the eye and application of drops
4 personality changes; amoral behaviour	Careful explanations to relatives will be needed
3 General cachexia – weight loss, pressure sores, infections with rising metabolic rate and fever	Keep as mobile as possible initially, Skin care and pressure area care. Care of the patient with fever

For **craniotomy**, see pre and post operative care on p 107.

Note: Undesired effects of treatment are that radiotherapy causes tiredness, loss of white cells and immunity and possible blood clotting defects. Loss of hair is usual – but will grow again. Also many chemotherapy agents are highly toxic and not easily tolerated.

Terminal care may be very distressing for the patient, their family and junior nursing staff. Full discussions are needed.

Parkinson's disease

Sometimes known as paralysis agitans or 'the shaking palsy'.

Cause Unknown, but there is some evidence of a familial disorder. It is classified as degenerative and part of ageing. Known associations are earlier encephalitis and prolonged treatment with chlorpromazine.

Effects, signs and symptoms

Cells in the mid brain known as the substantia nigra produce dopamine. This is a chemical transmitter that works in balance with acetylcholine mainly in the basal ganglia of the mid brain, known as the corpus striatum.

Degeneration of the substantia nigra cells reduces the amount of dopamine and there is an imbalance of the two chemical transmitters. The mechanism of this imbalance is not clear but signs and symptoms are associated with a loss of strength, control and co-ordination of motor impulses originating mainly from the cerebellum that normally pass through the corpus striatum.

The patient presents with slowing down and progressive weakness of movement, tremor and rigidity of motion (including facial expression). The effects may begin on one side but eventually both sides will be involved. The slowing and weakness contribute to a typical shoulder drooping.

The tremor starts in the hands and fingers and a typical rolling movement of the thumbs and fingers is observed (pill rolling). In the earlier stages the tremor can be controlled with strong will power but this is gradually lost.

Rigidity may affect the gait, producing a typical shuffling action. Arms remain close to the body and do not swing. The mask like face betrays hidden emotions and intellect which may be normal. Eventually, chewing, swallowing and speaking are affected. There is often 'drooling' of saliva from the corner of the mouth. Finally, respiratory muscles are affected and chest infection is the usual cause of death.

There is some disturbance of autonomic function, with increased saliva and sweat. They have severe constipation.

Psychological effects may be due to frustration although in some cases, behaviour itself is affected by the disorder and dementia may be seen. Memory is lost and some become obsessional (often about bowels).

Diagnosis Clinical history and examination

Treatment Is aimed at restoring the balance of the chemical transmitters.
1 Dopamine is given in the form levodopa (not used if drug induced disease). Higher brain concentrations are achieved by giving levodopa with carbidopa.
2 Anticholinergic agents – most commonly used are orphenadrine and benzhexol.
3 All anti-Parkinsonism drugs have a lot of undesired effects – see British National Formulary for regimes and effects.
4 Surgery is better for unilateral disease but is sometimes done for bilateral with an interval between the two operations. Stereotaxis is used for the accurate placing of a lesion in the thalamus of the brain

Suggested nursing response

Assessment	Care
1 Reaction to drugs	Drugs are commenced after meals. Dosages, timing and actual drugs may need adjustment until stabilization is achieved
1 levodopa – anorexia; nausea and vomiting; hypotension; behaviour changes	
2 anticholinergic – nausea; tachycardia; blurring of vision; constipation; lost concentration	

continued overleaf

continued from previous page

Assessment	Care
2 Degree of loss of mobility – gait; drooling; incontinence due to slowing; eventual feeding problems; finally effects of chest infections	Work in harmony with physiotherapy. Maintain mobility and exercises as long as possible. Advise to take periods of rest as fatigue increases frustration. In late stages retraining for incontinence, care of the mouth and care of the patient with chest infection will be necessary
3 Observe for depression, frustration and feelings of isolation	May need psychiatric help. Listen to anxieties carefully. Arrange communication. Introduce to Parkinson's Disease Association

Congenital abnormalities of the nervous system

The most likely to be met by the general nurse are **hydrocephalus** and **spina bifida**.

Cause Not always known, but strongly associated with maternal factors
  1 Viral infections, especially rubella
  2 Exposure to X-rays
  3 Some drugs and possibly dietary factors
Research continues to establish proof.

Hydrocephalus

Is an accumulation of excessive amounts of cerebrospinal fluid in the ventricles of the brain and may be due to
  1 Obstruction of flow through the third and fourth ventricles and into the arachnoid space as a result of malformation.
  2 Failure of the absorption system of cerebrospinal fluid from the arachnoid space which may be a result of blockage in the arachnoid space itself (e.g. adhesions following meningitis).

Effects, signs and symptoms The ventricles of the brain enlarge and because the cranial bone sutures are not fused, the head will be enlarged. (There is an adult form in which the head cannot swell but raised intracranial pressure will occur.) The fontanelles will bulge and scalp veins are engorged. Pressure on the mid brain causes the eyes to look downwards (sun setting of eyes).

Raised intracranial pressure causes irritability and vomiting. Later, drowsiness and mental retardation will occur, If untreated, the baby will die from chest infection as coma develops.

Diagnosis – investigations
  1 Clinical examination
  2 Regular measurement of head circumference
  3 Brain scanning

Treatment
  1 Correction of any malnutrition
  2 Surgery – insertion of a shunt and valve (Pudenz or Spitz-Holster). The shunt is from the lateral ventricle into either the right atrium of the heart or the peritoneal cavity. It may need to be replaced as the child grows

Suggested nursing response
Before surgery
  1 Help with feeding to restore nutrition (may need nasogastric feeding)
  2 Great care of the skin over the skull to prevent sores which could cause infection
  3 Strong assurance to parents who will be frightened and possibly feeling guilty about an abnormal baby

Surgery see Fig. 2.5.7

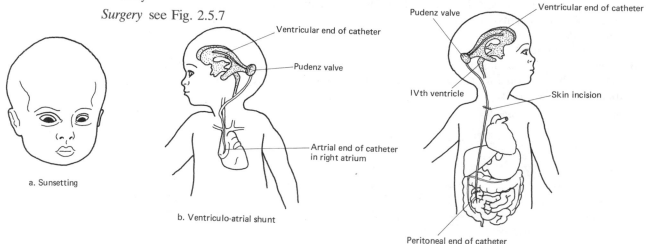

a. Sunsetting

b. Ventriculo-atrial shunt

c. Ventriculo-peritoneal shunt

Fig. 2.5.7 Hydrocephalus and its treatment

After surgery
1 Assess for shock and haemorrhage
2 Assess for infection
3 Position the head to prevent pressure on the valve
4 Assess for rising intracranial pressure if shunt becomes blocked
5 Return to normal feeding regime as soon as possible

Parents will need guidance on how to detect rising intracranial pressure and care of the valve, but should encourage normal development. The dangers of infections and conditions leading to dehydration should be explained. Parents should be involved in the post operative care as soon as possible.

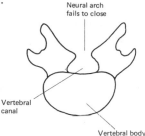 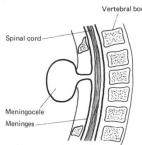 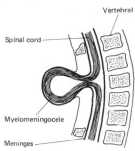

Fig. 2.5.8
Spina bifida cystica

Spina bifida

Is a failure of development of vertebrae in which the arch fails to close, allowing the prolapse of the contents of the vertebral canal.

Spina bifida cystica Is the one which gives most problems

Meningocele Meninges only protrude and lie on the surface of the back. Skin may not cover the whole and there is danger of rupture and meningitis
Myelo meningocele Meninges, spinal cord and nerve roots prolapse into a sac. Skin covering is poor and, with a thin arachnoid, rupture and meningitis is even more likely.

Lesions are usually in the lumbosacral region and may lead to a flaccid paralysis below the waist, including the bladder and bowels.
A meningocele is accessible for early surgery (soon after birth).
A meningomyelocole may involve extensive surgery to repair the defect, fashion ileal loop conduit for the incontinence and orthopaedic correction of deformities.

Suggested nursing response
1 The baby is nursed in the prone position
2 Prevention of infection – aseptic, non adherent dressings over the lesion (and operation site if surgery). Assess for rising metabolic rate (pyrexia)
3 Strict nappy care to prevent urinary tract infection

Extensive surgery involves detailed and sensitive discussions with surgical teams and parents. Agreement between nursing staff and the surgical team will help when junior staff are faced with difficult questions from anxious parents.

Results of surgery are not always very good.

For those who do or do not have surgery, help from the community nursing team and voluntary organizations will be needed for families. The Spina Bifida Society and Disabled Living Foundation give good advice and encouragement.

Trauma affecting the spinal cord

Although these may be considered relating to the loco-motor system in the sense that they are dealt with by orthopaedic departments, the nursing problems and care are more related to the effect on the peripheral nerve transmissions.

Fractured spine and dislocation of vertebral joints

Causes
1 Direct violence, 'whiplash', or jarring upwards
2 Pathological – a complication of osteoporosis which may be due to nutritional defects or be drug induced (long term use of corticosteroids)

Effects, signs and symptoms The broken bone may or may not be displaced but in all cases there will be pain and inflammation around the fracture site, which may give transient changes of sensation below the site if the spinal cord is compressed. More serious is that displacement and dislocation will damage the spinal cord giving loss of sensation and complete paralysis below the site of the injury.

High cervical damage will cause paralysis of all four limbs (tetraplegia or quadriplegia) and paralysis of the diaphragm is common as the phrenic nerve is occluded. Lower cervical damage will still cause tetraplegia but respirations are not affected. Lumbar cervical damage causes paralysis below the waist – paraplegia.

In both paraplegia and tetraplegia, autonomic pathways are affected too. Control of blood pressure, defaecation, micturition and sexual function will be lost.

Diagnosis – investigations
1 Clinical history and examination
2 Neurological assessment for loss of sensation and reflex activity
3 Spinal X-rays

Treatment
1 May need surgical reduction of any displacement
2 Immobilization by careful positioning and sometimes plaster of Paris cast of head and shoulders
3 More common – apply skeletal skull traction and nurse on a Stryker frame
4 Rehabilitation for daily living starts as soon as possible, even if paralysis is permanent
5 Assisted ventilation (positive pressure respirator) if respiratory difficulty

Suggested nursing response – first aid
1 Avoid moving the patient unless absolutely necessary until help arrives
2 For cervical injury, a cervical collar may be applied carefully, but still avoid moving until necessary
3 Give artificial respiration if needed
4 Give careful assurance as fear will be increasing the degree of shock
5 If transfer is delayed, immobilize limbs with bandages and apply padding between bony prominences

Remember the patient will not be able to feel if bandages are tight (nor other injuries below the lesion)

In addition, all the following care for the paraplegic patient

Lumbar lesions – paraplegia

1 Observe flaccid paralysis of legs. Some may still get spasms due to reflex activities	Limbs must be positioned carefully to avoid lesions which may stimulate spasm. Diazepam may be used
2 Assessment of micturition – distension should be avoided	A single catheter or continual drainage is used. Attempt to obtain reflex bladder emptying with training. Some patients develop techniques such as suprapubic compression for expression of urine. Long term indwelling catheter may be necessary
3 Observe for urinary tract infection – raised metabolic rate; pyrexia; tachycardia. Inspect urine and regular culture for micro-organisms (*Note*: burning and frequency of micturition may not be present)	Strict catheter care to prevent urinary tract infection. Unless oliguria, give 3–4 litres fluid daily. Care of patient with urinary tract infection – antibacterial drugs for extended periods

Ultimately, renal failure due to repeated urinary tract infection may be the cause of death. See 2.4 for care in *chronic renal failure*.

Suggested nursing response for the paralysed patient

Assessment	Care
Cervical lesion – tetraplegia	
1 Correct positioning on Stryker frame. Weights on skeletal skull traction (4–9 kg or more). Repeated X-rays until fracture is reduced	Nurse in extended position. The head, neck and trunk must always be in the same plane – not twisted. Aseptic dressings to skull tongs
2 Observe all pressure areas for redness – particularly danger with loss of sensation	Turn the patient at least 2 hourly, starting as soon as possible (even in the Accident Centre). Strict care with bed making to avoid creases. Ingenious use of appliances to relieve pressure but remember to maintain the position
3 Assess all limbs for return of reflex activity and spasm which may lead to contraction deformity	Protect from any lesion which may stimulate reflex contraction such as pressure sores. Spasm is sometimes controlled by prescribed diazepam
4 Assess for 'spinal shock' – sudden loss of all nervous activity due to loss of continuity with higher centres; falling blood pressure; respiratory arrest; loss of temperature control; bladder and bowel distension	Maintain the airway and ventilation if necessary. Maintain body temperature – may have hypothermia or hyperpyrexia. Introduce catheter with strict aseptic techniques
5 Absence of call to stool – some patients can still evacuate the bowel by straining	May need manual evacuation – initially by nursing staff, but later taught to the patient. Suppositories and enemas may be needed
6 Sex – some men may be able to obtain erection, but ejaculation of semen is usually absent. Women do not have sensations of sexual intercourse but are able to conceive and have normal pregnancy	May need very sensitive counselling with their partner. An introduction to SPOD (sexual problems of the disabled) group may help, but some prefer not to discuss the problem with others

Rehabilitation for daily living should commence as soon as possible.
1 Physiotherapy would be directed to strengthening upper limbs and dexterity of fingers.
2 Occupational therapy would be aiming to enable the patient to live independently – feeding, washing, dressing and learning skills which will be used in new occupations.
3 The disablement resettlement officer would organize work training and help with finding work (not always easy).
4 The nurse should be positively encouraging the patient in all these efforts. There are psychological problems in dealing with angry, frustrated patients occasionally – an air of relaxation in which patients can freely express their anger and anxiety should be cultivated.

Prolapsed intervertebral disc

Cause
1 Trauma – strains on lifting, twisting (or both together); repeated minor strains
2 Degeneration   3 There is evidence of an inherited predisposition

Effects, signs and symptoms The fibrous band known as the annulus fibrosis holding the intervertebral disc in place is torn. This allows the disc to prolapse and press on to nerves. Symptoms depend on the site of the prolapse.

Cervical – pain in the neck, shoulder girdle and arms with stiffness (sometimes pain in the head). Loss of sensation in the arms

Lumbar – pain in the back (sometimes sudden, preventing the patient straightening the back). The pain may radiate down the thigh and leg (sciatica). Some muscle weakness will develop and there may be some loss of sensation. Tendon reflexes may be altered and this may cause an alteration of gait.

Diagnosis – investigations
1 Clinical history and examination
2 Straight leg raising increases pain by stretching the sciatic nerve
3 Plain X-ray
4 Myelogram

Suggested nursing response – myelogram
1 Nursing is as for lumbar puncture (p 101)
2 Radio opaque dye may contain iodine – check for any known hypersensitivity
3 Water soluble dyes are now used and enable the patient to sit up earlier (6 hours) and mobilize.

Treatment
1 Bed rest to reduce inflammatory reaction around the lesion
2 Sedation is often prescribed to encourage rest and relaxation
3 Traction
   1 Cervical traction
   2 Lumbar lesions – bilateral skin traction on the legs may be used
4 Surgical – laminectomy (removal of the lamina of a vertebra and resection of the protrusion)

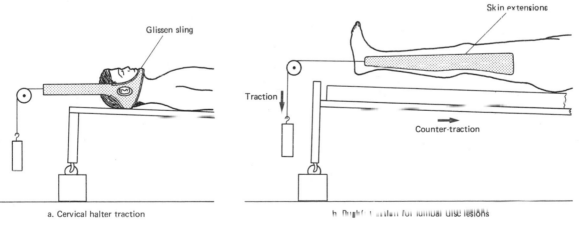

a. Cervical halter traction   b. Bright's traction for lumbar disc lesions

Fig. 2.5.9 Traction

Suggested nursing response
1 Assessment and care for the patient on bed rest – the bed must be very firm with orthopaedic boards
2 Maintenance of traction equipment on the patient
   1 Care of the skin where the appliance is attached
   2 Psychological support
   3 Help with sleep – may need analgesia and night sedation

Laminectomy – assessment and care are as for most operations

Special points to note

1 Nurse on a firm orthopaedic bed with slight reflexion of the knees to relax back muscles
2 Any turning should keep the head, trunk and legs in one plane
3 Strict asepsis with dressings as infection could reach the meninges.

Later – the patient may still need to wear a cervical collar or lumbar corset for some weeks (6–8 weeks) and even then will need to exercise with great care. Occupations involving heavy, difficult lifting may not be possible.

The eye

Functions	Structures involved
1 Focusing of light (reflected from objects) onto the nerve endings	The clear conjunctiva, cornea, aqueous humour, lens and vitreous humour are all concerned with clear focusing, but alteration of focus is by the changing shape of the lens caused by the action of the ciliary muscle. Ciliary muscle contracts, releases tension on suspensory ligaments, allows the lens to bulge for focusing on near objects (e.g. reading)
2 Controlling the amount of light entering the posterior chamber. (If you take photographs, you will know that you need just the right amount of light for a clear picture)	The iris will contract or relax according to the amount of light and the pupil will constrict or dilate accordingly. Dark conditions – dilated, allows more light rays to enter and stimulate a wider area of the retina
3 Light rays are converted into visual impulses for transmission to the brain	The retinal nerve endings, rods (for black and white vision) and cones (for colour vision). Cones are mainly found around the sensitive fovea of the eye where the best visual acuity is found. Cones need rhodopsin – formed by the activity of vitamin A

Note:

1 The eyes are continually scanning to visualize correctly – fixed eyes will not be able to see correctly as retinal cells need to be 'switched on and off'
2 Stereoscopic vision is achieved by focusing both eyes together. If one eye is closed, it is difficult to judge depth. (Try pouring a cup of tea with one eye covered!)

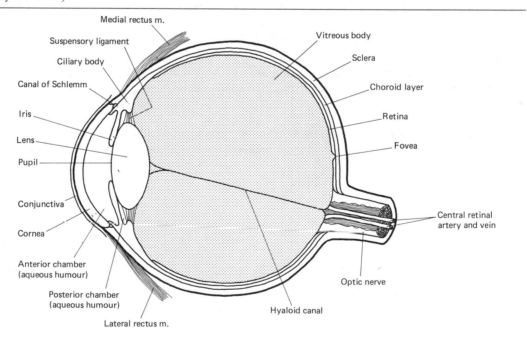

Fig. 2.5.10 Section through the eye

Conditions of the eye

Visual errors

Myopia – short sightedness
    The eye ball is too long   Distant objects blurred
    Light rays focus in front of the retina   Concave lens focuses further back

Hypermetropia – long sightedness
    The eye ball is too short   Near objects blurred
    Light rays focus behind the retina   Convex lens focuses further forward

(*Note for memory:* myopia is the short word, hypermetropia the long)

Presbyopia – ageing vision
  Lens cannot change shape
  Distant objects clearer, near objects blurred
  Convex lens will correct it

Astigmatism – the eye ball is abnormally shaped (ovoid) focusing at different sites from horizontal and vertical viewing. Cylindrical lens will correct

Nursing notes
Ensure that the patient's spectacles are available as needed. The nurse may need to clean them for some patients. Ensure the use of correct lens cleaning tissue to avoid scratching.

Contact lenses are often worn now – the nurse may need to remove them if the patient is unconscious. Application to an incapacitated patient may be necessary – gentle care needed.

Inflammatory conditions affecting the eye

Blepharitis is inflammation of the eyelid and may be general or localized. Redness, irritation and crusting are present
Hordoleum (known as a stye), is infection of the follicle of an eyelash
Chalazion is infection of a meibomian gland

Nursing notes
Blepharitis Clean with warm moist pads frequently; remove crusts carefully; apply antibacterial ointment
Hordoleum and *chalazion* Apply warm moist heat and antibacterial ointment. Chronic chalazion may need excision under local anaesthetic

Conjunctivitis – inflammation of the conjunctiva

Cause
  1 Virus
  2 Bacteria – staphylococci, pneumococci, gonococci
  3 Allergy
  4 Injury
  5 It is often secondary to other infections and is part of coryza (the common cold)

Effects, signs and symptoms Inflammation may be seen as redness over the surface of the eye. The patient complains of a sore 'grittiness' when opening and closing the eyes and usually feels miserable and ill.

Diagnosis – investigations
  1 Clinical examination   2 Swab taken for culture and sensitivity

Treatment Antibacterial ointment

Nursing notes
Conjunctivitis should be regarded as infectious by direct or indirect contact. All cloths, towels, instruments should be confined to use on the one inflamed eye. Strict washing of hands before and after any treatment is important. Ointments should be reserved for the individual patient.

Warm saline is ideal for bathing and irrigation of the eye may be necessary. Dark glasses should be worn but the eye is not padded or covered.

Keratitis – inflammation of the cornea

Cause
  1 Corneal ulceration following abrasion by a foreign body or injury
  2 Viral infection (Herpes simplex) – often gives the appearance of a dendritic ulcer
  3 It may be a sequel to a patient being unconscious with open eyes and careless abrasions of the surface of the eye

Effects, signs and symptoms
Inflammation may be seen as redness around the cornea. The patient will complain of pain in the eye and loss of vision. Excessive tears are formed and the eyelids may go into spasm.

Severe inflammation may lead to perforation with loss of aqueous humour and infection entering the eye ball. The iris is often inflamed with pus in the anterior chamber (hypopyon). The patient usually feels very ill and depressed.

Diagnosis – investigations
  1 Clinical examination and history
  2 Swabs for culture but viruses are not easily detected

Treatment
  1 Application of local heat
  2 Eye kept closed

3 Antibacterial agents may be given by drops, ointment, by subconjunctival injection or systemically

4 When iritis is present, a mydriatric drug (e.g. atropine 1%) may be given to prevent adhesions

5 If sensation is lost, eyelids are fused in tarsorrhaphy

6 If severe damage, corneal grafting may be needed later

Nursing notes

Prevention of corneal abrasion, early removal of foreign bodies and treatment for ulceration is important.

The general nurse may be helping a doctor or a specialized, trained ophthalmic nurse with the treatments. Careful administration of drops and ointments is important. Heat may be applied by an electric eye pad or hot spoon bathing.

If metabolic rate is raised, the patient should be nursed in bed, temperature controlled and glucose drinks given

Uveitis

Inflammation of the uveal tract which consists of the iris, the ciliary body and the choroid.

Anterior uveitis – iritis iridocyclitis

Posterior uveitis – choroiditis

Pan uveitis – combined anterior and posterior

Cause

1 Trauma

2 Infection

3 Associated with rheumatoid arthritis and other systemic diseases

Effects, signs and symptoms Inflammation may appear similar to keratitis with redness around the cornea, but the cornea itself is clear. The iris may go into spasm and cause a constricted pupil. The patient complains of pain in the eye, blurring of vision and photophobia. Pus may be seen in the anterior chamber (hypopyon).

Obstruction of the drainage of aqueous humour may cause glaucoma. Retinal detachment may be a complication of choroiditis.

Diagnosis – investigations

1 Clinical examination   **2** Swabs for infection

Treatment

1 Mydriatics – to prevent adhesions between the iris and the cornea, and to relieve pain

2 Corticosteroids may be given locally or systemically

Nursing notes

Early treatment is vital if eyesight is to be preserved. Note the use of corticosteroids and any undesired effects.

The patient will need bed rest in a darkened room and should wear dark glasses for some time to follow.

Sympathetic ophthalmitis

Inflammation of the uveal tract in one eye may involve the uveal tract of the other. The injured eye is called the exciting eye and the uninjured eye is called the sympathetic eye.

Enucleation (removal) of the exciting eye may be necessary. Steroid therapy is needed for the sympathetic eye.

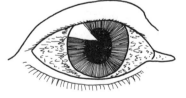 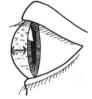

Fig. 2.5.11 Glaucoma

Glaucoma

Raised intra-ocular pressure leads to tension inside the eye which can obstruct blood flow to the optic nerve leading to progressive blindness.

Acute glaucoma

Acute blockage of the flow of aqueous humour through the canal (of Schlemm). Sudden onset of symptoms with severe pain radiating from the eye. Nausea and vomiting may occur and the patient becomes generally ill.

The anterior chamber can be seen to be bulging, the pupil is fixed and dilated. Vision decreases rapidly and if not treated within 4 hours, some patients may lose the sight completely and permanently.

Medical treatment Miotic drugs are used to constrict the pupil – this opens the angle towards the canal. The drugs used are eserine ¼–½% or pilocarpine 1–2%. Acetazolamide (Diamox) IM or IV acts as a diuretic and reduces the production of aqueous humour.

Surgical treatment Drainage operations and iridectomy – removal of part of the iris allows drainage even when the pupil is dilated.

Chronic glaucoma

A gradual rise in intra-ocular pressure often occurring in ageing. There may be no symptoms until vision becomes very bad. It may be treated with miotic drugs.

Nursing notes

Acute glaucoma Early treatment is very important. Advice for medical help and transfer for hospital care may be needed.

Again, the general nurse is mainly involved with helping specialists, but should understand the importance. Remember the care of the very ill patient in bed with diminished vision.

Chronic glaucoma Elderly patients need observation for indications of failing vision – especially those in long-stay geriatric wards.

Cataract

Opacity of the lens which may be congenital or may be due to the ageing process, diabetes mellitus or a penetrating eye injury. The effect is clouding of vision.

Treatment is by surgical extraction. Many methods are used now, learn the one used in your locality, but read about others too. Surgery is followed by fitting the patient with spectacles or contact lens for focusing.

Suggested nursing response to ophthalmic surgery

Details cannot be given in this text of all surgery but lens extraction is given as an example of the principles involved.

Before surgery
1 Carefully orientate the patient to his environment
2 Always approach with a word of greeting
3 Careful explanation of all procedures is necessary, including the expected procedures on return from surgery including the call bell system
4 Assessment of total condition is made. It is very important to observe for respiratory tract infections (disturbing cough); heart conditions (hypertension); diabetes mellitus
5 Swabs are taken to ensure that the eyes are free from infection
6 Prophylactic antibacterial drops may be prescribed
7 Eye lashes are usually trimmed

After surgery
1 Most operations are performed under local anaesthetic to reduce the danger of vomiting
2 Information about the outcome of the surgery is needed early to reduce anxiety
3 Many patients are sedated
4 Prescribed analgesia must be given on time
5 The patient is gradually sat up and told of the call bell system again. He is advised against reaching for articles initially, touching his eyes or dressings or trying to get out of bed
6 Dressings are carried out by specialists and specialist trained nurses, including suture removal
7 Early mobilization depends on the individual surgeon and the operation performed
8 Dark glasses are worn during the day
9 Eye pads or shields may be applied at night time
10 Prescribed drops may still be needed

Detached retina

More commonly occurs in patients with myopia (long eye balls) as the retina is thinner but it may occur as a complication of choroiditis, or following cataract extraction. The patient complains of flashing lights (tearing of the retina) followed by loss of vision – as if a curtain came across. Further loss of vision may follow if untreated. It is a painless condition.

Surgical repair is necessary. Again, many different operations are performed by different surgeons. For example, sealing the retina by cryo-surgery (intensely cold probe) or by laser beams; refashioning the sclera to the contours of the retina

Nursing notes

Before any surgery is performed, the patient has a period of complete bed rest with careful head positioning to allow the retina to fall into place. Even after surgery, a period of complete bed rest is needed.

Earlier fears that the patient had about loss of vision may now be less acute.

Trauma to the eye

Foreign bodies Loose particles may be removed by irrigation or a moist swab. Fixed particles require specialist removal

Perforating injuries

Suggested nursing response – first aid
1 Sterile pad over the eye
2 Do not attempt to remove any article
3 Transfer to hospital quickly – keep head still

Surgical treatment is again specialist. Enucleation (removal of the eye) may be necessary to prevent sympathetic ophthalmitis.

Nursing is as for ophthalmic surgery.

The shock and psychological trauma of eye injuries may be profound. Sensitive handling is important.

Chemical burns

Usually due to acids or alkalis splashed into the eye.

Suggested nursing response – first aid
1 Thorough irrigation with plenty of water
2 Transfer to Accident Centre quickly

Irrigation is continued and then follows treatment as for keratitis, uveitis or conjunctivitis.

Congenital defects

The only general defect considered in this text is strabismus – squint.

Strabismus (squint) Is due to a weakness in an eye muscle allowing one eye to deviate when stereoscopic vision is attempted. The deviating eye may lose its vision eventually. Correction is carried out as soon as possible.

Covering up the good eye and help from an orthoptist, plus parental perseverance may correct it without surgery.

Surgery involves refashioning or siting of the eye muscle and may need to be repeated.

Suggested nursing care for partially sighted or blind patients

Use nursing process in order to cover as many aspects as possible.
1 *Assess*
  1 The degree of blindness of the patient
  2 What he can and cannot do
  3 The degree of independence that they have
2 *Plan*
  1 The environment in which they are to be nursed: the position of furniture, food on the plate etc; the way to the toilet and day room; a good call bell system; all staff to be aware of the need for tidiness
  2 Activities to retain their enjoyment of independence: radios, tape recorders (speaking books) with head-phones; Braille or Moon books for reading
3 *Implement 1* Careful greeting of the patient to avoid startling, and saying good-bye.
  2 Care of the eyes if required (some patients could still put their own drops in).
  3 Show a sense of humour (many blind patients do say 'I see what you mean').
4 *Evaluate* Be prepared to change any care to meet the patient's feelings for assurance and independence

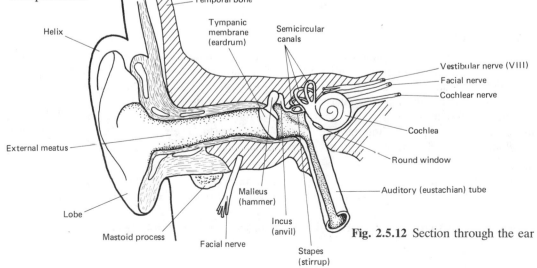

Fig. 2.5.12 Section through the ear

The ear (see Fig. 2.5.12)

Functions	Structures involved
1 The conduction of sound waves from the outside air to the nerve endings	The pinna funnels the waves into the external auditory canal which is lined with a thin coat of wax to aid resonance. Sound waves hitting the tympanic membrane cause it to vibrate which in turn causes the ossicles in the middle ear to move (first the incus, then the malleus and finally the stapes). The foot-plate of the stapes is situated in the oval window of the internal ear. Vibration of the stapes causes waves to be formed in the perilymph. The perilymph movement causes vibration of the membranes which in turn causes waves in the endolymph which can be detected by the nerve endings of the organ of Corti (cochlear apparatus)
2 The maintenance of balance and sensation of our position in space	Movement of perilymph and endolymph in the semicircular canals causes movement of the nerve endings in the vestibule of the inner ear (vestibular apparatus)
3 The transmission of impulses to the brain of both hearing and balance	The vestibulo-cochlear nerve is one of the cranial nerves. Synapses occur in the brain stem, mid brain and thalamus before transmission to the cerebral cortex Hearing – impulses are transmitted to the temporal lobe of the cerebrum Balance – various parts involved. Main centre is probably in the parietal lobe

Conditions affecting the ear

Inflammatory conditions

Otitis externa is inflammation of the external ear including the external auditory meatus. The outer layer of the tympanic membrane may be inflamed

Cause Bacterial infection – often secondary to infections of the outside skin. Dandruff may be a predisposing factor.

Effects, signs and symptoms Inflammation causes swelling and redness in the auditory canal which being embedded in bone increases pressure on nerve endings. The patient complains of intense earache and irritation.

Treatment
1 Analgesia
2 Gentle packing of the ear with impregnated ribbon gauze in some centres
3 Antibacterial drops to the ear
4 Keep the ear dry

Nursing notes
Early recommendation for treatment is important to save the patient a lot of pain and discomfort. Advise patients to keep the auditory canal dry.

Probing and packing of the ear should only be done by a specialist nurse or doctor. Ear drops should be gently warmed before instilling.

Advise the patient on care of the hair and hygiene.

Otitis media is inflammation of the middle ear.

Acute otitis media

Cause
1 Viral infections
2 Bacterial infections
    1 Spread up the eustachian (auditory) tube from throat infections. Organisms – haemolytic streptococci; staphylococci; pneumococci
    2 From external ear if the ear drum is perforated
    3 Rarely, a complication of fractured skull

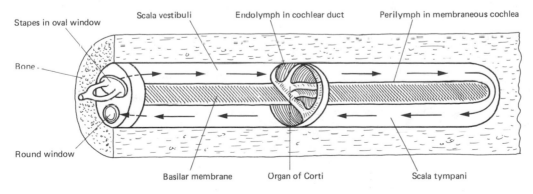

Fig. 2.5.13 The bony and membranous cochlea uncoiled

Effects, signs and symptoms The inflammation causes intense swelling of tissues in the middle ear, with the tympanic membrane bulging and appearing red when examined through an auroscope. The drum may perforate.

The pain may be minimal or very severe. It is particularly severe in young infants who may bang their head against a cot side in an attempt to relieve pain.

The ear may discharge pus with blood in it. The discharge is sometimes offensive smelling.

The metabolic rate may rise considerably in an infant and febrile convulsions may occur.

Diagnosis – investigations
1 Clinical examination – using auroscope
2 Swab of discharge for culture
3 Throat swab

Treatment
1 Analgesia
2 Local heat pad for pain relief
3 Antibacterial drugs according to culture but should be started on broad spectrum antibacterial drug immediately. Children are usually given amoxycillin or erythromycin systemically
4 Myringotomy is performed to relieve pressure and drain pus
5 Nasal and throat decongestants may improve drainage through the eustachian (auditory) tube

Suggested nursing response

Assessment	Care
1 Degree of pain experienced – some would keep a pain chart	Prescribed analgesia (aspirin is popular). Local warm pad applied
2 Drainage of material from the ear – note the nature, colour and smell of it	Careful wool padding and aural hygiene (preferably by a specialist nurse). The ear is not 'plugged'
3 Raised metabolic rate – rising temperature, pulse, feeling ill and tired	Prescribed antibacterial drug. Rest in bed. Maintain body temperature. Give glucose drinks
4 Observe for complications (see below)	Care of the patient with meningitis or encephalitis (p 101)

Secretory or serous otitis media

Is a condition of childhood due to blockage of the auditory tube. The secretions in the middle ear become thick and tenacious ('glue ear') and deafness occurs due to interference with ossicle vibration.

Myringotomy, drainage and the insertion of a fine tube known as a grommet is the treatment. Repeated visits to Out Patients and further treatment may be needed.

Chronic otitis media There is usually a perforation of the tympanic membrane, and chronic discharge of purulent material from the ear. Soft, keratinized tissue growing into the middle ear is known as cholesteatoma and interferes with the ossicle vibration.

Progressive deafness can occur. Sometimes the facial nerve may be involved and produce a facial palsy with drooping of the eyelids and mouth on the affected side.

Mastoiditis All forms of otitis media may lead to infection of the mastoid air cells with the accumulation of pus causing erosion and pain. More dangerous, is the close proximity to the meninges and the brain.

Foreign bodies in the ear

Are usually removable by gentle syringing.

Wax in the external auditory canal

Increased amounts do not need removal unless they cause symptoms.

Deafness, earache, vertigo and tinnitus may occur. The patient should be examined by a doctor before syringing is attempted.

Suggested nursing response for syringing of the ear
1 Must not be done without medical examination first
2 Solution should be at body temperature (37°C)
3 Fluid is never directed at the tympanic membrane, only to the upper surface of the canal
4 Gentle syringing is usually as effective as more forceful attempts, and safer!
5 Dry mop the ear on completion
6 The patient is advised to keep the canal dry

Menières disease

Cause Not known

Effects, signs and symptoms There is an increased amount of endolymph in the inner ear. Both balance and hearing are affected. The patient usually complains of sudden attacks of vertigo – acute dizziness as if the room is spinning. It may be so distressing that the slightest movement of the head causes vomiting (as in sea sickness).

There is progressive deafness as the cochlear apparatus is affected. Some complain of tinnitus – abnormal roaring or sounds (including ringing) in the ear which may be continuous. This is made worse when there are other extraneous noises such as a baby crying.

Diagnosis – investigations
  1 Clinical history   2 Audiometry and caloric tests   3 X-rays and scanning

Treatment
Medical Adjusting salt intake sometimes helps. Hyoscine, antihistamines and phenothiazines (e.g. chlorpromazine) are helpful
Surgery Different ENT surgeons try different operations. Radical operations to destroy the vestibular apparatus result in loss of hearing too.

Suggested nursing response
  1 Nurse patients in a quiet room with subdued lighting
  2 Avoid any sudden movements when approaching them
  3 Give a prescribed antiemetic – prochlorperazine (Stemetil) is very popular
  4 Vertigo may last for several hours – patience and assurance are needed by patients, relatives and staff

Note: Vertigo and tinnitus may be caused by some drugs. Two important ones are streptomycin and aspirin.

Surgery on the ear

Before operation
  1 Audiometric tests will be carried out and records should be kept
  2 Assurance and explanation of what will happen after surgery
  3 Medicated shampoo, shaving of hair well around the ear and hair fixed away from operation site

After operation
  1 Patients are nursed flat. Vestibular disturbances may cause nausea and vomiting
  2 Observe for indications of infection; rising intracranial pressure; damage to the facial nerve (facial palsy)
  3 Ear packs and dressings should be removed by specialist trained nurses or surgeons

Types of deafness

Congenital Usually nerve deafness and usually affecting higher pitched sounds. It may be due to chronic otitis media (conductive)
Adult
  1 Conductive deafness which usually results from inflammatory conditions of the ear affecting transmission of sound.
  2 Nerve deafness which may be congenital or may result from injury, infection or the ageing process.

Suggested nursing response

Congenital Early recognition is important as hearing aids are available even for nerve deafness. Specialist teaching may be required for the child to achieve true potential. The nurse needs to be alert when playing with children.

Adult
  1 Communication is the main problem, but close to that is the psychological frustration of the deaf adult.
  2 Speech should be only slightly louder but very clear with emphasis on consonants 't's and 'd's. Give visual clues by facing the patient and using hands. Many can lip read clear speech. Try to learn a sign language if you meet them continually.
  3 Spend time listening to patients' anxieties and frustrations.
  4 Encourage patients to seek surgical opinion about their deafness.
  5 Encourage the use of hearing aids. Help patients to clean and maintain them.
  6 Provide books and visual recreation activities in the wards.

2.6 Locomotor conditions

The locomotor system

This system will be considered as follows.

1 **Bone and bones**
2 **Joints**

1 Bone and bones

Functions	Structures involved
1 Providing a framework and support for the whole body. Influencing the body image	The skeletal framework consists of the axial skeleton (skull, ribs and vertebral column) and the appendicular skeleton (the limbs and limb girdles)
Bone growth is influenced by the growth hormone (pituitary gland)	
2 Providing protection for underlying tissues	The skull protects the brain. The rib cage protects the heart and lungs. The vertebral column protects the spinal cord. The pelvic girdle protects pelvic organs
3 By providing attachments for muscle and acting as levers, bones are needed to provide movement	Muscles are attached to bone through elastic tendons which are inserted on the outer surface of bones
4 Bone is a store for calcium. If serum levels of calcium fall, calcium can be released from the bone matrix. High levels of calcium will cause an increased storage. This mechanism is controlled by parathormone from the parathyroid glands	Bone tissue is composed of a series of Haversian systems in which osteocytes make a matrix of calcium, phosphate and organic material which is recognized as bone
5 Manufacture of erythrocytes, many leucocytes (not lymphocytes) and thrombocytes	Bone marrow or myeloid tissue (see 2.2.)

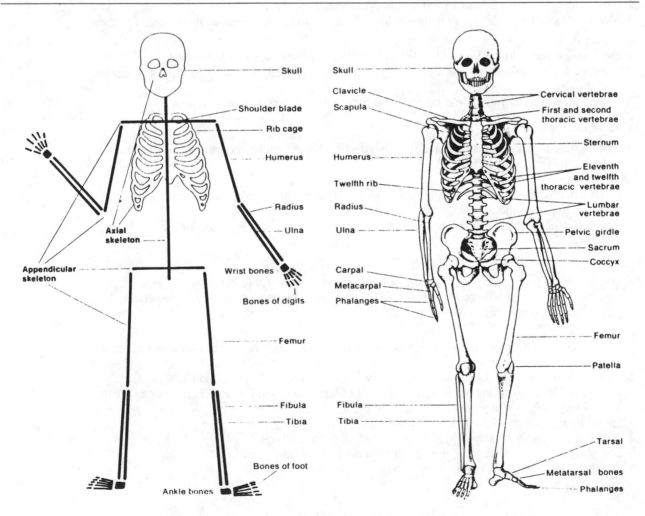

Fig. 2.6.1 The skeletal system

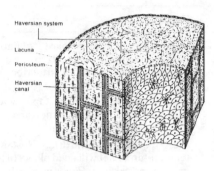

Fig. 2.6.2 Haversian system

Bone formation

Periosteum is the support membrane on the outer surface of bone and provides the blood supply there

Osteoblasts are bone forming cells. They manufacture bone matrix in ossification centres from collagen and mucopolysaccharides. Calcium is added to give strength.

Osteoclasts Erode matrix away to give the medullary cavities, reducing the weight and density of individual bones

Osteoblasts build – osteoclasts shape

Factors affecting bone formation

1 Nutrition for osteoblasts and osteoclasts to function. All osteocytes need glucose and amino acids in large quantities. Bone is very much a living tissue
2 Vitamin D is essential for calcium metabolism
3 Correct amount of parathormone to influence calcium metabolism
4 Growth hormone (and to some extent thyroxine in children) for normal development of long bones
5. An adequate blood supply and drainage

Note: There are no lymphatics in bone, therefore freedom from infection is vital too.

Conditions affecting bone and bones

Osteomyelitis

Inflammation of the bone tissue.

Cause Infection is usually staphylococcal. It may be introduced in compound fractures or orthopaedic surgery. It may be haematogenic – spread in the blood stream from an infected area on the skin (e.g. a boil or furuncle).

Nursing note
Osteomyelitis is comparatively rare now because of the scrupulous care given for compound fractures and in orthopaedic surgery. The condition is included here to emphasize the reason for such care.

Effects, signs and symptoms The common site for local infection is in the diaphysis of long bones. Pus is formed and enters the canals and spaces of the bone. Accumulation under the periosteum may cause it to elevate and be stripped, interfering with the blood supply to part of the bone, which will necrose (die). The dead bone tissue is called a sequestrum and becomes congested with purulent material. A sinus may form to the skin surface.

The patient complains of severe pain and tenderness over the area. The slightest movement increases the pain. Metabolic rate may be markedly raised with pyrexia, tachycardia and a feeling of tiredness and misery. The toxaemia and possible septicaemia may be life threatening. Unfortunately, in children, it may cause a lot of deformity. Eventually, with guarding of the area and repeated long term hospitalization it may affect intellectual development.

Diagnosis – investigations
1 Clinical examination and history. (Nursing history – note any trouble with boils.)
2 Swab for culture

Treatment
1 Rest in bed and local rest for the limb
2 A plaster of Paris splint may be made
3 High doses of antibacterial agents are given – clindamycin or flucloxacillin for 6–12 weeks
4 Surgical drainage of sequestrum

Suggested nursing response

Assessment	Care
1 Degree of local pain and tenderness	Immobilize the limb in a plaster of Paris back splint or on a Thomas splint. Careful moving and positioning. Apply local heat for relief. Prescribed analgesia regularly
2 Observe draining sinuses or open wound following drainage of sequestrum	Strict asepsis with dressings. Open wounds need packing to facilitate granulation and prevent reformation of a sequestrum
3 Raised metabolic rate. Observe pyrexia, tachycardia and malaise	Prescribed antibacterial drugs. Rest. Maintain body temperature. Diet will need plenty of glucose, protein and calcium. Fluids need to be given. Mouth care if dehydration occurs
4 Response to long hospitalization: boredom; frustration; acceptance	Divertional therapy. Time to listen to anxieties. Children need help and encouragement for learning. Prepare for problems when discharge is imminent. Parents need guidance too

Later, physiotherapy will be needed to restore strength to immobilized or weakened muscles.

Osteoporosis

Decreased density of bone tissue due to reduced activity of osteoblasts. Bone is worn away by the osteoclasts, producing cavities and cysts. Ultimately, pathological fractures may occur.

The cause is not known, but it does occur in Cushing's syndrome. It tends to occur in elderly ladies and may be due to the lowered level of oestrogen.

The pathological fracture is usually the first symptom – classically back pain produced by a 'collapsed' vertebra. Anabolic steroids may be prescribed and increased calcium in the diet will help.

Nursing notes
1 One cannot stress enough the importance of careful moving and particularly lifting of patients with osteoporosis to avoid pathological fractures.
2 Advice to elderly patients should be given
   1 Avoid heavy lifting
   2 Careful posture and movements but exercise regularly. (Exercise is thought to stimulate osteoblast activity.)
   3 Beware of the danger of falling

Osteomalacia (adult rickets)

A softening and weakening of bones due to insufficient calcium deposit in the tissue. It may be due to calcium deficiency in the diet, or inadequate vitamin D for calcium metabolism. It is sometimes due to excessive loss of calcium in urine.

The patient complains of pain in the bones and 'bowing' of long bones may be seen. Very low calcium levels in serum cause tetany (carpopedal spasm).

Treatment is to give increased calcium in the diet. Intravenous calcium gluconate would be given for tetany.

Paget's disease (osteitis deformans)

Chronic changes in bone structure. More common in the elderly and sometimes seen as a sequel to disorders of the prostate gland.

The patient complains of skeletal pain and headache (as the bones of the skull are affected). They are often seen with an apparently large cranium. Apart from pain and headache relief there is no specific treatment.

Tumours of bone

May be primary or secondary (metastases) from other primary growths (especially, bronchus, breast and prostate gland).

Primary – benign An area of dense bone forms (a nidus) and may be symptomless. If it impinges on other structures or causes pain, surgical excision and packing with chips of bone is carried out.

Primary – malignant

Osteo sarcoma (In cartilage, chondrosarcoma)

Cause Not known

Effects, signs and symptoms A nidus may form but again produce no symptoms. They are often found on X-rays for other investigations. Gradually persistent bone pain will develop and local inflammation may be seen.

There is no lymphatic spread. There is however, rapid haemorrhagic spread and metastases in the lungs have often formed before the primary growth is diagnosed. Weight loss may be significant and is ominous.

Diagnosis – investigations

1 Careful clinical examination
2 X-rays
3 Bone scanning
4 Blood for serum alkaline phosphatase (increased)
5 Biopsy of the nidus

Treatment

1 Radical removal of the tumour is needed – amputation of the limb, including the joint near to the trunk. e.g. hind quarter amputation for osteosarcoma involving the femur.
2 Chemotherapy – intermittent treatment to spare bone marrow. Drugs commonly used are vincristine, methotrexate and adriamycin

Suggested nursing response

Assessment	Care
1 Degree of pain and discomfort (including phantom pains following amputation)	Prescribed analgesia and explanations (See *nursing care for amputation* (p 137))
2 Responses to chemotherapy – undesired effects include	
1 alopecia – hair falling out	Assurance of regrowth. Provide wigs
2 stomatitis – inflamed mouth	Mouth care
3 bone marrow depression – sore throat and fever and a tendency to bleed	Care for infection

Early diagnosis may give good results but, sadly, many will need terminal care with increasing cachexia, respiratory tract infections and pain before death.

Counselling of relatives needs to be discussed with the whole team of doctors, nurses and therapists and will inevitably be guarded about prognosis.

Fractures

Breaking of the continuity of bones.

Causes 1 Direct violence
2 Indirect violence
3 Sudden excessive strain (e.g. cough fracture)
4 Pathological

Effects, signs and symptoms

A closed fracture or simple fracture No wound leading to the site. The break may be simple or more complex.

An open fracture or compound fracture A wound leads to the site, either due to the blow itself or the broken end of bone has been driven through the skin from inside. Infection is always a complication of compound fractures (either aerobic organisms or anaerobic bacteria). Clostridium welchii (gas gangrene) or Clostridium tetanii (tetanus) are found in soil and dirt.

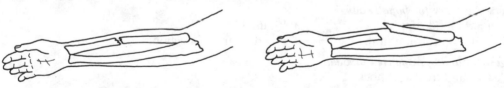

a. Closed fracture
b. Open fracture
Fig. 2.6.3 Types of fracture

An old mnemonic for remembering the signs and symptoms of all fractures is:

Pain	**d**eformity	**s**welling	**i**mmobility	**u**nnatural movement	**c**repitus (grating sound)
Please	**d**rop	**s**ixpence	**i**n	**u**ncle's	**c**ap

(The grating sound may be reported by the patient but should not be tested as more damage is caused.)

Blood loss can be severe and shock will occur due to pain (neurogenic), blood loss (hypovolaemia) and emotion. Inflammation always occurs and the metabolic rate will be increased but pyrexia does not show until later. Fat globules released from bone marrow may cause fat emboli which may affect lungs, or go through the pulmonary circulation to any organ including the brain. Globules may enter the urine through the kidney.

Effects of particular fractures

Shoulder girdle and upper limbs

Clavicle (collar bone) The shoulder on the affected side droops. The patient finds pain relief by supporting the elbow.

Humerus The whole arm is immobilized. Fractures near to the elbow may compress nerves travelling near to the joint, either directly or as a result of the swelling.
Colles's fracture A fracture of the radius (and often the ulna) at the wrist produces 'dinner fork' deformity.
Scaphoid Fracture of the scaphoid at the base of the thumb needs great care to avoid loss of thumb movement.

Pelvic girdle and lower limbs
Pelvis Danger of rupture of the urethra, bladder and intestines.
Femur Head or neck of femur fractures are more common in elderly patients. The main danger would be long immobilization.
  Shaft fractures may cause severe bleeding. Considerable shortening of the limb occurs as muscles pull the broken ends of bone across each other.
Tibia and Fibula Fractures of single bones do occur when no shortening will be seen and minimal deformity. Realignment for fracture of both bones may be difficult.
Pott's fracture Fracture of the fibula and tip of the tibia (internal malleolus) in the ankle

Diagnosis – investigations
1 Clinical history and examination   2 X-rays

Treatment
1 Reduction – traction and manipulation to obtain normal bone alignment
2 Open reduction – surgical opening of the fracture site to obtain realignment
  Open reduction for compound fractures is important also to:
  1 expose the tissues to oxygen which will kill anaerobic bacteria.
  2 remove any necrosed or damaged tissues on which micro organisms can multiply.
  3 thoroughly clean the site of dirt and soil.
3 Immobilization – until healing occurs
  1 Plaster of Paris cast splinting
  2 Traction – skeletal or skin
  3 Internal fixation by metal plates, screws, nails and pins
  4 Cast bracing
4 Rehabilitation for daily living, with physiotherapy being introduced as early as possible
5 Compound fractures – a course of antibacterial drug is commenced. Tetanus toxoid is given in Accident Centre and anti-gas gangrene serum may be needed

Healing of bone
1 Fibroblasts invade blood clot and inflamed tissue to form granulation tissue and cartilage.
2 Osteoblasts (mainly from the periosteum) form new bone-like tissue which surrounds the site like a collar, known as a callus. Although appearing dense, it is not strong enough for stress and weight bearing.
3 Osteoblasts and osteoclasts continue to build up and refashion the bone until ossification is complete. Upper limbs 6–8 weeks. Weight bearing limbs 10–12 weeks.

Factors necessary for bone healing
1 A good blood supply   3 Vitamin D
2 Protein and calcium in the diet   4 Freedom from infection

Suggested nursing response – first aid
1 Assess and treat for shock
2 Cover all wounds with sterile dressings
3 Do not attempt to reduce the fracture
4 Immobilize in the most comfortable or found position, using splints and bandages. (Check a first aid manual for individual fracture bandaging)
5 Apply slings for the upper limb if it can bend at the elbow
6 Send written information with the casualty to Accident Centre

Suggested nursing response – fractures

Assessment	Care
1 Degree of shock: pain; blood loss; blood pressure recording; skin cold and clammy; fear and restlessness	Avoid any unnecessary moving. Give prescribed analgesia. Intravenous infusion of plasma or dextran initially, followed by blood. Keep the patient warm but not over heated. Continual assurance
2 Evidence of wounds – even a small puncture wound is dangerous	Prepare for open surgery: check time of last meal; clean operation site as far as possible; ensure consent is given. Give prescribed antibacterial drugs, including tetanus toxoid. Maintain dressings – aseptic technique when changing

continued next page

3 Evidence of inflammation: tachycardia, later pyrexia, feels ill and tired for a few days

Maintain rest, temperature control. Glucose drinks when tolerated. A patient may be very ill for some days

4 Evidence of fat embolism: chest pain in pulmonary embolism; behavioural changes if brain involved; a fine rash of red spots which are known as petechiae; fat globules in urine

Care as for pulmonary embolism but anticoagulants may not be used. Explanation to relatives. Prognosis is not always good and counselling may be needed

5 Ability to take adequate nutrition and vitamin D – may have anorexia, nausea or vomiting at times or may have other injuries

Encourage high protein, high carbohydrate diet with added calcium. Encourage sun bathing if possible

6 Immobility problems
  1 constipation
  2 pressure sores

  3 boredom, irritability

  4 urine stagnation

High fibre diet. Suppositories may be needed
Change of position. Regular cleaning and relief of pressure. Reinforce need for good diet
Provide diversional and occupational therapy. Group patients of similar interests together. Encourage open visiting
Encourage fluids and stress need for bladder emptying to be complete

Nursing response for patients with a plaster of Paris cast

Assessment	Care
1 For pressure sore under the cast: numbness of a part, tingling sensations, burning sensation or persistent pain	Inform surgeon at once. Prepare to relieve the pressure by cutting the cast
2 For obstruction of the circulation due to the cast being too tight or to late swelling of the site (note especially the elbow): cold and pale (or even blue); excessive swelling; loss of movement; numbness or pain; negative 'blanching' test	Prevent first by careful application of the cast; careful placement of the limb in elevated position; encourage exercise of fingers or toes as soon as possible. Inform at once if it occurs. Prepare to relieve by cutting the cast

Initially, a plaster of Paris cast is wet and in drying out, heat is created. Drying should not be accelerated. Special need to avoid abnormal pressure by waterproof pillow supports should be stressed to junior nurses.

Dry plaster may cause abrasions at the edges or by flaking bits in the bed. Regular inspection of the skin and good bed making technique is required.

Nursing response for patients on traction

Assessment	Care
1 If skeletal traction, observe wound sites of pins. Swab for culture if infection seen	Aseptic dressings are applied. Try to keep them dry
2 Check all traction equipment: Thomas splint ring should press into groin but should not chafe; Pearson knee attachment (see Fig. 2.6.4); all cords and pulleys should move freely; weights should be checked; slings under the limb are checked for position	Report any sore areas. Light talcum powder applied to reduce chafing. Keep clean and dry. Report any breakdown of systems
3 Check the correct position of the bed and patient to ensure counter traction is maintained	Careful positioning of patient. May need explanations

Physiotherapy for joint movement (e.g. knee) may be started as soon as possible.

Internal fixation See care of patients having orthopaedic surgery. Mobilization is achieved much earlier.

Cast bracing Is a new technique being introduced in some orthopaedic centres. It involves the application of two weight bearing casts (plaster of Paris or new synthetic materials) joined by gliding action hinges. They provide fracture immobilization but weight bearing and walking can be undertaken much earlier with the help of crutches.
The patient needs advice about
1 the correct use of crutches.
2 protecting the casts from contamination.
3 watching for swelling, skin discolouration, abrasions or numbness.
4 elevating the limb when not walking for venous return.

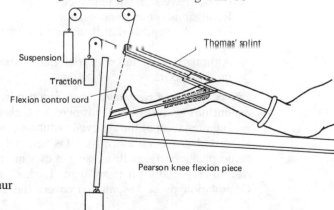

Suspension
Traction
Flexion control cord
Thomas' splint
Pearson knee flexion piece

Fig. 2.6.4 Skeletal traction for fractured femur

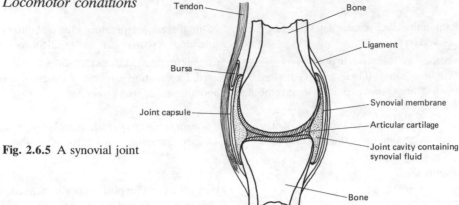

Fig. 2.6.5 A synovial joint

2 Joints

Functions	Structures involved
Providing articulation or bending of limbs and extremities. Freely movable joints are called synovial and include ball and socket, hinge and gliding joints	Hyaline cartilage on end of bone. Synovial membrane secretes oily synovial fluid. Capsule and ligaments holding the ends of bone together

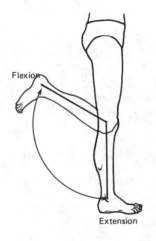
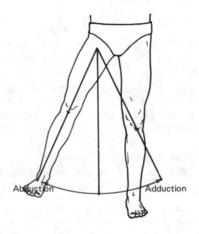
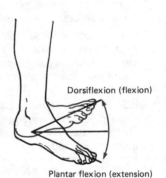

Fig. 2.6.6 Types of movement

Other joints are:
1 partially movable joints e.g. intervertebral joints between vertebral bodies with discs
2 fixed joints e.g. the sutured joints in the skull

Conditions affecting joints

Arthritis

Inflammation of joints. There are many different conditions in which arthritis is part of the disease. In this text, only rheumatoid arthritis, septic arthritis and osteo-arthritis (osteo-arthrosis) will be considered.

Rheumatoid arthritis

Is really an inflammatory condition of connective tissue as well as specific joint disease.

Cause Not known

Cause factors
1 It is much more common in women
2 It does have familial tendency
3 Remissions occur in pregnancy
4 Research suggests that it may be an auto immune disorder in which there is rejection of the synovial membrane – but again the reason is not known.
5 Although associated with cold, damp conditions, they probably aggravate the condition rather than cause it.

Effects, signs and symptoms There is a prodromal illness (before the arthritis is seen) in which the patient has tachycardia, slight pyrexia, feels tired and complains of limbs aching.
Inflammation of the synovial membrane occurs. The arthritis classically occurs in the peripheral joints and as many are involved it is cally polyarthritis. The joints of the hand (interphalangeal and carpo-phalangeal) are distressing as they interfere with daily living. The joints are hot, swollen and painful, especially on movement. Lack of movement leads to muscle wasting between them. Granulation tissue (a pannus) covers the cartilage. Bone inside the joint capsule is gradually

destroyed. Tendons and ligaments are damaged and the whole joint becomes unstable and often dislocates.

The patient may present with an unusable hand with gross distortion of knuckles. Larger joints are also affected – the ankle and knee are very susceptible.

Associated conditions

Rheumatic nodules Painful subcutaneous swellings on bony prominences

Bursitis Inflammation of a bursa e.g. tender swellings in front of the knee joint (house-maids' knee)

'Stiff' lungs Rheumatoid disease in the lungs reduces their elasticity and may interfere with breathing

Arteritis Peripheral arteries become inflamed and reduce the blood supply to hands and feet. The patient has cold extremities

Anaemia May be due to chronic inflammation or bone marrow may be affected

It can be appreciated that this chronic condition may last for many years and patients have psychological problems coping with it. Depression and anxiety are common.

Diagnosis – investigations

1 Clinical examination and history
2 X-rays of the joints and lungs
3 Blood for haemoglobin estimation, plasma protein estimations (globulins are increased) and full blood count. The presence of rheumatoid factor is determined by a Latex fixation test.

Treatment

1 Complete rest in bed
2 Iron supplements or blood transfusion for anaemia
3 Analgesia is achieved by using aspirin which has anti-inflammatory effects too
4 Anti-inflammatory drugs – aspirin (acetylsalicylic acid), phenylbutazone, indomethacin
5 Gold salts – myocrisin (action not understood)
6 Corticosteroid drugs (anti-inflammatory effect) – prednisolone, adrenocorticotrophic hormone. (Occasionally steroids may be given into the joint itself – intra-articular.) All antirheumatic drugs have undesired effects. Refer to the British National Formulary for a full guidance.

Surgery Replacement surgery of many joints has now been done quite successfully
Physiotherapy is needed to achieve
1 correct positioning for immobilization splinting   *2* exercises to prevent muscle wasting
Occupational therapy is needed to help patients cope with daily activities such as dressing, cooking and feeding as well as craft work to develop muscle groups.

Suggested nursing response

Assessment	Care
1 Raised metabolic rate in acute phases – pyrexia, tachycardia, malaise, fatigue	Rest in bed (but care of positioning affected joints). Temperature controlled by light clothing. Glucose drinks encouraged
2 Degree of anaemia – skin pallor; tachycardia, palpitations; fatigue	Encourage high protein diet with plenty of iron. Some recommend goats' milk instead of cows' milk as there is a suspicion of hypersensitivity
3 Degree of pain and tenderness in the joints	Give prescribed analgesia. (Aspirin, if tolerated, can be given 3–4 hourly.) Put joints in padded splints. Avoid extremes of heat and cold – both aggravate the pain
4 Rheumatic nodules	Light covering may help
5 Observe for chest infection	Care as for chest infection. Good posture for ventilation is important
6 Arteritis – cold hands and feet	Some patients like cotton or woollen mittens and socks
7 Tolerance of drugs – observe for undesired effects *1* aspirin – gastric erosion; allergic rashes or asthma; tendency to bleed	Give after meals to avoid gastric erosion. Report and do not give until seen by a doctor if problems occur
2 indomethacin and phenylbutazone – gastric erosion; aplastic anaemia (sore throat, bruising) Indomethacin may be given by suppository to avoid gastric erosion	
3 gold salts – dermatitis; stomatitis; renal damage; bone marrow depression	Given in carefully monitored doses. Deep intramuscular injections
4 corticosteroids (see 2.8)	
8 Co-operation with physiotherapy and occupational therapy	The nurse is involved in positively encouraging the patient in exercises and practices
9 Psychological needs – may be depressed or anxious	Sit and listen to fears and anxieties. May need psychiatric help. Relatives need counselling and support too

Septic arthritis

Infection of a joint.

Cause

1 Bacterial invasion, usually as a complication of other injuries
2 Bovine tuberculosis (now very rare)

Effects, signs and symptoms The acute inflammation in the joints causes swelling, redness, severe pain and loss of function. Aspiration of synovial fluid will show pus and organisms can be cultured. There is danger of infection entering the bone and some stiffness of the joint usually occurs.

Nurses are more likely to meet elderly patients with stiff joints from past infections. Modern antibacterial therapy and surgery have reduced the incidence of acute disease but the danger is still there.

Metabolic rate may be quite significantly raised and the patient will feel very ill.

Diagnosis – investigations

1 Clinical examination and history
2 X-ray of the joint
3 Aspiration of joint synovial fluid under aseptic conditions

Treatment

1 Rest of the joint in a splint. (The Thomas splint was designed for arthritis of the knee joint)
2 Antibacterial drugs

Suggested nursing response

Assessment	Care
1 Degree of inflammation in the joint. Pain may be severe	Rest the limb in a splint. Apply local heat for relief. Give prescribed analgesia
2 Raised metabolic rate – pyrexia, tachycardia, malaise	Bed rest. Maintain body temperature. High carbohydrate diet and fluids
3 Response to long term immobilization (may need some weeks for resolution) Rehabilitation exercises – physiotherapy is introduced carefully.	Diversional therapy

Osteo-arthrosis

(The term osteo-arthritis is becoming redundant as inflammation is not the primary problem.) Osteo-arthrosis is the degeneration of a joint – mainly the articular cartilage on the bone surfaces, due to prolonged wear and tear.

Cause It is regarded as part of the ageing process. Factors that accelerate the disease are previous injury, abnormal gait for any reason and, most of all, obesity.

Effects, signs and symptoms As cartilage is eroded, the underlying bone is exposed. Irritation of bone causes increased growth of bone which protrudes in spurs and ridges producing the reduced movement, the creaking and pain. Broken spurs may further irritate the joint and increase the pain. The joint will eventually become deformed. Large, weight bearing joints (especially the hip joint) are mainly affected but other joints exposed to excessive wear may be involved (Bony outgrowths on the knuckles are called Heberden's nodes.)

The main problems facing the patient are that increasing pain tends to make them less active and they tend to increase weight which, of course, increases the joint damage.

The pain may be continual and increase the 'psychological' ageing of people. Reversal of this, following treatment, is sometimes quite dramatic.

Diagnosis – investigations

1 Clinical examination and history
2 X-ray examination
3 Blood tests to exclude rheumatoid factor

Treatment

1 Rest, pain relief and reduction of weight may be all that is necessary for early cases.
2 For intractible pain, surgery is undertaken
   1 Osteotomy – removal of bony spurs
   2 Arthrodesis – fixing the joint by fusing the bones together. Stiffness is better than pain!
   3 Arthroplasty – refashioning of the joint
   4 Total hip replacement is the main operation for osteo-arthrosis now.

Suggested nursing response for total hip replacement

Before surgery

1 Assessment and preparation (usually of an elderly patient). Obese patients will have been advised on weight reduction (but this is not easy)

2 Observe for indications of cardiac disease, respiratory disease, renal disease and neurological disorders, which may affect the response to anaesthetic and post operative immobilization
3 Blood is tested for cross matching and ordered for transfusion
4 The skin is cleaned thoroughly and shaved. Orthopaedic surgeons still like scrupulous skin preparations with antiseptic solutions to reduce the danger of contamination by skin micro-organisms.
5 Physiotherapy for breathing exercises, coughing and also leg exercises will be given
6 Prophylactic anticoagulants are often prescribed to prevent deep vein thrombosis

The operation The acetabulum is replaced by a cup. The head of the femur is usually replaced by a metal prosthesis to fit into the cup. Various types of prosthesis are used. Some use cement to hold the cup in place (some patients have reaction to this), some modern ones do not need cement.

There may be considerable blood loss during the operation but not necessarily. The hip joint remains unstable after surgery as the capsule of the joint has been opened – there is danger of very easy dislocation of the joint for a few days after the operation.

After the operation

Assessment	Care
1 Positioning of the leg	Leg is kept in abduction with the aid of a special pillow to prevent dislocation. Great care to avoid adduction when turning the patient. Careful support needed for the use of bed pans. Avoid flexion of the hip
2 Positioning of the patient to prevent chest infection and to allow good cardiac action	Gradual and careful lifting into a semi-recumbent position for good ventilation
3 Observe wound and drains – check volume of drainage	Vacuum drainage is maintained. Strict asepsis with all dressings. Drainage and sutures are removed on individual surgeon's instructions – usually drainage in 48 hours and sutures 7–10 days
4 Pressure areas – should be inspected frequently	Relief of pressure. Patient may be able to lift from the bed with the aid of a trapeze (monkey pole). Hygiene. Introduce diet as soon as possible
5 Urine output – suppression due to shock and retention due to immobility and positioning	Urgent care of (possible) renal failure. Assistance first. May need a single sterile catheter for relief
6 Degree of pain – many patients belittle post operative pain in comparison to their previous problems	Prescribed analgesia. Paracetamol may be sufficient in some cases. Avoid narcotics if possible
7 Wound, chest or urinary tract infection. 1 record temperature, pulse, respirations 2 observe sputum and urine (reaction to cement may appear as inflammation too)	Care for infections. Antibacterial drugs as prescribed. Increased fluids. Further need for early introduction of normal diet as soon as possible
8 Deep vein thrombosis – tender, swollen calf	Prevent by exercises. Care for deep vein thrombosis

Mobilization is very much a matter of the surgeon's preferences according to the surgery performed. Physiotherapists will have introduced exercises and these must be continued. Most patients can walk with crutches or a walking frame within one week of surgery.

Trauma of joints

(*Note:* Many joint injuries involve bone fractures too)

Sprain The tearing of ligaments and stretching the joint capsule. The patient complains of severe pain when it occurs and pain that worsens with movement or weight bearing.

Suggested nursing response – first aid
1 Rest the limb
2 Apply cold to the part for early pain relief and minimize swelling
3 Remove possible tight clothing with care

The joint is X-rayed in the Accident Centre and immobilized with adhesive strapping (occasionally plaster of Paris cast).

Ligaments may take some time to repair and joints are very often unstable after a sprain.

Dislocation The displacement of the bones in a joint. Partial displacement is called subluxation and may be caused by a fall or severe wrench. There is pain, swelling, loss of movement of the joint and obvious deformity in most cases.

Congenital dislocation of the hip is a condition of the new born infant – there is sometimes a shallow acetabulum and hormonal laxity of the joint capsule. It should be discovered and corrected on first examination.

Suggested nursing response – first aid
1 Immobilize the limb in the position found   2 Do not attempt to reduce the dislocation

Reduction of a dislocation demands skill on the part of the surgeon to avoid further tissue damage, including damage to nerves and blood vessels. General anaesthetic may be required. Immobilization in strapping or plaster of Paris cast will be for 2–6 weeks.

Repeated dislocations or severe joint damage initially may indicate the need for surgical repair.

Internal derangement of the knee joint

The most common is a torn semilunar cartilage.

Cause A twisting rotation of the joint while the foot is anchored. (Common in football players as studs in their boots anchor the foot as they twist.)

Effects, signs and symptoms The tearing injury causes pain and in some cases, the joint locks in position. Swelling will occur. In those where locking does not occur, further use of the joint will increase the pain.

Prolonged pain on movement causes the patient to 'guard' the joint by increased rest, but there is often muscle wasting when this happens–a factor which can affect post operative recovery.

Diagnosis–investigations
1 Clinical history and examination for a characteristic 'clicking' of the joint
2 X-ray
3 Arthroscopy may be done

Treatment
1 Initially, rest with local heat application for the pain
2 Prescribed analgesia
3 Surgical excision–meniscectomy is performed

Suggested nursing response–first aid
The knee is usually in a bent position. Immobilize it by tying it to the other leg (may be placed across the opposite leg). Do not attempt to change the locked position or straighten the limb.

Meniscectomy–care as for orthopaedic surgery
Before operation Meticulous skin shaving, hygiene and application of preparation lotions.
     Physiotherapy–straight leg raising is taught but is difficult.
After operation The limb is usually immobilized in a Robert Jones bandage or plaster of Paris
     cylinder cast.

The operation is quite painful–give prescribed analgesia. Physiotherapy for restoration of muscle power (quadriceps exercises) starts as soon as tolerated–the nurse needs to encourage the patient to contract the quadriceps muscles frequently through the day. As many are active sportsmen, they need assurances that full activity should be possible within 5–6 weeks.

Disorders of the feet

Talipes–'club foot' is a congenital fault of development. It requires repeated orthopaedic surgery
     and immobilization periods for correction.
Hallux valgus–'bunions' is an acquired deformity of the metatarso-phalyngeal joint of the big
     toe–usually caused by wearing faulty footwear. Keller's operation is used to correct it by
     removing the end of the metatarsal bone.

Nursing note
It should be stressed that, apart from the obvious interference with normal walking, any sores on the feet, fractures involving the foot and surgery involving the foot cause a great deal of pain.

Amputation of a limb

Indications
1 Peripheral artery disease (arteriosclerosis) with gangrene–a complication of diabetes mellitus
     and ageing
2 Prolonged ischaemia of the limb after arterial thrombosis or embolism
3 Crush injuries in which the blood supply has been occluded (see acute renal failure) to prevent
     metabolites entering the circulation
4 Infection by *Clostridium welchii* (gas gangrene)
5 Chronic osteomyelitis
6 Malignant neoplasm (e.g. osteosarcoma)

Amputation may be traumatic but recent advances in micro surgery have led to replacement of severed limbs.

Suggested nursing response–first aid
The severed limb should be placed in a clean, plastic bag, kept as cool as possible (but not in direct contact with ice) for transfer to Accident Centre.

Bleeding should be controlled and sterile dressings applied over the stump.

Surgical removal

Before surgery Psychological assessment and preparation is very important. A careful explanation of the need for surgery will be given.

A careful assessment of the effects on the patient's body image and daily living activities will help the nurse to develop a positive approach. Listening to the anxieties can be met with encouragement of what they will be able to do. An introduction to a (well selected) amputee may help. The family will need to adopt this positive approach too.

Physical assessment and preparation is as for other general surgery. Skin preparation should again be thorough as bone is involved. Blood for emergency transfusion is prepared.

Surgery The site is chosen to give a good blood supply for tissue healing and also to enable good fitting of a prosthesis.

After surgery

Assessment	Care

1 Reactionary haemorrhage
  1 direct vision of the stump (a 'split' bed will help)
  2 measure the contents of the vacuum drain
	Apply tourniquet. Send for medical help. Have blood ready for transfusion. Possibly prepare for return to theatre

2 Possible infection which will delay healing and could cause secondary haemorrhage. Observe for – pyrexia, tachycardia, malaise, dehydration and wound inflammation (also for chest and urine infection)	Strict asepsis with all dressings. Antibacterial agents are sometimes given prophylactically or will be prescribed when first indications appear
3 Correct positioning of the stump to prevent contraction	Extension is maintained initially with the help of sand bags. Later, the patient can control and may spend part of the day in the prone position
4 Correct fashioning of the stump for prosthesis fitting	Elasticated bandaging is re-applied up to four times daily to mould the stump into a cone
5 Measurement for prosthesis is done by an expert limb fitter	Arrange
6 Careful mobilization	Work with the physiotherapist. Help the patient to balance first, then introduce crutches and walking. When limb or a temporary pylon is fitted, walking with sticks and eventually aim to walk without aids
7 Pain – initial post operative pain and phantom pains – as if the limb is still there	Prescribed analgesia. Careful explanation to the patient
8 Psychological acceptance of amputation – altered body image; loss of previous skills; frustrations with rehabilitation programme; periods of depression (often masked by jollity)	Positive encouragement. Wearing of normal clothes and shoes as soon as possible. Praise for newly acquired skills. Listen to fears and anxieties. Provide diversional therapy

Again, it is important to involve the team of medical, nursing, physiotherapy and occupational therapy staff along with social workers and the patient's family in the rehabilitation programme.

New occupations may be needed but many amputees would be able to continue to work in their previous jobs, depending on the skills required. The disablement resettlement officer may well use existing job facilities before organizing complete retraining.

2.7 Skin conditions

The skin

Functions	Structures involved
1 Protection from water	Keratinized epithelial tissues of the epidermis. Sebum (oily secretion of sebaceous glands) is waterproof
2 Protection from micro-organisms	Keratinized epithelium. Sweat from sweat glands is slightly antiseptic. Commensal bacteria inhabit the skin surface and form an additional control on other organisms
3 Protection from ultra violet light	Melanin is secreted by melanocytes in the basement membrane of the epidermis. Secretion is genetic, influenced by exposure to ultra violet light and controlled by hormones

continued overleaf

continued from previous page

Functions	Structures involved
4 Maintaining body temperature for correct homeostasis in cells (Enzymes in the body are temperature specific – they only work at about 39°C)	Temperature regulating centre in the hypothalamus controls vasodilation and vasoconstriction. In vasodilation peripheral blood vessels in the dermis dilate (skin becomes red) so that heat radiates away from skin surface. In vasoconstriction the blood vessels constrict, less blood passes through the skin surface, so less heat is lost. *In heat* Sweat glands will be stimulated to secrete more when vasodilation occurs. Heat is lost by evaporation of sweat. *In cold* Erector pilli muscles contract to lift the hairs and increase the amount of warm air next to the skin surface.
5 Sensitivity to touch, pain, temperature, and pressure	Touch – Meissner's corpuscles, Ruffini's corpuscles, Krause's end bulbs, and free nerve endings. Pain – free nerve endings. Temperature – free nerve endings. Pressure – Ruffini's corpuscles and Pacinian corpuscle. The mechanism of nerve endings in the skin is still being researched
6 Synthesis of vitamin D (required for calcium metabolism)	Ergosterol in the basement membrane is converted to vitamin D by the action of ultra violet light
7 Excretion of waste products	Sweat contains water, sodium and chloride ions and some urea
8 Storage of fat	Adipose tissue
9 Provision of movement and shape to the body – very important in body image	Areolar – loose (elastic) connective tissue. Adipose tissue
10 Some absorption can take place through the skin but not in normal circumstances	

It is believed by some people that the scent of sweat from some glands acts as an aphrodisiac (or love stimulant)!

Conditions of the skin

Dermatitis – inflammation of the skin

Some use the terms dermatitis and eczema to mean the same thing, others prefer to consider eczema as endogenous – due to internal factors and dermatitis as exogenous – due to external factors. The effects of the two are similar.

Eczema

The common type is atopic and usually starts in infants.

Causes
1 Genetic tendency to allergy (associated with allergic rhinits and asthma)
2 Stress factors

Dermatitis

Causes
1 Any external physical or chemical agent. For example
   1 Physical – abrasive dusts; heat and cold extremes; ultra violet light
   2 Chemical – acids, alkalis, antiseptics

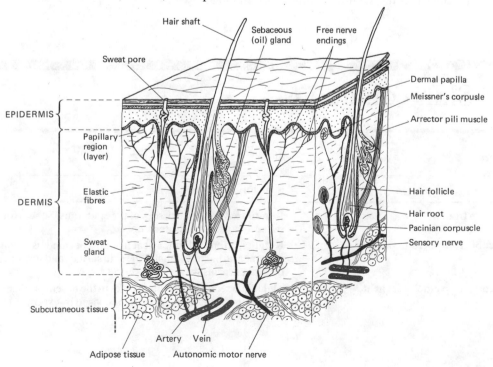

2 Frequent contact with detergents and grease solvents such as petrol reduce the ability of sebum to resist assault by these agents.
3 Allergic (usually more acute in onset)
   1 Allergens include nickel, cosmetics, plants, moulds and drugs
   2 Stress factors as in eczema

Effects, signs and symptoms The inflammation causes redness (erythema) and oedema. Small blisters (vesicles) and elevations of the skin (papules) appear. These may rupture and serum will weep from them (exudation). There is intense irritation eventually. The patient will scratch causing the rash to spread and will allow secondary infection. Scaling and thickening (lichen formation) of the skin will follow, causing even more irritation, scratching and spread.

In eczema, the rash is more diffuse and affects both sides of the body. In dermatitis, it tends to be more localized to the area of contact initially.

The patient may become generally weak and ill if the condition is widespread and persistent.

There is invariably a psychological reaction by the patient. They are very self-conscious of their altered body image and can become depressed or anxious. Anxiety in endogenous eczema may increase the symptoms further.

Diagnosis – investigations
1 Clinical history and examination. This includes a careful nursing history to establish the possible cause and how long the problem has existed
2 Sensitivity testing for the offending substance or allergen

Treatment
1 Removal of the cause
2 Wet dressings with calamine lotion for soothing
3 Steroid skin preparations
4 Antibacterial agents if secondary infection occurs

Suggested nursing response

Assessment	Care
1 Skin rash – type and irritation, area involved, distribution, for secondary infection	Careful assurance of the patient to reduce anxiety. Application of wet dressings. Application of steroid skin preparations – follow instructions carefully – apply sparingly. See British National Formulary for preparations used and the possible undesired effects
2 Psychological factors – evidence of anxiety causes and of anxious or depressed reaction	Individualized care – one nurse to care for one patient is the ideal. Listen to the patient's problems. Give counselling and encouragement that recovery is probable
3 Evidence of allergic reaction to any factors in the ward (e.g. flowers)	Remove the allergen if possible. Report to the physician

Acne vulgaris

Causes
1 Abnormal sensitivity to hormonal changes in puberty
2 Associated with seborrhoea (increased amount of sebum in the skin – described as 'greasy' skin)

Effects, signs and symptoms Plugs of keratinized protein block the exit of sebum onto the skin. Commensal micro-organisms on the skin cause infection which appears as pustules or comedones (known as 'black heads').

The major problem is the acute embarrassment experienced by the patient.

Suggested treatment and nursing care
1 Careful hygiene – regular washing with soap and water and regular hair washing to remove dandruff
2 Exposure to ultra violet light – natural sunlight ideal
3 Aseptic expression of comedones with a comedone extractor
4 Advice on diet reducing fat and carbohydrate intake
5 Antibacterial drugs if indicated

Impetigo

A contagious infection of the skin.

Cause Usually staphylococcal invasion of skin damaged by scratching or shaving.

Effects, signs and symptoms Vesicles and pustules will appear, followed by crusting which causes more scratching and extension of the rash.

In babies, extensive disease can be life threatening.

Suggested treatment and nursing care
 1 Thorough control of spread of infection
   1 to others – using own washing flannels and towels
   2 to themselves – advise to avoid touching and scratching
 2 Antibacterial ointments are applied as prescribed – chlortetracycline is usually used
 3 Crusts may be removed with mild antiseptic solutions

Furuncles and carbuncles

A furuncle is commonly known as a boil and is really a small abscess on the skin. They are usually associated with seborrhoea (greasy skin) and diabetes mellitus. Any pyogenic (pus forming) organism may cause boils.

Nursing notes
Treatment and care is to apply a protective dressing after antiseptic cleansing. Application of heat may accelerate the 'pointing' of a boil but not too hot to damage surrounding tissues.
    Prevent spread of infection when the boil is discharging.
A carbuncle involves a much bigger area of tissue, with multiple 'tracts' of infected material surrounded by inflamed and necrosed tissue.
    The patient may be very ill with a carbuncle.

Suggested treatment and nursing
Wide excision of the necrosed tissue and drainage of the infected material is needed, followed by moist packing of the cavity to allow granulation to occur. Aseptic dressings will be needed for some time, and antibacterial drugs will be needed systemically. The patient may need admission to hospital.
All patients with furuncles and carbuncles should have urine tested for glycosuria to eliminate diabetes mellitus.

Cellulitis

Inflammation of the skin and the underlying tissues.

Cause Invasion by micro-organisms through a minute break in the skin surface.

Effects, signs and symptoms The area is red, swollen, tender and eventually feels 'spongy' to touch. Eventually an abscess will form at the site. There is danger of toxaemia and metabolic rate may be raised.

Suggested treatment and nursing care
 1 Rest the part and care for the febrile patient if necessary
 2 Apply local heat and give prescribed analgesia
 3 Give a prescribed antibacterial agent

Infestations of the skin

Lice
Pediculosis capitis – head lice
  ▶ eggs are called nits and are attached to human hair
  ▶ like to live on clean and short hair
  ▶ damaged by good combing of the hair and then cannot lay eggs
  ▶ killed by application of Malathion or Carbaryl
Pediculosis corporis – body lice
  ▶ eggs laid in clothing
  ▶ disinfestation of clothing
  ▶ patient has a bath and puts on clean clothing

Scabies
  ▶ caused by a mite – acarus scabie
  ▶ direct contact with infested person
  ▶ burrows appear as dark lines (made by female who lays eggs in them)
  ▶ itching and scratching causes infection
  ▶ treatment is by (i) bathing, (ii) application of benzyl benzoate, (iii) bathing again 24 hours later

Psoriasis
Cause Not known but appears to be genetic. Acute episodes are associated with stress and local tissue response to injury.

Effects, signs and symptoms The rate of upward movement of epidermal cells from the basement membrane is increased. Raised, red plaques appear with silvery scales of keratinized cells. Air spaces cause the silvery appearance.
    Commonly appears on the outer (extensor) surface of the elbow and the front of the knee (possibly following minor abrasive injury). Pin point haemorrhage can be seen if the lesion is

scraped. Finger nails may have pin point pits in them. Lesions may be small and inobtrusive or may be very extensive (possibly whole skin surface).

Extensive disease could cause hypothermia and dehydration. The usual problem is cosmetic and psychological. Depression is common.

Suggested treatment and nursing care
1 Tar preparations – including coal tar bathing
2 Careful application of dithranol – only applied to the affected lesion – may cause irritation of normal skin
3 Extensive disease or intractible disease may be treated by PUVA – Psoralen (orally or topically) followed by ultra violet light treatment
4 Careful involvement of the patient, his family and sensitive handling by nursing staff is important in the psychological care. The disease is not infectious and nurses should handle psoriatic skin normally (gloves not indicated)

Tumours of the skin

Warts are not true tumours, but are due to a virus infection of the skin. Plantar warts on the sole of the foot are called verrucae. They may be removed by cryotherapy (application of extreme cold), application of caustic silver nitrate, salicylic acid or diathermy.

Nursing notes
Warts are infectious and individual toilet articles should be used. People with plantar warts should be advised not to attend swimming baths until clear of the infection.

Moles are benign tumours. They may be fleshy or pigmented by melanocytes. Fleshy moles may be removed by cautery, pigmented ones are either left alone or should be totally excised. Moles that increase in size must be reported for expert opinion in case malignancy has occurred.

Squamous cell carcinoma of the skin is most common in elderly patients. They metastasize early, and the areas have usually been subjected to repeated irritation by infection, chemicals or trauma.
Treatment is by excision or radiotherapy or both.

Basal cell carcinoma – also known as **rodent ulcer** or **basal cell epithelioma** is the most common tumour of skin. Growth is slow, beginning as a small papule (raised skin) which spreads outwards, leaving an ulcer in the centre which does not heal. It is related to people exposed to sunlight. A common site is on the face. Metastases are rare.
Treatment is usually by radiotherapy or surgical excision if possible.

Malignant melanoma is the most malignant tumour but also the rarest. The majority arise in pigmented moles or naevi and on skin exposed to sunlight and injury for some time. They appear as black nodules on the skin but may be missed if not easily seen. They metastasize quickly with lymphatic involvement and haemorrhagic spread causing death.
Treatment is by wide excision including the lymph glands draining the area.

Nursing notes
The importance is of course early diagnosis for any hope of success. Observations of moles on patients on long term care is important – any increase in size or darkening should be reported.

Ulcerations of the skin

Pressure sore – decubitis ulcer

Cause Prolonged pressure on the skin

Cause factors Patient – malnutrition; ageing; debilitating condition (e.g. anaemia, diabetes mellitus); incontinence; unconsciousness, paralysis or loss of sensation
Nursing – poor bed making; poor lifting technique and positioning; excessive rubbing and use of soap and water; bed pans left in position too long

Effects, signs and symptoms
Pressure interferes with the blood supply to the area involved. The area becomes inflamed, appears red and is tender. Continued pressure causes necrosis of tissues deep to the skin surface, but again red inflammation may be the only sign to be seen. Eventually this will appear as blackened tissue. The skin surface will be broken, either by abrasion or as the dead tissue (known as slough) breaks away, leaving the ulcer in the form of a crater.

The crater may extend far into the surrounding tissues beyond the broken skin surface. The ulcer is subject to infection and serious wasting and energy loss will occur.

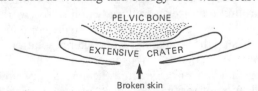

Fig. 2.7.2 Extent of damage with decubitus ulcer (pressure sore)

Treatment

1 Aseptic, non stick dressings to enable granulation tissue to develop
2 Relief of pressure to prevent further damage
3 Some may need antibacterial drugs topically or systemically
4 Some may need extensive plastic surgery

PRESSURE SORE RISK CALCULATOR

SCORING SYSTEM KEY: TOTAL SCORE OF **14** AND BELOW = 'AT RISK'				
A Physical condition	**B** Mental condition	**C** Activity	**D** Mobility	**E** Incontinent
Good 4	Alert 4	Ambulant 4	Full 4	Not 4
Fair 3	Apathetic 3	Walk/Help 3	Slightly limited 3	Occasionally 3
Poor 2	Confused 2	Chairbound 2	Very limited 2	Usually/Urine 2
Very bad 1	Stuporous 1	Bedfast 1	Immobile 1	Doubly 1

Fig. 2.7.3 The Norton scale

Suggested nursing response

Assessment	Care
1 Use Norton scale for calculating risk factors (**low score = high risk**)	Help to improve physical condition by good nutrition and treatment. Stimulate mental condition – try to maintain alertness. Mobilize patients – lift and move carefully. Control incontinence
2 Inspect pressure areas at least two hourly	Change position *at least* 2 hourly. Relieve pressure with nursing aids (sheepskins, ripple beds). Keep the area clean and dry. Apply a waterproof barrier such as silicon or zinc and castor oil if the patient is incontinent. Do not rub or massage
3 Assess the size, shape and depth of the ulcer, and look for any changes. Note the presence of slough, purulent material. Observe for evidence of healing	Strict aseptic techniques for dressings. Apply non stick preparations. Many proprietary products are available (such as silastic foam) which enable granulation without the cavity closing too soon. Waterproof protection films such as 'Op site' help healing and prevent contamination. Care of pressure areas must continue. Cleaning of the ulcer and removal of slough should be done before any application. Lotions used should be discussed with medical staff and some would insist that they should be prescribed

Gravitational ulcers

May be described as **varicose ulcers** when due to varicose veins or **arteriosclerotic** when due to arteriosclerosis.

Varicose ulcers – (see 2.2 for *varicose veins*)

Cause

1 Minor trauma of tissues poorly drained by venous return (tissues are usually oedematous)
2 Often following scratching of eczematous skin

Effects, signs and symptoms The ulcer extends in devitalized tissues with irregular edges. They invariably become infected – commonly by coliform organisms such as pseudomonas.

The patient may complain of soreness and the irritation of surrounding skin. Mobility is further reduced which will make venous return from the part even worse.

Suggested nursing management

1 Improve venous drainage by using support bandaging, elevating the leg when resting, encouraging walking and avoiding standing (but if unavoidable, exercising the toes)
2 Thorough cleansing of the ulcer with hydrogen peroxide or sodium hypochlorite solution.
3 Massage of the tissues around the ulcer to reduce lymph stasis (work away from the ulcer)
4 Application of impregnated dressing bandages which usually contain zinc oxide and may also contain a counter irritant to stop the scratching. Antibacterial solutions may be applied topically or systemic treatment may be needed if serious infection.
5 Firm psychological support and encouragement as healing is very slow. Self contamination of dressings may be an indication of serious loneliness or psychological state.

Arteriosclerotic ulcers

Are caused by the shedding of necrosed skin following an arterial occlusion. They are very painful and do not respond well to treatment. Amputation of the limb may be necessary.

Burns

Causes
1 Dry heat (Moist heat causes a **scald**)
2 Electrical – strong current causes burns on entry and exit, also deep tissues are damaged
3 Radiation – e.g. ultra violet light (including sun burn), infra red light, gamma rays and X-rays
4 Intense light – laser beams
5 Chemicals – strong acids and alkalis

Effects, signs and symptoms

Superficial – partial thickness – first degree The epidermis is red (inflamed), blistered or destroyed. Nerve endings remain and intense pain is experienced, possibly leading to neurogenic shock

Deep – full thickness – second degree The epidermis and dermis are destroyed. Nerve endings may be destroyed and pain may be less severe. As skin is destroyed, plasma exudes and severe fluid loss may lead to hypovolaemic shock. Fluid loss is estimated by Wallace's rule of nines.

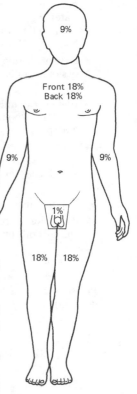

Fig. 2.7.4 Wallace's rule of nines

Partially as a result of burning, partly as a result of dehydration, red cells are destroyed (haemolysis) and haemoglobin may be released. This may block the glomerular filter of the kidney and cause renal failure. Renal failure may also be caused by shock and septicaemia.

Skin destruction allows the entry of micro-organisms and severe infection with toxaemia and septicaemia may occur. Metabolic rate will rise severely and energy demands greatly increased when infection is present.

Apart from the inhalation of hot air, fumes and smoke causing respiratory damage, many patients with severe burns elsewhere develop respiratory effects possibly due to shock or toxins.

For no apparent reason, many patients with burns develop acute gastric, duodenal or intestinal ulcers. Patients with severe burns are initially shocked and ill, then very much afraid of disfigurement and go through periods of deep depression.

Diagnosis – investigations
1 Assessment of the depth and extent of burns is necessary.
2 Blood is taken for cross matching as transfusion may be necessary.
3 An important test is the haematocrit which will be raised due to dehydration.
Haematocrit – the ratio of cell volume to plasma volume in blood.

Treatment
1 *Treatment for shock*
   1 Analgesia for neurogenic shock.
   2 Intravenous fluids (mainly plasma or dextran) for hypovalaemic shock.
   3 Blood is usually given when available.
2 *Treatment of skin destruction*
   1 Exposure method allows dry crust (eschar) to form and granulation occurs underneath.
   2 Closed method uses the application of non stick dressings under strict aseptic technique. Antibacterial impregnated dressings help to prevent and treat infection. Slough and debris must be gently cleared away before dressings are applied.
   3 Skin grafting is needed for extensive full thickness burns as the epidermis cannot regenerate sufficiently.
3 *Treatment of infection* Antibacterial agents may be given intravenously.
4 *Treatment of renal failure* See 2.4 for renal failure.

Suggested nursing response – first aid
1 Put out any fire on the patient's clothing.
2 Make sure that electricity is switched off before approaching (If high voltage electricity, keep 20 metres away as current may jump or 'arc' to burn you.)
3 Reassure the patient.
4 Minor burns and scalds – cool as quickly as possible (hot flesh burns underlying tissues).
5 Chemical burns – apply lots of cold water to dilute the chemical and cool the area.
6 Extensive burns – remove tight articles of clothing, rings or watches. Cover the area with a sterile dressing.
7 Do not give anything by mouth as shock may cause vomiting and loss of consciousness could lead to inhalation pneumonitis.
Transport to Accident Centre urgently.

Suggested nursing care for extensive burns

Assessment	Care
1 Degree of shock and dehydration – blood pressure lowering; restlessness; tachycardia. Later oliguria. Catheter may be introduced to monitor fluid balance. Central venous pressure line	Care of the intravenous infusion. Place in most comfortable position. Low BP – feet raised and head and shoulders raised. Give prescribed analgesia. Continual assurance
2 Extent and depth of burnt skin – later, presence of slough, infected material and dead tissue	Gentle cleansing and removal of slough, dead skin and purulent discharge. Application of non stick dressings. Gentle bandaging. Some are nursed exposed instead of having dressings applied
3 Evidence of infection – pus in the wounds; raised metabolic rate (a shocked patient will not have pyrexia)	Care to prevent infection by strict reverse barrier nursing and using strict aseptic technique for dressings. Give prescribed antibacterial agents. Rest. Glucose may be needed intravenously. Maintain body temperature
4 Nutritional state – there will be serious nitrogen (protein) loss and healing will use up protein and glucose rapidly	Intravenous feeding should be started early using amino acids, lipids and glucose or fructose preparations. Nasogastric feeding may be needed. When possible, the patient should be given as much as 20 mega-joules per day

See 2.4 for nursing of patient in renal failure

5 Psychological reactions – fear and anxiety; altered body image; depression	Careful discussions with the patient reinforcing good progress. Listen to anxieties. Care of scar tissue – an introduction to camouflage cosmetics is very helpful for morale. Guidance on clothing may be needed. May occasionally need professional psychiatric help. Involvement of the family is needed

Please refer to the British National Formulary for individual non stick proprietary dressings and learn the ones used in your local department.

2.8 Endocrine conditions

The endocrine system

This system of ductless gland will be considered by individual glands.

1 **Pituitary gland (hypophysis)**   4 **Supra-renal (adrenal) glands**
2 **Thyroid gland**   5 **Pancreas**
3 **Parathyroid gland**

The gonads (sexual glands) will be studied in 2.9.

1 The pituitary gland (hypophysis)

There are two parts of the gland:
  1 Anterior – adenohypophysis
  2 Posterior – neurohypophysis
Both are closely related to the hypothalamus, the adenohypophysis through a portal vein system and the neurohypophysis through nerve fibres.

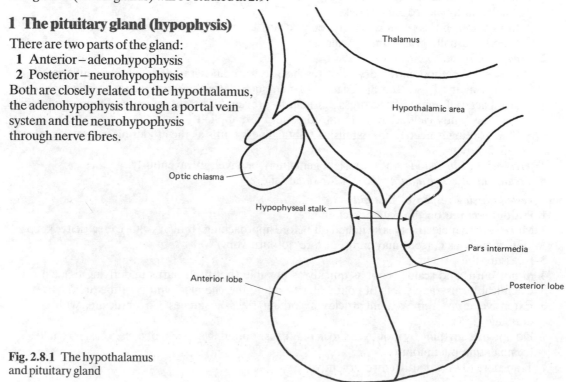

Thalamus

Hypothalamic area

Optic chiasma

Hypophyseal stalk

Pars intermedia

Anterior lobe

Posterior lobe

Fig. 2.8.1 The hypothalamus and pituitary gland

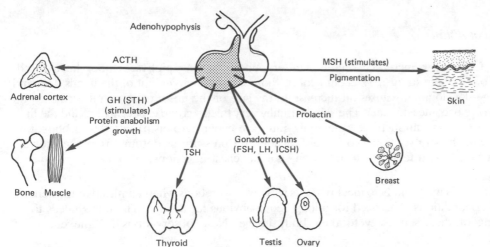

Fig. 2.8.2 Hormones produced by the anterior pituitary gland

Functions	Structures involved
Adenohypophysis	

1 Release of growth hormone (somatotropin) which:
  1 promotes the growth of bone and connective tissues
  2 reduces cell glucose catabolism (break down)
    (antagonizing insulin action)
  3 increases fat catabolism in the cells
	Anterior cells under the influence of a growth hormone releasing hormone from the hypothalamus

2 Release of trophic hormones – those that control the activities of the other glands	Anterior cells under the influence of releasing hormones from the hypothalamus
1 thyrotrophin or thyroid – stimulating hormone (TSH)	Thyrotrophin releasing hormone
2 adrenocorticotrophic hormone (ACTH)	Corticotrophin releasing factor in response to the corticosteroid levels in the blood passing through the hypothalamus
3 follicle-stimulating hormone (FSH) In the female – follicle growth and oestrogen secretion in the ovary. In the male – sperm formation in the testes.	Follicle-stimulating hormone releasing hormone (FSH-RH)
4 luteinizing hormone (LH) in female – ovulation, corpus luteum formation and progesterone secretion	Luteinizing hormone releasing hormone (LH-RH)
5 interstitial cell-stimulating hormone (ICSH) in male – secretion of testosterone in the testes	
6 prolactin – stimulation of milk formation in the breasts and maintenance of corpus luteum	Prolactin release factor in response to high levels of oxytocin in blood. (During pregnancy, inhibition factors are released by the hypothalamus in response to ovarian hormone levels)
3 Release of melanocyte stimulating hormone – influences skin colour	Release mechanism is not known. The cells releasing the hormone are in the area between the two hypophyses – known as the pars intermedia
Neurohypophysis	
1 Release of antidiuretic hormone (ADH) – controls water reabsorption in renal tubules More ADH = more reabsorption Less ADH = less reabsorption	Production is in the hypothalamus. Storage is in the posterior cells. Release is controlled by nerve receptors in the large thoracic veins and the hypothalamus known as osmo-receptors. Changes in the osmotic pressure, the plasma volume and stress affect the release
2 Release of oxytocin – controls uterine contractions and ejection of milk in lactation	Production in the hypothalamus. Storage in the posterior cells. Release by nervous stimulation of the nipples

Conditions of the pituitary gland

Tumours

These are usually benign but may alter functions of the gland or structures close to them. If secretory cells are involved, over secretion of hormones will result. If non secretory cells are involved, the tumour may interfere with secretory cell function and under secretion occurs.

Pressure on the optic chiasma interferes with vision and many cause loss of vision in one half or quarter of the visual field.

Treatment is by removal (hypophysectomy) either through a craniotomy or through the frontal sinuses.

Increased activity of the adenohypophysis (anterior pituitary)

Usually due to an adenoma (tumour).

Gigantism Caused by increased secretion of growth hormone before puberty and afterwards. Some giants have large muscles and may be fit for some time, but many tend to die early through infections. They may suffer from pressure effects of the tumour.

Acromegaly Caused by increased secretion after puberty when epiphyseal lines have fused. Patients are often of big stature. Thickening of the bone causes enlargement of the hands, feet and jaw. Cartilage development causes an increase in the size of the nose, ears, costal cartilage and larynx (the voice becomes deeper). The skin is usually very thick – noted especially around the lips.

They may also have an increased metabolic rate (see hyperthyroidism), altered carbohydrate metabolism with hyperglycaemia, gonad disfunction and pressure symptoms from the growing tumour. They do have a tendency to infection – notably chest infections.

Nursing notes

The general nurse is more likely to meet patients with over secretions when admitted to the general ward for other conditions. The need for a long bed is obvious for a giant. The nurse needs to be understanding of their sensitivity to their body image. Note observations for the effects of acromegaly.

Treatment is by surgical removal of the gland (hypophysectomy), implanting a radioactive isotope such as $Yttrium_{90}$, or cryosurgery (application of cold liquid nitrogen). Bromocriptine reduces growth hormone levels.

Replacement hormones will be needed – hydrocortisone, thyroxine, oestrogen or testosterone are given.

Decreased activity of the adenohypophysis

Pituitary dwarfism is due to a deficiency of growth hormone in a child. All structures may be normally formed but out of proportion. In some cases, arms and legs are stunted. Mental development is normal.

Frohlich's syndrome may be due to damage to the hypothalamus or the pituitary by an invading tumour. It often develops at puberty.

Syndrome consists of *1* obesity *2* drowsiness, *3* sexual immaturity and *4* diabetes insipidus

Simmonds' disease Reduced size (atrophy) of the pituitary or its destruction by

 1 tumours
 2 fractured base of the skull
 3 hypophysectomy
 4 Sheehan's syndrome – thrombosis of blood vessels in the gland following shock (as in postpartum haemorrhage)

Some of the tumours may appear in childhood – growth ceases, resulting in dwarfism and the skin becomes wrinkled (wizened appearance).

In adults, there is general wasting of body tissues with severe weight loss. Anorexia is common. Body hair becomes sparse. There is reduced size of breasts and genitalia, loss of sexual function. Hypoglycaemia and hypotension occur. There is great danger from trauma, infection or stress as adrenocorticotrophic hormone is not produced.

Treatment is to give replacement hormones such as hydrocortisone, thyroxine, testosterone or oestrogen.

Nursing notes

Simmonds' disease is fortunately rare, but an important sequel to profound shock or head injury. Observations are important. Early diagnosis enables treatment for most patients.

The patient will need great encouragement through a lot of psychological stress as well as physical.

Decreased activity of the neurohypophysis (posterior pituitary)

Diabetes insipidus

Is due to an under secretion of antidiuretic hormone.

Causes

 1 Idiopathic – no reason known   **4** Hypophysectomy
 2 Pituitary tumour   **5** Meningitis
 3 Fractured base of skull

Effects, signs and symptoms Reduced amount of antidiuretic hormone or failure of the renal tubules to respond to it, prevents adequate reabsorption of water. The patient passes grossly large quantities of urine (polyuria), (over 20 litres in 24 hours by some patients).

This leads to severe dehydration and thirst (polydipsia) with the patient needing to drink corresponding amounts of fluid.

Diagnosis – investigations

 1 Clinical history
 2 Careful records of fluid intake and output
 3 Water deprivation test – no fluids given for 8–12 hours. If diabetes insipidus – polyuria continues with weight loss, dehydration and electrolyte levels rise in serum

Nursing note

The patient needs careful supervision and observation. Severe dehydration may cause shock with hypotension and collapse.

Vasopressin test – positive responses to vasopressin.

Treatment Vasopressin (antidiuretic hormone) is given as lypressin nasal spray or desmopressin nasal spray or intramuscular injection.

Suggested nursing response

Assessment	Care
1 Fluid balance – intake and urinary output carefully measured	Provide 2 or 3 jugs of fluid on locker and replace regularly when used. Provide more than one urinal or bed pan for use if the patient is in bed
2 Assess for dehydration and possible shock – headache, anorexia, nausea; weight loss; loss of skin elasticity; blood pressure	Report to medical staff. Increase fluid intake

Response to prescribed treatment is very good but needs to be continued. A lot of relief is found but encouragement is still needed.

Hypophysectomy See 2.6 for craniotomy

Nasal route

Before operation

1 Nasal swabs are taken for culture of organisms
2 Antiseptic nasal cream applied
3 Prophylactic antibacterial drugs may be given
4 Corticosteroids may be given before surgery
5 Careful explanation and reassurance are needed for the patient and their family

After operation

1 Assess for evidence of rising intracranial pressure. Activity is reduced to avoid increased pressure – blowing of the nose and sneezing should be avoided.
2 Assess for leakage of cerebro spinal fluid in the nose. Gentle swabbing of running nose with sterile swab.
3 Assess for indications of infection – see care of patient with meningitis
4 Assess for adrenal insufficiency (low blood pressure, nausea, vomiting and extreme weakness). Corticosteroids may prevent this.
5 Cortisone replacement therapy may be given intravenously initially but then orally. Dosage is gradually reduced to a minimum maintenance dose.
6 Thyroxine is usually started orally 2–3 days after surgery.

2 The thyroid gland

Functions	Structures involved

1 Manufacture, storage and secretion of thyroid hormones
  1 Thyroxine T_4
    Tetra iodo thyronine / 4 iodine atoms
	Thyroid hormones combine with a globulin for storage in the colloid material.
	Released into blood, they combine with a blood protein (protein bound iodine – PBI) for transport to tissues

2 Tri iodo thyronine T_3 / 3 iodine atoms	
Thyroid hormones – control metabolic rate; influence physical and mental growth of children; activate nervous systems; influence vitamin A formation; affect glucose absorption in the intestine; lower serum cholesterol	Growth of gland and activity – thyroid-stimulating hormone (TSH) from pituitary
2 Manufacture and secretion of calcitonin – decreases the blood serum calcium level (antagonized by parathormone)	Released from special 'C' cells in the gland

Note also:

1 The abundant blood supply from carotid artery branches (inferior and superior thyroid arteries)
2 The proximity of the trachea and the recurrent laryngeal nerve
3 The parathyroid glands embedded in the poles of the gland

Conditions of the thyroid gland

Goitre

Enlargement of the thyroid gland.

Causes

1 Iodine deficiency in the diet
2 Substances blocking the uptake of iodine by the thyroid

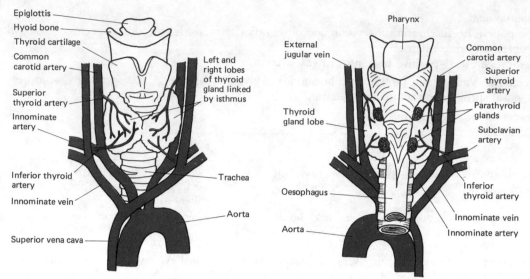

Fig. 2.8.3 The thyroid and parathyroid glands

Iodine deficiency→low thyroxine levels→increased thyroid-stimulating hormone→increased gland size.

Blockage (drugs for hyperthyroidism, salicylates, lithium)→low thyroxine production→increased thyroid-stimulating hormone→increased gland size

The swelling is painless but may cause pressure symptoms or cosmetic embarrassment.
It is not associated with hyperthyroidism.

Prevention–introducing iodine into the diet (iodized table salt)

Treatment

1 Potassium iodide prevents enlargement
2 If hypothyroidism, adults may need thyroxine
3 Surgery if gross disfigurement or pressure symptoms such as dyspnoea or dysphagia

Hyperthyroidism or thyrotoxicosis or Graves' disease

Increased secretion of thyroid hormones.

Cause

1 Not known in some cases
2 An emotional shock may activate the disease
3 There is evidence of an antibody–long acting thyroid stimulating substance (LATS) but the mechanism of its formation is not known.

Effects, signs and symptoms

1 Increased metabolic rate
    1 The skin is hot and sweating is profuse
    2 The pulse rate is increased even when sleeping
    3 There is a large appetite but loss of weight
    4 Activity is increased and tremors may occur
2 Increased nervous activity–restlessness, agitation and apparent anxiety states
3 Exophthalmos–protrusion of the eye ball is due to increased tissues behind the eye but the mechanism is not understood

Long standing disease may eventually lead to cardiac arrhythmia, enlargement and heart failure.

Diagnosis – investigations

1 Clinical history and examination
2 Regular pulse chart and sleeping pulse recordings
3 Circulating thyroid hormone levels
4 Radio isotope ^{131}Iodine uptake test–increased uptake in hyperthyroidism
5 Thyroid-release hormone (TRH)/thyroid-stimulating hormone (TSH) relationship test–in hyperthyroidism, TRH will *not* cause an increase of TSH

Treatment

1 Antithyroid drugs, carbimazole or propylthiouracil. Cardiac arrhythmias are controlled by propranalol
2 Radio isotope ^{131}Iodine therapy (mainly used for older patients)
3 Thyroidectomy

Suggested nursing response

Assessment	Care
1 Increased metabolic rate – hot, sweaty skin (but usually good complexion); tachycardia, palpitations; electrocardiography for arrhythmias; sleeping pulse; appetite; weight loss; over activity	Provide washing facilities. Light clothing. Well ventilated room. Encourage rest – reduce stimulations – possible sedation. Give prescribed propranalol for cardiac arrhythmias. Encourage high protein and carbohydrate diet. Fluids encouraged, but avoid coffee and tea if possible
2 Increased nervous activity – restlessness, agitation, anxiety state. Also embarrassment about exophthalmos	Relaxed approach by staff. Sedation may be prescribed. Listening to anxieties and explain the condition to the patient and their relatives. Spectacles (possibly tinted) may help to disguise eye ball protrusion
3 Undesired effects of antithyroid drugs (see National Formulary for full range) – indications of infection (pyrexia) if white cell count is diminished (leucopenia); skin rashes in hypersensitive patients	Report to physicians. Withhold drug until seen. Care of infection. Control of body temperature. Many need calamine lotion for skin rash

Thyroidectomy

Before surgery

1 Medical treatment with antithyroid drugs and propranalol would be given prior to surgery
2 Lugol's iodine is given to reduce the vascularity of the gland (about 2 weeks prior to surgery)
3 Careful explanation of the operation and assurance about the scar healing is necessary
4 Skin cleansing and shaving are as for general surgery

Surgery

1 About 80% of the gland is removed
2 The parathyroid glands must be left
3 Closure with clips or sutures. Suture line along natural crease of skin
4 Most surgeons would include a vacuum drain to the bed of the gland

After surgery

1 Sit the patient up as soon as possible with the head and neck well supported
2 Sips of water to relieve a dry mouth and throat – normal diet resumed as soon as tolerated

Observe for complications	Care required
1 Haemorrhage – check vacuum drain and back of the neck. Difficulty in breathing or swallowing indicate pressure from bleeding or haematoma	Inform surgeon. Prepare for return to theatre. Open clips and allow blood or clot to be evacuated
2 Thyroid crisis – rare but dangerous! Excessive thyroid hormone released into the blood stream – acute rise in metabolic rate with severe tachycardia and hyperpyrexia, restlessness and death from heart failure	Urgent – report immediately. Propranalol is given for tachycardia. Cooling fans and light clothing or even tepid sponging. Corticosteroids may be given
3 Recurrent laryngeal nerve damage – hoarseness of the voice persisting; dysphonia (difficulty speaking); laryngeal stridor (noisy difficult breathing)	Reassurance – permanent damage is rare. If both cords are paralyzed and breathing difficulty, tracheostomy may be needed
4 Carpo-pedal spasm (tetany) – painful muscular contractions, especially of the hands and feet and possible cardiac arrhythmia which may occur up to a week after surgery. (Tetany is due to damaged parathyroid gland and loss of blood calcium)	Intravenous injection of calcium gluconate is given. Later, oral calcium and vitamin D may be given
5 Hypothyroidism (myxoedema) – usually appears later	Thyroxine is given

The drain is removed within 24–48 hours. Clips and sutures are removed in 3–5 days. (Quote your local practice in examination answers.)

Advice should be given about jewellery or clothing to disguise the wound in early days, but healing is usually very clean.

Exophthalmos may remain after surgery.

Hypothyroidism

Decreased secretion of thyroid hormones. Congenital type affecting children is **cretinism** – there is stunted growth and mental subnormality if not treated early. Early indications may be sluggish responses, feeding problems, enlarged tongue, subnormal temperature, bradycardia and constipation.

Treatment is by giving thyroxine

Nursing note

Early recognition of the condition by nursing staff and response to mothers' anxieties may prevent serious disorder by starting treatment as soon as possible.

Myxoedema

Cause

1 Part of the ageing process (thyroid gland becomes smaller with age)
2 Auto immune disease (Hashimoto's disease)
3 Result of radioactive ^{131}Iodine treatment
4 Result of thyroidectomy
5 Forgetting to take thyroxine!
6 Goitres with iodine deficiency

Effects, signs and symptoms

Lowered metabolic rate

1 The skin is cold, coarse and dry. Hair is thin and easily falls out
2 There is increased sensitivity to cold
3 Temperature, pulse and blood pressure are all below normal
4 Appetite is poor, but weight increases. Constipation is common

Lowered nervous activity

1 The patient is slow mentally
2 There is a tendency to deafness
3 Lethargy and apathy develop

The signs and symptoms may appear very slowly and insidiously – as much as five years before diagnosis is made, as they correspond with normal ageing in the early stages.

Nursing note

It is important to observe patients in long stay wards for indications of myxoedema.

Many patients are admitted to the wards with severe hypothermia in winter months and are then found to have myxoedema.

Diagnosis – investigations

1 Clinical history and examination
2 Nursing history from the patients' relatives is helpful
3 Blood for thyroid hormone levels

Treatment Thyroxine sodium: the commencing dose is 50–100 micrograms, or for elderly patients 25 micrograms. This is increased gradually to a maintenance dose of 100–300 micrograms daily. Patients need reminding to continue for life. Withholding of the drug will not reveal problems for some time.

Suggested nursing response

Assessment	Care
1 Lowered metabolic rate	
1 cold, coarse, dry skin, thin hair	Avoid excess use of soap. Oily lotions for cleaning would help. Great care needed with combing and brushing hair
2 increased sensitivity to cold, low temperature, bradycardia	Nurse in a warm room. Provide extra bed clothes. Accept limited activity – do not 'drive' them
3 poor appetite, constipation	Provide high fibre, high protein but reduced carbohydrate and fat diet. Prescribed laxatives, suppositories or enemas may be needed
2 Lowered nervous activity – mental dullness, lethargy, apathy and deafness	Patient approach by the nurse. Inform relatives who may be exasperated and assure of improvement with treatment. Provide communication aids. Face to face speaking. Possibly hearing aid
3 Hypothermia – subnormal temperature (below 35°C) recorded by a low reading rectal thermometer or oesophageal probe. Below 33°C, cardiac arrhythmia, confusion and coma are life threatening	Reheating is slow unless below 33°C when careful rapid warming in an intensive care unit is needed. 33–36°C – apply blankets – the reflective 'space' blanket is popular. Aim to increase by 0.5°C per hour. Nurse in a warm room

See also *care of the elderly patient* 2.15

3 The parathyroid glands

Function	Structures involved

Manufacture and secretion of parathormone which controls plasma calcium levels by:
  1 mobilizing calcium and phosphate from bone if calcium levels fall,
  2 reducing the excretion of calcium in the kidney,
  3 promoting intestinal absorption of calcium.
Note: The balance of calcium salts in the plasma is necessary for
  1 normal muscular contraction including the heart muscle
  2 blood clotting
  3 normal nerve impulse transmission
	Cells of the four glands – release is in reponse to a fall in the plasma calcium level

Conditions of the parathyroid glands

Hyperparathyroidism – increased secretion of parathormone

Primary Usually due to benign adenoma but may be due to overgrowth (hyperplasia) or, rarely, cancer

Secondary Increased loss of calcium through damaged kidneys or malabsorption stimulates over activity

Effects, signs and symptoms Excessive serum calcium causes weakness and eventually muscle paralysis. Bowel distension causes pain and constipation occurs with reduced peristalsis.

Anorexia, nausea and vomiting may cause the patient not to drink, increasing the concentration of calcium in urine, resulting in ureteric calculi. Calcium is withdrawn from bone tissue, leaving brittle bones which may fracture easily.

Nervous tissue damage may cause behaviour changes.

Treatment is by surgical removal for primary disease. Vitamin D may be given for secondary disease.

Nursing notes
Careful observation of muscle weakness and cardiac monitoring may be needed. Great care is needed when lifting and moving patients to avoid pathological fractures.

The surgery would be performed in a specialist unit, but the principles are very similar to those for thyroidectomy.

Hypoparathyroidism

Reduced secretion of parathormone. It is usually a sequel to damage in thyroidectomy but it may occur spontaneously when, for no apparent reason, the glands become very small (atrophy).

Effects, signs and symptoms
Tetany Low serum calcium levels causes increased muscular excitability and nerve activity. Spasmodic contractions of muscle groups occur – classically those of the wrist and ankle causing carpo-pedal spasm.

The patient may complain of tingling sensations as sensory nerves are activated. Laryngeal spasm may obstruct the airway. Epilepsy may occur. Behaviour changes may be noted.

Treatment is by giving calcium gluconate intravenously and orally, but maintenance is kept by giving vitamin D.

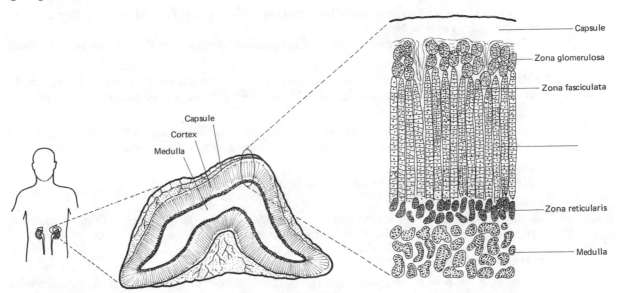

Fig. 2.8.4 The adrenal glands

4 The supra renal or adrenal glands (see Fig. 2.8.4)

Functions	Structures involved
1 Manufacture and secretion of corticosteroid hormones	Cells of the cortex. Influenced by adrenocortico trophic hormone (ACTH)
Glucocorticoids *1* balance the building up (anabolism) and breaking down (catabolism) of protein. Protein is broken down to amino acids and converted to glucose in the liver (gluconeogenesis). *2* balance the action of insulin on glucose *3* influence the distribution of body fats	
Mineralocorticoids – main one being *aldosterone* which increases the reabsorption of sodium ions in the renal tubule. Sodium takes water with it and increases the blood volume	Cells in the outer part of the cortex known as zona glomerulosa. Release is in response to reduced blood flow to the kidney, renin release, angiotensin formation. Angiotensin stimulates production of aldosterone
Sex hormones – androgens, oestrogen and progesterone. The sex hormones determine the masculinity or femininity of the individual, influencing hair distribution, breast formation, genital development and behaviour	Cells in the deeper part of the cortex known as zona reticularis
2 Manufacture and secretion of adrenaline and noradrenaline. Noradrenaline causes wide vasoconstriction and increases blood pressure. Adrenaline causes increased heart rate; dilation of bronchi; release of glucose from liver and muscle glycogen; increased metabolic rate	Cells of the medulla. Release stimulated by nerve endings of the sympathetic nervous system originating in the hypothalamus in response to stress, fright, trauma or inflammation

Nursing examinations
Fear stimulates your hypothalamus to cause increased release of adrenaline which releases more glucose for your brain cells to work!

Conditions of the supra renal glands

Addison's disease

Causes
1 May be due to atrophy of the gland for no apparent reason – possibly auto immune reaction
2 Tuberculosis of the glands
3 Rarely, tumours of the glands

Effects, signs and symptoms Reduced activity of the cortex leads to reduced levels of hormones. Gluconeogenesis is impaired and hypoglycaemia occurs. The patient feels tired, tends to lose weight and complains of anorexia and nausea. There is a loss of sodium and water from the body causing a low blood pressure.

There is a classic 'bronze' pigmentation of the skin due to increased release of ACTH which behaves like melanocyte stimulating hormone.

There is a marked inability to cope with stress – including minor infections, trauma or exposure.

Acute adrenal failure – Addisonian crisis

There is a sudden loss of sodium and water with a fall of blood pressure causing shock. Renal failure may occur due to hypovolaemia.

There may be extreme weakness and debility with vomiting. If untreated, coma and death will follow.

Treatment of crisis Intravenous saline is given very quickly, cortisol is given intravenously (hydrocortisone). The patient's feet should be raised. Recovery may be quite dramatic.

Nursing notes
Observations for acute adrenal failure are important – debility, indications of shock including blood pressure recording. If any doubt, send for medical help as life is threatened.

Treatment of Addison's disease
1 Hydrocortisone   2 Fludrocortisone (mineralocorticoid drug)

Nursing notes
The patient will need a steroid card and advice on increasing the dose if infection occurs. Some will carry an emergency ampoule of hydrocortisone for injection if crisis should occur.

Cushing's syndrome

Is mainly caused now by the prolonged use of corticosteroid drugs and is due to the increased circulating levels of the hormones.

Effects, signs and symptoms

1 *Glucocorticoid*

   1 Increased breakdown of protein (catabolism) leads to muscle wasting, osteoporosis with pathological fractures (collapsed vertebrae) and delayed wound healing.

   2 Increased gluconeogenesis (antagonising insulin) produces diabetes mellitus with glycosuria, polyuria and polydipsia.

   3 Altered fat distribution to the face, shoulders and abdomen.

2 *Mineralocorticoid* Increases sodium and water retention causing oedema (fat and oedema in the face gives moon shape). Fluid retention also increases blood pressure.

3 *Sexual* Altered androgen and oestrogen levels bring about change to opposite gender. Women tend to have more hair including facial hair (hirsuitism), smaller breasts and an enlarged clitoris. Men tend to have less hair, enlarged breasts (gynaecomastasia) and smaller genitalia. Voice changes and behaviour are affected too.

Treatment is by adjusting drug dosage if possible.

Suggested nursing reponse

Protein break-down

1 Measure muscle wasting by upper arm circumference
2 Remember the patient's weakness of muscle power
3 Very careful lifting and moving to avoid fractures
4 Old scars and ulcers may break down

Diabetes mellitus

1 Test urine daily for glycosuria
2 May need control by diet

Fluid retention	*Sexual changes*
1 Care of oedematous skin	1 May need sexual counselling
2 Reduced sodium intake in diet	2 Spouse may need a lot of support
3 Observe blood pressure	

Condition of the medulla – phaeochromocytoma

A rare tumour which secretes adrenaline and noradrenaline. They are usually in the medulla of the suprarenal gland but may be found in other parts of the body.

Over secretion of adrenaline causes a very marked rise of blood pressure which may cause heart failure or cerebrovascular accident.

Treatment is by surgical removal.

5 The pancreas

See 2.3 for digestive functions.

Endocrine functions	Structures involved
1 Manufacture and release of glucagon.	Alpha cells in the islets of Langerhans
Glucagon causes the break down of glycogen to glucose – increasing blood glucose levels	Release is in response to a lowering of blood glucose levels
2 Manufacture and release of insulin.	Beta cells in the islets of Langerhans
Insulin promotes the movement of glucose across the cell membrane for metabolism within the cell – reducing blood glucose levels. Insulin stimulates glycogen formation in the liver	Release is in response to a rising blood glucose level, particularly after a meal
Insulin and glucose needs are dependent on the energy demands of the tissues.	

Conditions of the pancreas

Diabetes mellitus

Cause factors

1 Familial – strong evidence but gene not identified yet. It is more common in Western civilization where it may be as high as 10% of populations.

2 Related to ageing, obesity and stress although direct cause not established. (Often found in older patients in grief over the loss of a loved one.)

3 Treatment with corticosteroids (which antagonize insulin).

Effects, signs and symptoms The pancreas fails to secrete enough insulin or antagonists to insulin prevent glucose from entering the cell for increased energy demand.

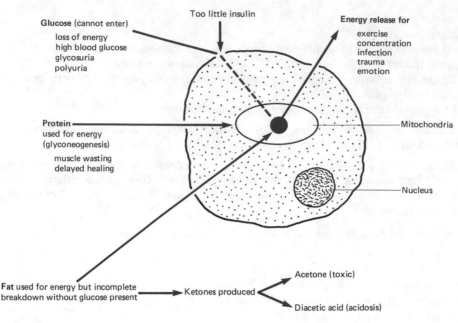

Fig. 2.8.5
Diabetes mellitus

Loss of energy The patient feels more tired and drowsy, unable to concentrate and may be irritable

High blood glucose Once above the renal threshold (average 10 m.mol/l) glycosuria will occur. There is increased glucose in the sweat and patients complain of pruritis

Glycosuria The glucose has an osmotic diuretic effect and increased volumes of urine are passed (polyuria). The fluid loss leads to dehydration and acute thirst (polydipsia)

Protein glyconeogenesis Muscle wasting and weakness may further reduce activity. Younger patients appear thin and feeble, older patients tend to put weight on but this is fat and not protein. Wound healing is delayed – minor abrasions, incisions and pressure sores may persist

Ketosis When energy demands increase further, fats may be used for energy, but ketones are produced as well. Keto-acidosis leads to vomiting, coma and death.

Diagnosis – investigations

1 Clinical history and examination
2 Ward urine test for glycosuria
3 Blood glucose levels (normal 3–5 m.mol/l)
4 Glucose tolerance tests

Suggested nursing response – glucose tolerance test

1 The patient is fasted from midnight.
2 In the morning, at the start of the test, 50 g of glucose in water is given.
3 Blood glucose and insulin levels are recorded after taking samples of venous blood every half hour. Both levels should normally return to the fasting level within two hours.
4 Glycosuria may be tested also but specimens may be difficult to obtain.

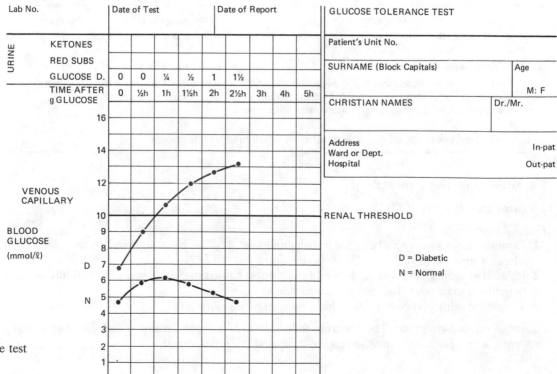

Fig. 2.8.6
Glucose tolerance test

Treatment

Consists of ensuring a correct balance between:
 1 Energy demands (daily living patterns)
 2 Glucose (carbohydrate) controlled diet
 3 Insulin requirements

When more work is needed, more glucose and more insulin are required.

 1 *Controlled carbohydrate diet* Between 100 g and 250 g per day are needed in divided portions according to work pattern, e.g. more for breakfast if work is heavy between then and lunch time.

Nursing note

Diet may need to be replaced by glucose drinks or intravenous glucose when the patient is not able to eat or is vomiting.

 2 *Other diet factors* Vegetable protein is preferred now to avoid fat content of meats. Fat control is vital too. High fibre improves absorption and peristalsis.

 3 *Insulin* is prescribed in small doses initially, gradually increasing and/or changing the type of insulin until stabilization is reached.
 1 Short but quick acting – soluble and neutral insulin
 2 Intermediate   – isophane insulin
 3 Long acting   – insulin zinc suspension

 4 *Oral hypoglycaemic agents*
 1 Sulphonylureas (e.g. chlorpropamide, tolbutamide) act by augmenting insulin action
 2 Biguanides (metformin) acts by increasing tissue utilization of glucose

All early onset patients need insulin and diet. Mature onset patients may only need the diet or the diet and oral hypoglycaemic agents. All need insulin to cover stabilization, serious infection, trauma or surgery.

Hypoglycaemia

May be caused by either, too much insulin, too much of a sulphonylurea, too little diet or very strenuous exercise when the muscles take up the glucose and more glycogen forms in the liver. The low blood glucose level affects the brain cells, producing hunger, sweating, mood changes (loss of temper), tachycardia and eventual loss of consciousness. Many patients have epileptiform fits.

Treatment is urgent

Oral glucose if still conscious   Intramuscular glucagon   Intravenous glucose

Suggested nursing response – first aid

If in doubt, treat as hypoglycaemia by giving glucose, prepare glucose injection or give prescribed glucagon

Suggested nursing response – prevention
 1 Always give glucose or a meal within 20–30 minutes of giving insulin.
 2 Advise the patient to carry extra glucose for strenuous exercise or when feeling hypoglycaemic.
 3 Many centres allow patients to experience a minor hypoglycaemic attack for them to detect warning signs and symptoms.
 4 Beware of long acting insulins in the night time. If inadequate carbohydrate has been taken, hypoglycaemia can occur in the early hours of the morning.

Ketoacidotic or diabetic coma

Causes
 1 Increased energy demands (especially infection)
 2 Inadequate treatment (sometimes neglect or carelessness by the patient)

Effects, signs and symptoms Ketones (acetone and diacetic acid) are produced by incomplete fat metabolism. Vomiting and gradually developing coma occur. Acetone is smelt in the breath. Ketones are present in the urine (ketonuria). Acidosis (lowered blood pH) leads to over breathing (hyper ventilating). By exhaling more carbon dioxide, carbonic acid dissociates in the blood in an attempt to correct the pH.

   High blood glucose (hyperglycaemia) leads to increased glycosuria; osmotic diuresis leads to severe dehydration. The skin is usually hot and dry. The patient will be very thirsty while still conscious.

Diagnosis – investigations
 1 Clinical history – usually more gradual onset but patient may be found in a coma
 2 Clinical examination – hot, dry skin, acetone on breath
 3 Blood glucose is high – over 10 m.mol/l
 4 Blood pH is low (below 7.4)

Treatment
 1 Intravenous or intramuscular soluble insulin or neutral insulin, to increase glucose metabolism and reduce fat metabolism

2 Intravenous sodium bicarbonate to correct the acidosis

3 Intravenous saline and dextrose to correct dehydration
(*Note:* Glucose is required for energy, and complete fat metabolism while insulin is being given)

4 Intravenous potassium is needed as, with insulin therapy, potassium may be lost from the blood into the cells (prevents cardiac arrhythmia).

Suggested nursing response

Assessment	Care
1 Rising ketone levels – nausea and vomiting, loss of consciousness; acetone on breath; ketonuria; over-breathing	Semiprone position to prevent inhalation of vomit. Nasogastric tube for aspiration. Give prescribed soluble insulin (usually according to blood glucose levels and ketonuria). Prescribed intravenous sodium bicarbonate or lactate
2 Rising blood glucose – glycosuria. (It is more usual now to test peripheral blood sample with a reagent strip)	Give prescribed insulin. Catheterization for testing of urine (and also accurate fluid loss measurement). Dressing to puncture sites
3 Evidence of dehydration – hot, dry skin; sunken orbits; rapid pulse, low blood pressure	Maintain intravenous infusion. Mouth care will be needed. Care of the skin
4 Progressive loss of consciousness – drowsiness; loss of consciousness	Care of the unconscious patient. Turning at least two hourly
5 Cardiac arrhythmias if low blood potassium – cardioscope monitoring	Prescribed potassium – great care needed when given intravenously – must be thoroughly mixed
6 Evidence of infection – raised temperature, tachycardia; cough, sputum; urine; diarrhoea	Maintain body temperature. Continue rest even when conscious. Prescribed antibacterial agents will be needed

Associated conditions or complications of diabetes mellitus

Every body system is affected in some way and the following are just examples of problems

Respiration Prone to chest infections including pulmonary tuberculosis

Circulation Arteriosclerosis in peripheral arteries leads to 'diabetic gangrene'. See 2.2. Prone to coronary thrombosis

Digestion Prone to gastrointestinal infections

Excretion Prone to urinary tract infections. Nephrotic syndrome (see 2.4) is very dangerous

Nervous Peripheral neuritis produces altered sensation. Cataract and retinopathy may lead to visual loss

Locomotor Bone fractures may take longer to heal. Immobilization increases danger of pressure sores

Skin Minor skin lesions heal slowly and may be infected. Prone to pressure sores if immobilized. May develop tissue damage at the site of insulin injections (less common with purified insulins)

Reproduction Pregnancy may be normal, but babies are often large and help with labour may include the need for caesarian section. There is an increased risk of the child being diabetic. Rarely, autonomic neuritis may cause impotence.

Psychological effects

1 Loss of self esteem – it may be difficult for a patient (particularly young one) to come to terms with a permanent condition and the need for care.

2 Fear – many may become anxious about complications and depression may occur.

3 Learning – there is no reason why normal schooling should not take place. Diabetics learn their own condition and control very well (if taught well!).

Suggested nursing response Advice and care are needed – for example

Infections The patient needs advice to avoid crowds or other patients with known infections. The diabetic diet is a good healthy one to help prevent infection – encourage

Skin lesions Prevent by scrupulous care of the skin. Great care of the feet is needed. Older patients may need a chiropodist to cut toe nails. All wounds should be dressed carefully

See also, *care of amputee following gangrene 2.6.*

Urinary tract Encourage a good fluid intake. Strict care of the perineal and genital area to avoid infection

Circulation Encourage exercise – many diabetic patients are thoroughly involved in sport, dancing and outdoor activities.

Psychology Introduce the patient to the British Diabetic Association and their magazine *Balance*, which gives useful information for normal living – articles by famous diabetics and recipes for diet variations.

Teaching for self care

1 Awareness and ability of the patient first. Try to plan within an active day

2 Plan progressive lessons in giving insulin; urine testing; blood testing; diet control and variations

3 Let them practice under supervision but gradually withdraw
4 Praise their good efforts

Diabetes mellitus and surgery

All patients will need insulin and glucose to cover the period of surgery. Observations for hypoglycaemia and keto-acidosis must be constant.

Following surgery There is increased risk of chest infection. Wound healing may be delayed and there is increased risk of wound infection.

Stabilization with glucose, diet and insulin will be needed, but many older patients can quickly resume oral hypoglycaemic drugs if they have no difficulty in following the prescribed diet.

2.9   Reproductive conditions

The male reproductive system

This system will be considered as follows.

1 The testes, epididymis and scrotum   2 The vas deferens and seminal vesicles   3 The penis
Conditions of the prostate gland and urethra **are in 2.4.**

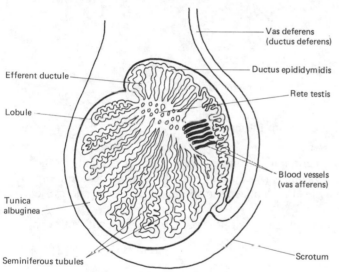

Fig. 2.9.1 Section through the male reproductive organs

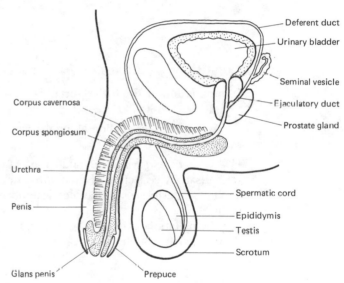

Fig. 2.9.2. Tubules of the testis and epididymis

1 The testes, epididymis and scrotum

Testes

Functions	Structures involved
1 Spermatogenesis – the production of sperm from germ cells. The process is called meiosis or reduction division as the number of chromosomes is halved from 23 pairs (diploid) to 23 (haploid)	Cells lining the seminiferous tubules. Sperm formation is stimulated by the follicle-stimulating hormone (FSH) from the pituitary gland
2 The manufacture and secretion of hormones – mainly testosterone Testosterone acts by: *1* producing masculinity through growth of male genitalia, body hair distribution, skeletal framework and behaviour *2* building up of body protein (anabolism) in the form of muscle and bone *3* mild effects on renal tubules – sodium and water reabsorbed, potassium excreted *4* inhibiting production of FSH and ICSH	Interstitial cells in the lobules of the testes (Leydig cells). Testosterone is released by stimulation from the hypothalamus, and interstitial cell-stimulating hormone (ICSH) from the pituitary gland, beginning at puberty

Epididymis

Functions	Structures involved
1 Storage of sperm – usually about 1–3 weeks	Long coiled tubes (about 5–6 metres long) embedded in a
2 Maturation of sperm	fibrous tissue. Connected to the testis at the head of the
3 Secretes about 5% of the seminal fluid	epididymis and to the vas deferens at the tail
4 Releases sperm for ejaculation when orgasm takes place	

Note: Complete maturation of sperm for penetration of the ovum is not complete until *capacitation* which may in fact take place in the female tract.

Scrotum

Functions	Structures involved
1 Provides a compartment for the testes and the epididymis	Pouch of skin, an inner double lining of serous membrane – the tunica vaginalis
2 Maintains the temperature of the testes for maximum spermatogenesis (slightly below body temperature)	The smooth muscle in the pouch known as the dartos muscle and the cremaster muscle attached to the testis will contract when cold to elevate the testes and reduce the size of the scrotal pouch

Note: The contents of the scrotum have many nerve endings and are therefore extremely sensitive to touch and pain. There is a large blood supply through the testicular artery and drainage by the vein, both travelling through the spermatic cord with the vas deferens.

Conditions of the testes, epididymis and scrotum

Inflammation of the testes – orchitis

Causes
  1 An ascending infection along the vas deferens from the urethra
  2 Mumps (parotitis)

Effects, signs and symptoms Sudden onset of inflammation causes severe pain and swelling in the scrotal sac. A collection of fluid in the tunica vaginalis (hydrocele) may develop and cause more swelling. Interference of the blood supply may lead to death of the spermatogenic cells and cause sterility.
  The metabolic rate is raised, with quite a high fever and with the pain, the patient will feel very ill. Urinary symptoms may be absent.

Inflammation of the epididymis – epididymitis

Causes
  1 Ascending infection from the urethra by a pyogenic organism (including gonococcus – sexually transmitted disease)
  2 Possibly a complication of prostatectomy

Effects, signs and symptoms Again, the inflammation causes acute pain, swelling of the scrotum and a possible hydrocele. The patient usually does have urinary symptoms which may be burning micturition with urethritis or frequency of micturition with cystitis. Sterility may again be a complication.
  Metabolic rate is raised with fever, tachycardia and malaise.
  As it is often difficult to differentiate, the doctor usually refers to a combination disorder – **epididymo-orchitis**.

Diagnosis – investigations
  1 Clinical history and examination
  2 Urine for culture and sensitivity
  3 Blood for virology

Treatment
  1 Analgesia for pain
  2 Antibacterial drugs unless mumps virus is responsible

Suggested nursing response

Assessment	Care
1 Degree of pain and swelling in the scrotum – visual observation. Note facial expressions carefully as some men will be too embarrassed to admit to scrotal pain	Give prescribed analgesic – some men need high doses of pethidine. Apply a scrotal bridge with padding to rest it on. Later, a large, padded scrotal suspensory bandage may be used. Apply local warmth but avoid over heating
2 Evidence of general inflammation effects – raised metabolic rate, pyrexia, tachycardia, malaise	Rest in bed. Maintain body temperature. Give plenty of fluids with added glucose
3 Serious anxiety about virility and possible sterility – also anxiety in his wife	Listen carefully to fears. May prefer to discuss with a male doctor or nurse. Careful counselling is needed

Most patients in fact make a good recovery in a few days and impotence and sterility are rare. If gonorrhoea is diagnosed, there will be a need for contact tracing of the sexual partner who will also need treatment.

Tumours of the testes

Teratomas – highly malignant tumour
Seminomas – mostly malignant but not as rapid in growth as teratoma. The cause is not known. They are more common in younger men. Expanding mass may be felt in the scrotum.

Treatment is by excision through an inguinal incision followed by radiotherapy.

Nursing notes
Early diagnosis is critical as teratomas metastasise quickly – advise any young man with scrotal swelling to see his doctor quickly. Surgical hazards are:
1 danger of infection from perineal area
2 severe pain following scrotal handling
3 psychological problems as impotence and sterility are almost inevitable after treatment.

Congenital disorder of the testes – undescended testicle

The cause is not known. It is a reasonably common disorder – 30–40 per 1000 baby boys. The testicle may
1 remain in the abdomen (true undescended) – usually removed as danger of malignancy
2 be held in the inguinal canal (ectopic)
3 be retracted into the upper part of the scrotum (retractile)

Surgery Repositioning of the testes is known as *orchidopexy*. The testes is anchored by a suture to the thigh or embedded in skin of the thigh. Treatment must be completed before puberty

Torsion of the testis The testis twists itself within the tunica vaginalis and there is danger of rapid loss of function of the testis. It is an extremely painful condition. It may be reduced manually or needs urgent surgical correction.

Hydrocele A collection of fluid in the tunica vaginalis which causes swelling in the scrotum which is often painless. It is removed if there is gross enlargement or interference with testes functions. Some old men, who could not undergo surgery, have them aspirated but there is danger of infection and haemorrhage.

Varicocele A dilation of the plexus of veins around the testis which may cause sub fertility by increasing the temperature in the testis. May be removed surgically.

2 The vas deferens and seminal vesicles
Vas deferens

Functions	Structures involved
The passage of sperm from the epididymis to the prostatic urethra during ejaculation. Ejaculation is a reflex muscular action which occurs with the male orgasm – there is muscular contraction in the seminal vesicles and prostate too. Sperm may remain in the vas deferens for over a month after ejaculation	Fibrous outer coat, smooth muscle coat (three layers) and epithelial coat. Extends from the tail of the epididymis through the inguinal canal (part of the spermatic cord) over the top and down the posterior surface of the bladder, joining the duct of the seminal vesicle and passing through the prostate gland as the ejaculatory duct

Seminal vesicles

Functions	Structures involved
1 Production of about 30% of seminal fluid (very rich in nutrients – especially fructose) Influenced by levels of testosterone	Pouches of glandular tissue in convolutions
2 Muscular contraction during ejaculation adds fluid towards formation of semen	Muscular wall which contracts on ejaculation

Semen is finally formed when the prostate gland adds a further 60% during ejaculation and a small portion from small bulbo-urethral glands. Semen is alkaline, one ejaculation gives an average of 5 ml containing up to 100 000 000 sperm per ml.

Conditions affecting the vas deferens and seminal vesicles

The only 'consideration' is that of male sterilization – **vasectomy**.

Vasectomy

Before operation
    1 Careful discussion and explanation with the man and his wife as reversal is very difficult. Usually the wife should consent too
    2 Washing and shaving of the scrotal area before surgery
Surgery
    1 Usually local anaesthetic, sometimes general
    2 Small incision in the neck of the scrotum
    3 Ligation of the vas to avoid reopening
After surgery
    1 Observe for haemorrhage, including late haematoma
    2 Observe for infection
    3 Will need repeated examinations of seminal fluid for up to 3 months to eliminate sperm from the vas or seminal vesicles

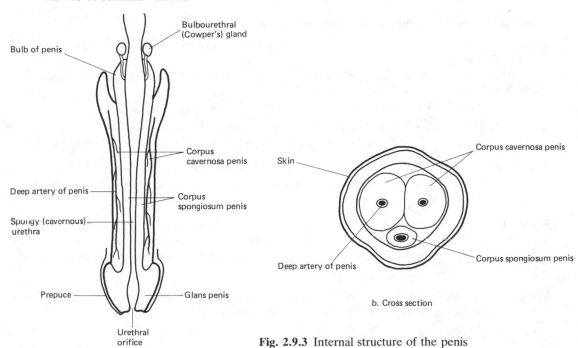

a. Coronal section

b. Cross section

Fig. 2.9.3 Internal structure of the penis

3 The penis

Functions	Structures involved
1 Contains the penile urethra for the passage of urine and semen during ejaculation	Inner lining of transitional epithelial tissue contained between the cylindrical masses of erectile tissue, ending in the meatus within the glans
2 Becomes erect for insertion into the female vagina during intercourse. During erection, the prepuce (foreskin) of the penis is retracted, exposing the very sensitive glans penis. Stimulation of the erectile tissues and glans leads to the reflex action of ejaculation	Blood enters the corpus cavernosa and corpus spongiosum to cause stiffening of those tissues during sexual stimulation

Conditions of the penis
Inflammation of the glans penis – balanitis

A bacterial infection between the prepuce and the glans. Local cleansing and hygiene needs to be taught.

Sexual intercourse should be avoided until all inflammation has settled. Antibacterial agents may be needed in severe infection.

Chancre

Is the infected ulcer that appears through infection by *Treponema palidum* in *syphilis*. Although most commonly seen on the penis, it may appear on other skin surfaces. It is highly infectious.

Treatment for syphilis and contact tracing is necessary. Procaine penicillin, tetracycline or erythromycin are the current antibacterial drugs mainly used for syphilis.

Carcinoma of the penis

Squamous cell carcinoma which usually starts as a small tumour which ulcerates. It is often painless and metastases of the inguinal glands is common.

Treatment is by radiotherapy, partial or total amputation, cytotoxic therapy, or combinations of these treatments.

Phimosis

Narrowing of the prepuce (foreskin) which may be caused by early attempts at retraction of the foreskin – parents may need guidance. It occasionally occurs as a congenital abnormality.

Treatment is by circumcision (removal of the foreskin).

Nursing notes

The nurse may be able to give advice to parents about the care of the male genitalia. The prepuce does not separate completely from the glans penis until the boy is two years old.

Circumcision is done on religious or hygienic grounds in babyhood. Post operative dressings are difficult – non stick vaseline gauze is preferred next to the raw surface of skin exposed.

Paraphimosis

Occurs in more adult men. The foreskin is retracted back over the glans and cannot be replaced. (*Note:* male catheterization technique – make sure that the foreskin is replaced as soon as possible.) The tight foreskin obstructs the venous return from the glans and it becomes distended making replacement even more difficult. It may be replaced under anaesthesia or it may need a dorsal slit of the foreskin. Circumcision may be needed.

Congenital defects of the penis
Hypospadias

The urethral meatus opens onto the lower surface of the penis. It is treated by 'plastic' repair surgery. Possibly more than one operation will be needed.

Epispadias

The urethral meatus opens onto the upper (dorsal) surface of the penis. Extensive reconstructive surgery including urinary by-pass may be needed.

Nursing notes

Children with these defects are obviously susceptible to urinary tract infection. Scrupulous nappy care needs to be taught and practised.

The surgery is specialized and details cannot be given in this text book.

The female reproductive system

This system will be considered as follows.

1 The ovaries
2 The uterine (fallopian) tubes
3 The uterus and cervix
4 The vagina and vulva
5 Normal pregnancy
6 Termination of pregnancy
7 The breasts

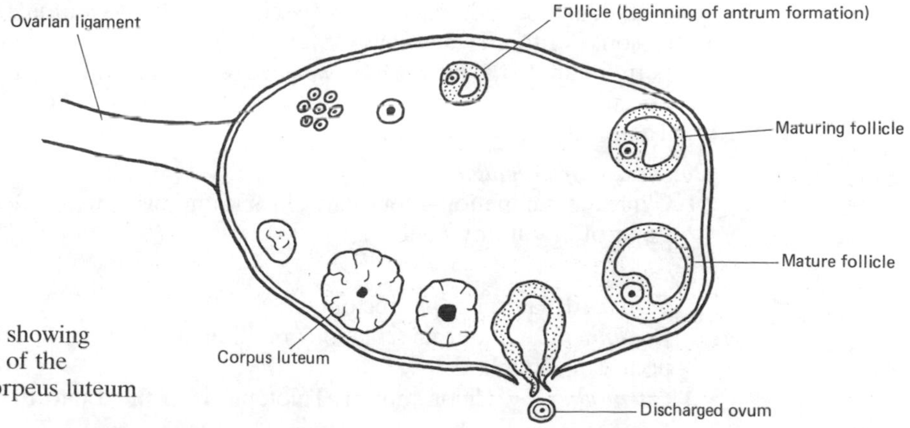

Fig. 2.9.4 Section through the ovary showing successive stages in the development of the ovarian follicle, the ovum and the corpeus luteum

1 The ovaries

Function	Structures involved
1 The production and release of the female gamete (the ovum) from follicular cells within the tissues by meiosis (reduction division) – 23 pairs (diploid) to 23 (haploid) chromosomes	Follicles develop and ripen on a cyclical basis (28 days) under the influence of the follicle-stimulating hormone from the pituitary gland. Completion and rupture of the follicle (ovulation) is brought about by luteinizing hormone (LH)
2 The manufacture and release of the feminizing hormones oestrogen and progesterone	
Oestrogen influences the development of the female genitalia, the breasts, the pubic hair and altered fat deposits to produce the rounded female appearance. It also influences feminine behaviour	Oestrogen is released by thecal cells around the follicles under the influence of both follicle-stimulating hormone (FSH) and luteinizing hormone (LH)
Progesterone prepares the uterus for pregnancy by increasing the secretion of water and stimulating the secretion of endometrial glands	Progesterone, in small quantities, is released by the developing follicles, but larger quantities are produced by the corpus luteum after ovulation

Note: Follicle-stimulating hormone and luteinizing hormone are released by the pituitary gland in response to blood levels of oestrogen and progesterone.

Follicle-stimulating hormone is present at higher levels at the beginning of the menstrual cycle to develop the follicle but minimizes when oestrogen level reaches a peak at ovulation.

Luteinizing hormone is present at higher levels through ovulation, but is minimal when progesterone level reaches a peak.

Contraceptive hormone preparations work by altering blood levels of oestrogen and progesterone to prevent ovulation.

Conditions of the ovary

For inflammation of the ovary (**oophritis**) – see **salpingo-oophritis** or **salpingitis** p 163.

Tumours of the ovary

Cysts may be small, benign swellings with no symptoms. Some are very large and may disturb function

Complications
1. Danger of torsion on twisting, commonly after exercise. In complete torsion, the patient complains of persistent acute abdominal pain
2. Haemorrhage may occur within a cyst, with symptoms of an acute abdominal pain again
3. Rupture of a cyst may lead to peritonitis
4. Infection of a cyst may occur following ascending infection or from an inflamed appendix
5. Malignancy is possible in all ovarian cysts

Dermoid cyst may contain many different tissues such as skin tissue (hair, sebaceous glands) teeth, intestinal tissue and nerve tissue.

All diagnosed cysts are removed because of the possible complications.

Laparotomy is followed by
1. Ovarian cystectomy – removal of the cyst but save the ovary in younger women and girls
2. Oophorectomy – removal of the ovary if blood supply has been affected (e.g. torsion)
3. Bilateral oophorectomy – in older women after the menopause in case of more cysts or metastases forming

Carcinoma of the ovary

Cause Not known. Most common between 40 and 60 years.

Effects, signs and symptoms The tumour grows, in some cases quite rapidly, but may cause very little disturbance in the early stages. Sometimes a hard pelvic swelling may be felt.

The peritoneum is infiltrated and small 'seed' growths may occur. The reaction is to produce excess fluid in the abdominal cavity – ascites. The first symptoms may be abdominal discomfort and distension. Peritonitis may cause severe abdominal pain. There is rapid haemorrhagic spread from the peritoneum to the liver. Gross weight loss, even further ascites, exhaustion and eventually coma may occur.

The prognosis is poor – only 30% survive 5 years with treatment.

Diagnosis – investigations
1. Clinical examination – not many clues in the history
2. Laparotomy if any doubt

Treatment
1. *Surgical* Bilateral oophorectomy
2. *Radiotherapy* External radiation or radium implants in the uterus to try to stop metastases in the pouch of Douglas
3. *Chemotherapy* Chlorambucil. Thiotepa (is instilled into the peritoneal cavity)

Suggested nursing response

Assessment	Care
1 Evidence of pelvic tumour – complaint of a lump	Report urgently
2 Presence and degree of ascites – abdomen may be quite tense	Diuretics may be used. Paracentesis abdominis is carried out under aseptic technique (but depletes proteins)
3 Evidence of peritonitis – acute abdominal pain; high core temperature; tachycardia; exhaustion	Bed rest. Prescribed analgesia (may need high doses of narcotics frequently and regularly). Maintain body temperature
4 Emaciated skin which is thin and breaks easily – note pressure areas and development of sores	Gentle hygiene. Care of pressure areas. Aseptic dressings to any wounds
5 Gross weight loss. Anorexia also leads to dry coated mouth	Encourage protein in diet, but difficult to enforce. Gentle mouth care
6 Psychological 　1 self conscious about ascites 　2 anxiety about pain 　3 fear of dying	Advise on clothing. Assurance about analgesia. Listen to fears. Discuss with the family. Involve spiritual leader (priest or minister)

See also *care after laparotomy,* and *care after radiotherapy.* Observe and care for undesired effects of drugs.

2 The uterine (fallopian) tubes

Functions	Structures involved
1 The gathering of the ovum expelled from the ruptured follicle of the ovary. The ovum is expelled into the peritoneal cavity – some are not gathered by the uterine tube	The fimbriae (finger-like projections) in the outer infundibular part of the tube are able to gather the ovum. The open end of the tube is continual with the peritoneum which is also draped over the tubes as they lie against the broad ligaments.
2 The moving of the ovum towards the uterus for implantation. Nutrient cells secrete fluid for maintaining the ovum as it travels	Columnar cells on the inner lining of the tube have cilia which waft towards the uterus. The tube is narrowest as it passes through the wall of the uterus.
3 Fertilization of the ovum takes place in the uterine tube – usually in the outer third – the infundibulum. Once fertilized, mitosis of cells is started and the structure is then known as a blastocyst	Parts of the tubes are the infundibulum (outer), the ampulla (middle), the isthmus (inner) and the interstitial (as it passes through the wall of the uterus)

Conditions of the uterine tube

Inflammation of the uterine tube is called *salpingitis*

Salpingitis

Causes
1 Ascending infection by micro-organisms, such as staphylococci, coliform bacteria and gonococci, which may follow childbirth, abortion or sexual intercourse (including rape).
2 Infection spread from appendicitis or peritonitis
3 Blood born infection in septicaemia

Effects, signs and symptoms Usually, both tubes will be inflamed, causing tenderness and acute lower abdominal pain. The swelling may be palpated by the doctor on vaginal examination. There may be a purulent vaginal discharge. The tubes may be filled with pus (pyosalpinx).

The metabolic rate is usually quite high, although some do not have a very high temperature in the early stages. There may be a urinary tract infection too.

Peritonitis is a common complication. There is the generalized abdominal pain with guarding. The patient is then very seriously ill, with severe toxaemia. Core temperature is high, severe tachycardia and exhaustion will be observed and there is a danger of dying.

Later, the resulting fibrosis may lead to blockage of both tubes – sterility will follow. Severe narrowing may allow sperm through for fertilization, but the blastocyst cannot pass the fibrosed tissue – see ectopic pregnancy.

Diagnosis – investigations
1 Clinical history and examination
2 Cervical swabs for culture and sensitivity
3 Careful nursing history may reveal any indiscretions to suggest the condition

Treatment
1 Surgery is not indicated
2 Laparotomy may be necessary to exclude other conditions – if salpingitis is found, only a swab would be taken

3 Antibacterial agents are given according to culture and sensitivity

4 Intravenous drugs may be needed if severe peritonitis

5 If gonococci are the cause, contact tracing is needed and avoidance of sexual intercourse until completely clear of infection

Suggested nursing response

Assessment	Care
1 Degree of and nature of abdominal pain – if bilateral or unilateral	Give prescribed analgesia. Careful positioning for comfort
2 Evidence of urinary tract infection – burning and frequency of micturition	Care of the patient with urinary tract infection. Give extra fluids. Antibacterial agents may be needed
3 Metabolic rate (especially high if peritonitis), pyrexia, tachycardia, exhaustion, dehydration, weight loss	Maintain body temperature. Give glucose drinks or intravenous regime. May need intensive nursing care for peritonitis. See 2.4.
4 Vaginal discharge – may be purulent and blood could be present	Careful cleansing and vulval toilet will be needed. Analgesia may be needed for soreness
5 Psychological state	Individual care for each patient
1 anxiety about possible sterility	Listen to feelings of anxiety. Guarded assurance – may need to be understood between whole health care team
2 guilt feelings if sexually transmitted disease or self attempts at abortion	Nurse may need to help the patient to express feelings here
3 deep grief feelings following rape	May need professional psychiatric help
4 fear of dying	Sensitive assurance

Ectopic pregnancy

Any fertilized ovum which becomes implanted outside the uterus. The most common site is in the uterine tube.

Causes

1 Fibrosis following salpingitis narrowing the tube and preventing movement of the blastocyst into the uterus.

2 Congenital abnormality of the uterine tube

Effects, signs and symptoms Mitosis continues in the blastocyst and the embryo starts to grow, embedded in the wall of the uterine tube. Eventually it will rupture.

A small rupture into the tube may produce a 'mole' as the embryo dies. The patient may experience pain and have a vaginal loss of blood, but symptoms then settle.

The more dangerous event is that the tube itself is ruptured, leading to severe haemorrhage into the peritoneal cavity. There may be bleeding into the vagina too. The patient complains of lower abdominal pain and appears shocked – restless, cold, clammy skin, low blood pressure and severe tachycardia. Air hunger – gasping for air may be seen.

There may be some peritonitis as well, but as surgery is undertaken and blood aspirated, this may not persist.

Diagnosis – investigations

1 Clinical history (pregnancy will usually have been diagnosed)

2 Examination

3 Blood taken for cross matching

Treatment

1 Start blood transfusion with **O** Rh negative blood

2 Urgent surgery with minimal preparation

3 Laparotomy, ligation of blood vessels, usually removal of the tube (salingectomy) and peritoneal toilet will be carried out

Suggested nursing response

Assessment	Care
1 Degree of shock – blood pressure falling; pulse rate rising; restlessness and anxiety; air hunger	Position according to blood pressure. Feet raised, but keep trunk slightly elevated – Jack-knife position (keeps blood in the pelvic cavity). Assist with urgent blood transfusion. Blood may need to be warmed. Oxygen may be needed
2 Abdominal pain – site and nature (if severe, it may affect the degree of shock)	Give prescribed analgesia (usually as part of immediate pre-medication for surgery)

continued next page

3 Husband and wife's anxiety	Careful assurance. Dramatic recovery follows successful
1 initially, about survival	surgery, but the danger is very serious
2 later, grief at loss of baby	Listen to feelings and allow a time of quiet togetherness!
3 anxiety about future pregnancy	Guarded assurance as there is a risk of damage in the opposite tube

The surgeon would carry out a salpingogram later to establish if pregnancy was possible.

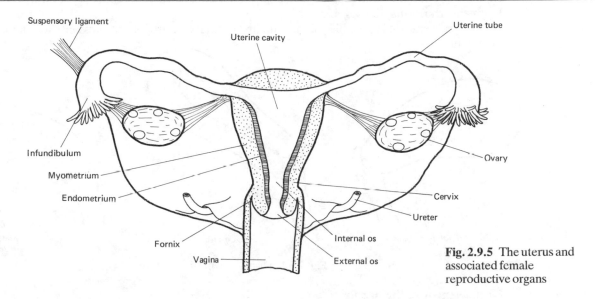

Fig. 2.9.5 The uterus and associated female reproductive organs

3 The uterus and cervix

Functions	Structures involved
1 Preparation to receive	The inner lining of the uterus in the endometrium. It thickens under the influence of oestrogen. It becomes more secretory under the influence of progesterone from the corpus luteum
1 the fertilized ovum (or blastocyst) which would also be maintained in the uterus	
2 the unfertilized ovum which will be expelled during menstruation	If fertilization has not taken place, the corpus luteum stops producing progesterone and the endometrium is shed
Implantation into the endometrium is prevented if a foreign body lies in the uterus – the principle of the intra uterine contraceptive device	
2 Provides a passage for sperm to pass through the uterine tube	Sperm enter the external os of the cervix and swim through to the infundibular part of the uterine tube
3 Allows the normal growth of the foetus in the pelvic and abdominal cavity	The walls of the body and fundus are very expansive to accommodate growth
4 Rhythmic, powerful contractions during labour for the delivery of the baby	The muscular wall (myometrium) under the influence of oxytoxin from the posterior lobe of the pituitary gland

The correct position of the uterus is important for uncomplicated menstruation and pregnancy. It should be anteverted (inclined forward) and anteflexed (bent forward).

It is maintained by the round ligaments (fibro muscular), the broad ligaments, utero-sacral ligaments and the anterior and posterior ligaments (all folds of peritoneum).

Peritoneum is draped all over the body of the uterus.

Conditions of the uterus and cervix

Menstruation problems

Pre menstrual tension – headache, irritability, depression, fullness feelings in the lower abdomen, tender breasts, backache are some of the symptoms reported.

They are thought to be due to the imbalance of oestrogen, progesterone and other hormones producing fluid retention and some hypoglycaemia.

Nursing notes

The nurse may need to advise a patient to seek help if the symptoms are severe. Diuretics are sometimes prescribed. Advice to control salt and fluid intake, but maintain glucose intake.

Dysmenorrhoea is painful menstruation which usually occurs in younger women, but rarely at the beginning of puberty. It is possibly due to the effect of progesterone increasing the tonus of the uterine muscles and usually lasts for only a few hours.

Nursing notes

Again, the nurse acts as a friend and adviser here. Analgesics may be prescribed. Some explanation of menstruation may be needed to allay some girls' fears.

Amenorrhoea is absence of menstruation. May be due to pregnancy, menopause, or congenital abnormality

Menorrhagia is excessive bleeding during menstruation

Metrorrhagia is bleeding between menstrual cycles and should always be investigated

Endometriosis Areas of functioning endometrium outside the uterus. They undergo the menstrual changes but cannot be evacuated. Cysts and adhesions form (e.g. chocolate cyst in the ovary). Dysmenorrhoea may be severe.

Surgical removal is possible. Some patients may have oestrogen suppressants which may cause menopause.

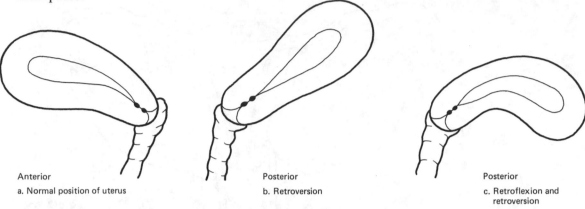

Anterior
a. Normal position of uterus

Posterior
b. Retroversion

Posterior
c. Retroflexion and retroversion

Fig. 2.9.6 Displacement of the uterus

Displacement of the uterus

Retroversion The uterus is inclined backwards. The cause may be chronic inflammation in the pelvic floor, with adhesions holding the uterus towards the back.

The patient may complain of dysmenorrhoea, backache, dyspareunia (painful sexual intercourse) or menorrhagia. It may be a cause of infertility.

Treatment is either by the use of a Hodge pessary or surgical shortening of the round ligaments and repositioning of the uterus in its anteverted position.

Prolapse – see conditions of the vagina, as uterine prolapse is usually due to weakness of the vaginal wall as well as the support ligaments of the uterus.

Tumours of the uterus and cervix

Fibroids are benign tumours in the wall of the uterus – *fibromyomata*. The cause is unknown.

Effects, signs and symptoms Submucous fibroids project into the cavity of the uterus – the patient usually complains of menorrhagia.

They may present as 'polyps' which protrude through the cervix. These may ulcerate and cause metrorrhagia.

Intra mural fibroids grow within the wall of the uterus and usually cause symptoms of pressure on other organs – bladder pressure would cause frequency of micturition, rectal pressure may cause constipation.

Subserous fibroids grow out of the uterus under the peritoneum, sometimes on pedicles. The patient may be found to have a pelvic lump but no other symptoms. They may become twisted (tortion) and lead to acute abdominal pain.

Diagnosis – investigations

1 Clinical examination and history

2 Blood should be checked for evidence of anaemia due to blood loss

Treatment Surgical removal by either myomectomy if the woman wishes to have children or hysterectomy (removal of the uterus)

Suggested nursing response

Assessment	Care
1 Evidence of anaemia – pallor, tiredness, tachycardia	Rest. High protein diet with iron content. Prescribed iron supplements
2 Evidence of pressure symptoms – frequency of micturition, stress incontinence, retention of urine, constipation, haemorrhoids	Careful explanation. Increase fluid intake to avoid urinary tract infection. Catheterization if really necessary. High fibre diet. Prescribed suppositories or aperients
3 Vaginal discharge – there may be an offensive, smelling discharge or blood loss between periods (metrorrhagia)	Vulval toilet and hygiene. Provide sanitary towel

Preparation for myomectomy or hysterectomy is as for abdominal surgery.

Carcinoma of the cervix

Cause is not known but there is some evidence of a relationship with early and promiscuous sexual intercourse.

Effects, signs and symptoms Carcinoma of the cervix is described in five stages.

Stage 0 The pre-invasive state. The patient has no symptoms and there are no obvious signs. Discovery is of suspicious cells in the cervical smear test.

Stage I The tumour presents as a mass or ulcer limited to the area of the cervix. The patient may complain of irregular bleeding (especially after intercourse) and an offensive vaginal discharge. In older women, there will be post menopausal bleeding.

Nursing note

The nurse as a health educationalist should recommend regular cervical smear tests to women at risk. The cure rate is very high at this stage.

Stage II There is infiltration of the surrounding tissues of the cervix.

Stage III Infiltration of the vagina and pelvis wall may lead to increasing pain as nerve endings become involved. In older women, infiltration may be quite rapid.

Stage IV Infiltration involves the bladder, rectum and usually metastases of the lymph nodes and liver. Prognosis at this stage is extremely poor.

Diagnosis – investigations
  1 Clinical history and examination   2 Cervical smear test   3 Cone biopsy

Treatment
  1 A cone biopsy may remove all cancer tissue
  2 Radiotherapy – radium or caesium implants are applied
  3 Extensive surgery is needed if wide infiltration has occurred and may be followed by radiotherapy
  4 Some surgeons perform a radical surgical excision of the uterus, the uterine tubes and ovaries, pelvic glands, tissues around the uterus and most of the vagina (Wertheim's hysterectomy).

Suggested nursing response
  1 Radioactive implants are used
  2 Staff need to wear film badges (avoid involving any pregnant nurse)
  3 Indwelling catheter as oedema of the urethra may cause retention
  4 Vaginal pack to hold implants in position
  5 Applicator threads should be showing
  6 Removal may be painful – prescribed analgesia is given before the procedure
    Although staff should avoid long periods in the vicinity, normal conversation and care should continue.

Wertheim's hysterectomy
  1 Extensive surgery – nursing care of a shocked patient
  2 Peritoneum involved – may lead to paralytic ileus after surgery – will need nasogastric aspiration and intravenous fluids
  3 Indwelling catheter and vaginal pack needed
  4 Possible danger of urinary tract infection

Advanced disease – problems include
  1 Emaciation, anorexia, pressure sores
  2 Pain and frequency of micturition, possible uraemia
  3 Incontinence of faeces
  4 Offensive vaginal discharges and soreness
  5 Severe pain
  6 Fear, depression
  7 Family distress

Apply your nursing model for a full care plan.

Carcinoma of the body of the uterus

Usually arises in the endometrium. It occurs more commonly in older women after the menopause, when it causes post menopausal bleeding and is therefore reported early.

Diagnosed by curettage scrapings. Total hysterectomy and bilateral salpingo-oophorectomy is indicated as spread to the ovaries may be rapid. This may be followed by radiotherapy or radiotherapy alone may be used. Prognosis is not good

Cervical erosion

Correctly **cervical ectropian** or **eversion**. Growth of columnar cells on the vaginal portion of the cervix. A reddened area covered with mucus forms around the external os which may cause

1 mucopurulent vaginal discharge

2 bleeding – between periods and after intercourse

3 irritation and discomfort

Treated in out-patients by cryosurgery usually or by cautery. The patient needs to wear pads for 2–3 weeks and avoid intercourse which may cause bleeding.

Nursing note

The nurse should advise patients to report any cases of unusual vaginal discharge, bleeding or discomfort. Many women may be embarrassed or afraid of what may be discovered, but in many cases the cure rate is very high.

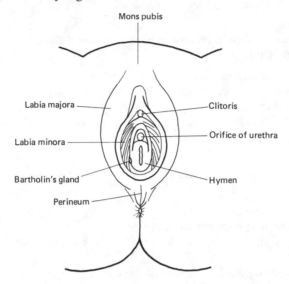

Fig. 2.9.7
External female genitalia

4 The vagina and vulva

Vagina

Functions	Structures involved
1 Receives the erectile penis and semen during sexual intercourse	A collapsible, tubular organ with mucous membrane on the inner surface, in folds or rugae and a smooth muscular coat. All embedded in fibrous connective tissue. Posterior fornix behind the cervix. Anterior fornix in front of the cervix
2 Dilates to allow the passage of the baby in childbirth	
3 Allows the flow of the shed endometrium during menstruation	

Note:

1 In virginity, protection from infection by mucous membrane fold – the hymen.

2 Protection from infection is given by the action of Doderlein's bacilli – commensal bacteria that produce lactic acid from glycogen. The low pH(4) prevents other bacteria from growing.

Vulva

Functions	Structures involved
1 Provides stimulation for glandular secretions, vaginal preparation and sexual excitement to allow penile penetration	The clitoris is made of erectile tissue. Bartholin's glands secrete fluid
2 Provides the entrance for the penis and exit for the baby and menstrual flow	Labia majora and minora or lips provide the opening to the vaginal orifice
3 The opening on to the surface of the female urethra	Urethral meatus between clitoris and vaginal orifice

Conditions of the vagina and vulva

Inflammation of the vagina – vaginitis

Causes

1 Monilial – *Candida albicans* (a mould) – known as 'vaginal thrush'. It is associated with pregnancy, diabetes mellitus, oral contraceptives and broad spectrum antibacterial drugs.

2 *Trichomonas vaginalis* – transmitted during intercourse

3 Streptococcal or coliform organisms in women past the menopause – known as senile vaginitis

Effects, signs and symptoms The local inflammation causes soreness, vaginal discharge and often irritation of the skin and vulva too. Ulcers may form in senile vaginitis. The vaginal discharge may be white, coloured by pus, brown and may be offensive smelling.

Diagnosis – investigations

1 Clinical history and visual examination   *2* Swabs taken for culture and sensitivity

Treatment

Monilial antifungicidal agent, e.g. nystatin cream or pessaries, nightly for 14 nights

Trichomonal Metronidazole 200 mg × 3 daily orally for 1 week or pessaries nightly for 2–3 weeks. (Partner needs treatment too and intercourse should be avoided)

Senile Oestrogen is given either orally or in pessaries, but danger of uterine bleeding. Antibacterial agents may be needed also

Suggested nursing response
1 Assess the nature of vaginal discharges
2 Assess the patient who may feel unclean or guilty
3 Give clear instructions about the insertion of pessaries or drugs to be taken for a prolonged period

Vulvitis

Inflammation of the vulva. May be part of vaginitis or part of a skin disease – boils may appear in or around the vulva.

The ulcerated infected sore of syphilis (chancre) is usually found in the vulva or vagina of the female.

The inflammation may be due also to allergic reactions to toiletries and deodorants. Pruritis (itching) of the vulva is distressing and disturbs sleep.

Nursing notes

In the majority of cases, good hygiene with warm baths and vulval toilet is sufficient.

The nurse needs to listen and observe carefully for problems of discharge, local lesions or general disease such as diabetes mellitus.

It may be necessary to educate some girls on good vulval hygiene.

Bartholin's abscess

An infection of a Bartholin's gland and duct (which becomes blocked) by coliform organisms, staphylococci or gonococci. The hot, red swelling over the gland may be quite painful and the patient may have a fever.

Bed rest, analgesia and antibacterial drugs may be given, but urgent surgical drainage may be needed when pain is severe. The gland is opened out, as if a pocket (marsupialization). This prevents formation of a cyst or further blockage.

Suggested nursing response
1 Vulval toilet is performed four hourly
2 Regular bathing and cleaning is continued
3 Antibacterial drugs course will be completed at home
4 Education to avoid infection is needed too

Carcinoma of the vulva

Usually occurs in older women. It starts as a small, hard painless ulcer but may spread rapidly to involve the inguinal glands. Chronic skin inflammation with white plaques becomes very irritable – stretching causes further break-down of cells.

Treatment is usually by radical vulvectomy with a wide excision of tissues and glands including the skin – obviously needing to heal slowly by granulation tissue

Suggested nursing response
1 Prevent infection of the wound – delays healing
2 Prevent urinary tract infection – there is a catheter in place initially
3 Allow healing by granulation by using non stick dressings
4 Later encourage movement to avoid skin contracture
5 Prevent boredom and frustration as healing and care may be prolonged

Prolapses through the vagina

Anterior wall – (upper) – cystocele (Causes difficulty passing urine (dysuria) and frequency of micturition.

Anterior wall – (lower) – urethrocele Causes stress incontinence of urine.

Posterior wall – (upper) – enterocele Small intestine involved. Causes discomfort in pelvic cavity.

Posterior wall – (lower) – rectocele Rectum and perineum involved. Causes difficulty in defaecation.

Total prolapse – procidentia The cervix protrudes at the vulva. The woman complains of a feeling of 'something coming down'.

Treatment
1 Surgical repair – *colporraphy* – described as anterior, posterior (or both)
2 If an elongated cervix is present, it may be amputated (Manchester repair)
3 After the menopause, hysterectomy may be performed
4 Surgery for prolapse is carried out through the vagina

Suggested nursing response for vaginal route surgery

Before surgery

  1 Strict hygiene and shaving of the pubic, vulval and perineal area must be performed
  2 Prolapsed uterus which has ulcerated will need treatment before surgery

Surgery The patient is in the lithotomy position. A urinary catheter is inserted at operation

After surgery

  1 A vaginal pack may be inserted but is removed within 24 hours usually
  2 Gentle vulval toilet 4 hourly for 2 days followed by saline baths as soon as she is able
  3 Soluble sutures are used
  4 The catheter is removed after 48 hours but the nurse needs to observe for retention of urine
  5 Advice to avoid heavy lifting, constipation and intercourse for three months

Suggesting nursing response for gynaecological surgery – abdominal route

Is as for laparotomy involving the pelvic cavity

Note:

  1 Highly sensitive area often increases the degree of pain experienced
  2 The peritoneum may be involved in the surgery giving a possibility of ileus or infection
  3 Careful observations are very important

5 Normal pregnancy

Full details of pregnancy and maternity care cannot be covered in this text. Three areas to be mentioned are

  1 Signs and symptoms of pregnancy
  2 Some physiological and psychological changes
  3 The stages of labour

Signs and symptoms of pregnancy

  1 Amenorrhoea – cessation of menstruation
  2 Breast enlargement – engorged veins, pigmentation of the areola, enlargement of areolar follicles (Montgomery follicles)
  3 Presence of chorionic gonadotrophin in the urine (produced by the placenta)
  4 Enlargement of the uterus – the fundus is palpated by the twelfth week of pregnancy

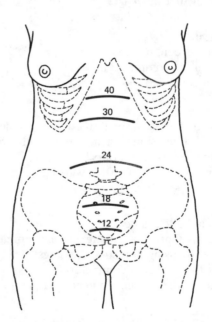

Fig. 2.9.8 Height of fundus in pregnancy

  5 Nausea and vomiting due to hormonal disturbance in the early months by some but not all mothers

Nursing notes

The nurse should advise the mother to seek medical confirmation and antenatal advice as early as possible.

Antenatal advice would include diet, exercise, vulval hygiene and avoidance of infections (especially rubella), drugs, alcohol and cigarette smoking.

The husband should be involved in discussions as early as possible. Couples often need counselling about their sexual relationships during pregnancy. Intercourse is possible with care.

Physiological changes

The skin Increased pigmentation of the areola and nipple of the breasts, the linea alba of the abdomen and sometimes generalized browning.

Circulation Cardiac output increases. Blood volume increases. Blood pressure normally falls slightly – *danger if it rises*. Anaemia may occur due to haemo dilation.

Respirations Vital capacity is increased but a very large uterus may cause breathing difficulty.

Digestion Reduced gastric acid secretion. Slower peristalsis.

Excretion Frequency of micturition.

Endocrine Tendency to glycosuria. Enlarged parathyroid glands increase calcium levels in the blood.

Nursing notes

Blood pressure is a very important clinical observation throughout pregnancy, to note pre eclampsia (see a midwifery text book).

Increased iron in the diet and iron supplements may be needed to prevent anaemia. Exercises and support bandages are used for varicose veins.

Slow rising, tea and biscuits before getting out of bed, may reduce morning sickness. Antiemetic drugs are a last resort.

Urinalysis is important to detect latent diabetes mellitus. Diabetic mothers tend to have large babies.

Calcium may be removed from bone if not increased in the diet – increasing milk product consumption is advised.

Psychological changes

Early stages A tendency for mood swings from elation to depression. There may be anxiety about the husband's reactions and feelings.

Later There is a feeling of euphoria ('wellness') until the impatience of waiting the last few weeks. There is some anxiety at some stage that 'the baby will be all right'.

Suggested nursing response

Good antenatal care and parentcraft classes should dispel most fears, but mothers (and fathers) need to be considered individually as well as in groups.

The stages of labour

1st stage

1 Onset of uterine contraction pains
2 Blood stained vaginal loss (show)
3 Rupture of membranes
4 Dilation of the cervix

Nursing note

May be a prolonged stage, with increasing anxiety and fatigue.

Sympathetic care by the nurse and support from a husband will help.

2nd stage Full dilation of the cervix, delivery of the baby by uterine contractions with help from mother 'bearing down'

Nursing note

A highly emotional moment for mother, baby and father. Some like to hold the baby on the abdomen even before the umbilical cord is severed.

Note: In emergency delivery, there is no hurry to cut the umbilical cord until sterile apparatus is available.

3rd stage The gentle delivery of the placenta, through further uterine contractions. There is danger of severe haemorrhage if placenta is not delivered clearly.

Nursing note

Injection of syntometrine (ergometrine and syntocinon) aids uterine contractions and prevents post partum haemorrhage

The puerperium

1 The return of the pelvic organs to their normal state
2 Lactation and breast feeding
3 Psychological adjustment to mother – baby and family

Nursing notes

Patient handling by the nurse and the husband may be needed to cope with unstable emotions in the mother.

Depression may become serious and need professional advice.

The need for early bonding is very important. Handling the baby herself, breast feeding or bottle feeding will help. Physical holding is encouraged even if the baby needs to be in an incubator for a time.

Maternity care and care of the newborn

From your syllabus, you are reminded that you should:

1 Be professionally aware of the physiological and social significance of childbirth and of the family as a unit of society.

Revision note Read more detail on the physiology of pregnancy. For social significance, see *infancy* in 2.14 and references throughout the text of the social needs relating to a family.

2 Understand the first aid measures necessary for immediate care of the mother and the baby before the arrival of a professional attendant.

First aid

1 Delegate a sensible person to call for an ambulance
2 Reassure the mother and ensure privacy
3 When baby is expelled, support with the head down, wipe mucus from the nose, mouth and eyes with a clean cloth or tissue
4 If spontaneous respiration does not occur, apply a stimulus as taught
5 Keep the baby close to the mother's body. Do not cut the umbilical cord, do not apply traction to remove the placenta
6 Massage of the fundus of the uterus may help to control any haemorrhage
7 Transport mother and baby in warm blankets to the maternity department

3 Build a foundation of knowledge and experience in the care of the mother and newborn child, to meet your roles as a health educator.

Revision note Consider advice that you would give to expectant mother for her daily living, for the safety of her baby and for a happy pregnancy.

4 Understand the roles of the midwife.

Revision note The roles of the midwife are
1 A practitioner of normal obstetrics qualified to make diagnoses and decisions.
2 A supervisor of pregnancy, labour and delivery of the baby.
3 An assessor of abnormal situations.
4 A deliverer of obstetric first aid when complications occur, until the doctor attends.

6 Termination of pregnancy – abortion

Induced abortion

May be criminal (back street) resulting often in overwhelming infection, haemorrhage and high mortality.

Legal abortions were introduced to stop criminal acts, to ensure that the physical and psychological health of the mother and baby was preserved and reduce the number of unwanted children. The techniques used are

1 Vacuum aspiration
2 Dilation and curettage
3 Intra amniotic, extra amniotic or intravenous instillation of prostaglandins. This method involves the induction of a miniature labour

Suggested nursing response

Emotions Sensitive communications with the patient. Handling the distress of labour if prostaglandins are used. Feelings of guilt or grief on completion.

Physical Observe for nature of pains. Assess for evidence of haemorrhage or infection. Ensure that evacuation of the uterus is complete – any retained products will be evacuated under general anaesthetic.

Legal Ensure that the certificate is completed correctly.

Conscientious objection The nurse should advise in advance that she objects to the procedure on conscientious grounds.

She should still give good nursing care before and after the procedure but is not required to be directly involved.

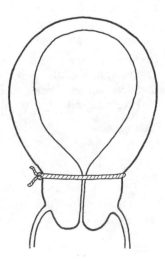

Fig. 2.9.9 Shirodkar's suture

Spontaneous abortion

As many as 25% of pregnancies may terminate spontaneously, usually within the first 12 weeks but can be any time. Many are thought to be because there are malformations of the foetus that make it incompatible with life. Others are due to an incomplete cervix, fibroids or hormonal (progesterone) deficiency (an incomplete cervix can be treated by a Shirodkar's suture).

Threatened abortion

Slight bleeding, cervix closed.

Suggested nursing response
Pregnancy can be maintained by:
1 Complete rest in bed with sedation
2 Avoid constipation, vigorous or strenuous exercise and smoking
3 Gradual but gentle mobilization
Intercourse would be discouraged, even when the threat appears to be over.

Inevitable abortion

Vaginal bleeding with clots, lower abdomen pain and external os usually dilated.

Complete foetus, placenta and amniotic sac are evacuated totally
Incomplete some products of conception are retained. Bleeding may persist and lead to hypovolaemic shock.
Ergometrine is given and evacuation under a general anaesthetic is performed

Nursing notes
There is likely to be considerable emotional distress and grief in both the mother and her husband. Sensitive handling and reassurance is important.
Advice about future pregnancies should be on an individual basis and should perhaps be delayed until grief has settled.

7 The breasts

Functions	Structures involved
1 Preparation for lactation. Breast development begins at puberty under the influence of oestrogen and progesterone	Breasts are attached to the pectoral muscle by connective tissue – the fascia. Lobes of connective tissue contain the secreting glands – the alveoli which drain into the ducts. Alveoli are arranged in lobules. Ducts converge into main lactiferous ducts. Dilations of the lactiferous ducts are the ampullae behind the alveola. Ducts finally end in the nipple (erectile tissues)
2 Lactation – the manufacture and delivery of milk for breast feeding of the baby	Alveoli develop more during pregnancy. After delivery (2–4 days) oestrogen levels fall, prolactin from the pituitary gland stimulates milk production. Suckling of the nipple evacuates the milk from the ampullae. Oxytocin is released from the posterior pituitary and causes contraction of the alveoli and milk is delivered along the ducts to the ampullae for further suckling
3 Provides an important part of the feminine body image	The shape and size are mainly due to the amount of fat and connective tissue supporting the alveoli

Note: Blood supply – branches from the axillary intercostal and internal thoracic arteries with drainage through similar venous routes.
Lymphatic drainage is into the axillary lymph nodes.

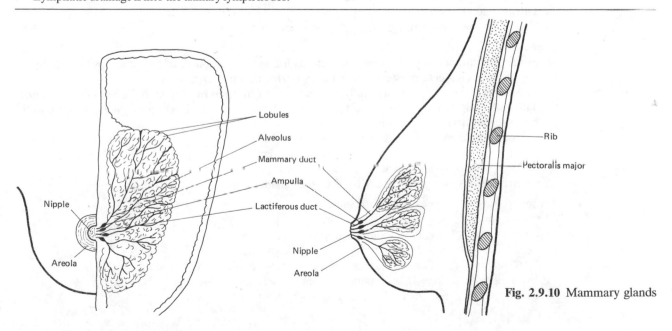

Fig. 2.9.10 Mammary glands

Conditions of the breast

Inflammation of the breast – mastitis

Acute mastitis Is usually associated with childbirth. A lactiferous duct may become blocked and milk may engorge tissues causing a 'sterile' inflammation. There is danger of staphylococcal infection entering from the nipple. Occasionally an abscess may form.

Suggested nursing response
Prevention
  1 Pre natal care of the nipples to prevent cracking and advice for good suckling
  2 Prevent contact with carriers of staphylococcal infections

Treatment
  1 A broad spectrum antibacterial agent is given (breast feeding will need to be abandoned – lactation is suppressed by Quinestrol)
  2 Surgical drainage and very gentle aseptic dressings are applied
  3 Nursing care of a patient with fever will be needed – control body temperature, rest, glucose drinks

Tumours of the breast

Benign tumours – Fibroadenoma Usually smooth and rounded. They are freely movable and clearly defined. Tender on pressure.
Removed by 'lumpectomy'.

Nursing note
The patient appreciates early assurance that it is a benign tumour.

Carcinoma of the breast

The most common malignancy in women. The cause is not known, but there is evidence of a family history in some cases. It is less common in women who breast feed their babies.

Effects, signs and symptoms Originates as a small lump or thickening of breast tissue.
    The lump is painless, ill defined and tends to be fixed.

Nursing note
Remember – examination techniques for women as part of the health education role.

Local infiltration alters the shape of the breast and may retract the nipple. Blockage of the small lymphatic ducts causes a change in the skin appearance (peau d'orange – orange peel).
    Ulceration through the skin surface may occur. Surprisingly, some women will not present for treatment until there is ulceration and a fungating mass in the breast.
    Lymphatic spread is to the axillary nodes which may be enlarged and tender. Occasionally enlargement would affect drainage from the arm. Blood spread may lead to metastases in the lungs, the liver and bones.
    Respiratory disorders, ascites and pathological fractures may occur.

Diagnosis – investigations
  1 Clinical examination
  2 Thermography – recording infra red heat from the body. Malignant areas give off more heat (hot spots)
  3 Mammography – special soft tissue X-ray examination
  4 Ultrasound examination
  5 Biopsy of the lump during surgery (frozen section)

Treatment
  1 Surgical – lumpectomy or simple mastectomy followed by a course of radiotherapy to include the lymphatics. (Radical mastectomy is rarely performed now.)
  2 The development of tumours can be slowed but not stopped by changing the hormonal balance. This may help women where the tumour has already metastasized – particularly when painful bone secondaries are present.
  3 *1* Oophorectomy – removal of the ovaries, or
     2 Hypophysectomy – removal of the pituitary gland (or destruction by radiotherapy), or
     3 Adrenalectomy – removal of the adrenal glands
  4 Oestrogen may be given orally to alter the balance.

Suggested nursing response for mastectomy
Before surgery
  1 Physical care of the skin, axilla, and arm movements
  2 Discussion with a breast care nurse should be arranged
  3 Introduction of a patient who has had a successful operation (but needs great care)
  4 Psychological care of the woman who fears cancer and her changed body image
  5 Involvement of her husband at all stages

Surgery Many surgeons now attempt to remove as little breast tissue as possible. Silicone implants are available for some patients if the skin can be kept intact.

After surgery
1 Assessment and care of the airway
2 Assessment and care for haemorrhage (not common) – most surgeons use a vacuum drain to prevent haematoma formation
3 Prevention of infection
4 Early positioning and mobility of the arm on the affected side to assist lymphatic drainage
5 The breast care nurse will introduce a soft prosthesis first

Radiotherapy
1 Assurance to the patient that side effects are minimal with modern treatment
2 The skin needs to be kept dry, free from perfumes and for some time after treatment, sun bathing should be avoided

Rehabilitation Breast care nurses are able to help patients to have a normal life by providing good, well balanced prostheses and advice about clothing, sexuality and daily living activities

Prognosis For early detection the prognosis is very good. For infiltration with few lymph glands it is quite good. For late diagnosis prognosis is poor because of metastases.

2.10 Psychological problems

There are few text books that agree on a simple analysis of psychological needs. The four areas in Model B (p 2) seem to be a useful basis for revision purposes, but it is also necessary to consider some mental illnesses.

Psychological needs

Psychology is the study of behaviour in an attempt to discern the individual needs and differences. The four main needs are defined as:
1 **Security**   – freedom from fear
2 **Esteem**   – perception of oneself
3 **Communication** – ability to relate thoughts and feelings
4 **Learning**   – intellectual development

Using nursing processes, it is possible to devise useful nursing roles for these needs

1 Security

Assessment
1 Any indications of fear or anxiety
2 Expressions by the patient and his relatives
3 Evidence of defence mechanism against fear
Examples – regressive behaviour; aggression towards staff; denial of anything wrong; extreme or inappropriate jollity

Care plan
1 Give opportunity to express fears
2 Constant assurance and encouragement
3 Diversional therapy
4 Giving information (but avoid conflicting views)

2 Esteem

Assessment
1 How the patient feels (esteem relates to feelings of 'wellness', body image and dress)
2 Indications of embarrassment or self consciousness
3 Something of the patient's status in life (family, work, intelligence)

Care plan
1 Encouragement as improvement occurs
2 Individual clothes – outdoor dress as soon as possible
3 Approach as an individual – name, rank – discuss work or ideas

3 Communication

Assessment
1 Difficulties in communicating – language and vocabulary differences
2 Blindness, deafness or dumbness

Care plan
1 Use language cards for foreign languages
2 Avoid jargon when talking to patients
3 Make physical communications by eye contact, holding hands
4 Use appropriate aids for the blind and deaf

4 Learning

Assessment
1 Previous level of the patient's intellect or skill
2 Intellectual development stage of children
3 Problems of memory in the elderly

Care plan
1 Give opportunity for learning by providing books, allowing television or even computers if appropriate
2 Organize play for children appropriate to their development
3 Help the elderly to use their long term memory by reminiscing with them

Mental illness

The objectives of the mental nursing experience require you to
1 show an understanding of psychological needs and differences
2 be able to deal with emergencies
3 be able to modify your behaviour towards patients in general wards who have a mental illness
4 recognize signs of mental disorder leading you to seek expert guidance

Neuroses or psychoneuroses

The patient usually has awareness of a problem and often has some insight into his reactions. Behaviour is usually socially acceptable

Includes: anxious states; obsessions; phobias; hysteria; anorexia nervosa; reactive depression

Psychosis

In acute phase, the patient is divorced from reality and may not have insight (but some do). Behaviour may be socially unacceptable and serious disorganization of personality often interferes with daily living (eating, sleeping etc.).

Includes: schizophrenia; manic depressive psychosis; endogenous depression; alcohol and drug dependence; personality disorders

The modern nursing approach is to treat the patient with a problem, rather than give them a diagnostic label.

The patient who is anxious

Cause Difficulty in coping with stress, often precipitated by some new factor.

Effects Usually manifests itself in physical symptoms which in themselves may increase fear and stress. These symptoms are: epigastric discomfort, indigestion, dryness of the mouth, diarrhoea; headaches, tremors, insomnia; palpitations, sweating attacks; frequency of micturition
   Some experience 'panic attacks' – gasping respirations; severe palpitations; epigastric pain; intense fear of dying

Suggested nursing response

Assessment	Care
1 Manifestations of anxiety state – physical symptoms	Carry out investigations to eliminate physical disorder and confirm clear results
2 Any factors which precipitate fear, such as hospital or particular objects or experiences	Eliminate factors as much as possible. Treat at home. Give prescribed tranquilizing drugs
3 Patient understanding of relationship between anxiety and physical disorders (psychosomatic)	Explain carefully and indicate loss of physical symptoms as anxiety is decreased
Any major factor such as family or marital problems may need further expert psychotherapy.	

The patient who has an obsession

Cause Anxiety. Usually a tidy, meticulous personality normally.

Effects May take the form of disturbing thoughts (to do something outrageous) or compulsive ritualistic actions (such as hand washing). The performance of the rituals temporarily relieves the anxiety. Later, life may become totally dominated by the rituals. Depression and suicide may follow.

Suggested nursing response

Assessment	Care plan
1 The nature of the obsession	Behaviour therapy is used. The ritual is discouraged, even allowing anxiety to increase – the patient realizes that the consequences of not doing the rituals do not bring about the feared result
2 The causes of deep-centred anxiety	Later development of trust between the patient and nurse may lead to the patient talking of his problems. Expert psychotherapy may be needed

The patient who has a phobia

A phobia is a fear of a given object or situation. For example, arachno-phobia (fear of spiders); agoraphobia (fear of open spaces). Phobias are manifestations of anxiety states

Effect
Patients will go to extreme lengths to avoid the object or situation.

Suggested nursing response

Assess	Care plan
1 The nature of the phobia	Behaviour therapy. Find a starting point where anxiety is tolerable (e.g begin with pictures of spiders) and gradually expose the patient to stimuli, but pointing out that fears are unjustified (desensitization). A careful relationship is needed
2 The patient's awareness of anxiety factors	Relaxation exercises and techniques for relieving anxiety
3 Effect of the phobia on the patient's family	Involve the relatives in the desensitization programme

The patient who seeks attention – hysteria

Hysteria is a way of meeting an anxiety conflict, by producing symptoms, and changing the patient's environment to suit themselves.

Effects
  1 Conversion hysteria – physical symptoms such as blindness, deafness and loss of voice.
  2 Dissociative reactions – altered conscious states.
    1 Amnesia – loss of memory
    2 Fuge state – removal to another place (without recollection of the journey)
    3 Somnambulism – sleep walking
    4 Multiple personality – separate personalities manifest
  3 May threaten suicide attempts to gain attention.
  4 There may be only partial awareness of what they are doing.

Suggested nursing response

Assessment	Care plan
1 Nature of hysterical behaviour – needs careful observation to detect when behaviour is manipulative	Behaviour therapy. Reward mature behavioural responses (ignoring immature responses). Direct attention seeking into acceptable activity and responsibility
2 The deep anxieties causing the hysteria	Establish nurse–patient relationship for discussion of fears
Expert psychotherapy and tranquilizers may be needed.	

The patient with anorexia nervosa

Primary A disturbance of body image, usually in adolescent girls – wishing to be 'thin'
Secondary A manipulative ploy for attention-seeking by losing weight

Effects Refusal to eat, emaciation, depression of vital functions (e.g. constipation). Hormonal upset leads to amenorrhoea. Restlessness and hyperactivity are common.

Suggested nursing response

Assessment	Care plan
1 Degree of starvation – body weight; muscle wasting; fluid balance	Bed rest in hospital and nutrition until body weight is restored to normal limits. (Needs a lot of patience!)
2 Underlying emotional or anxiety problems	Good nurse–patient support needed. May need expert psychotherapy for some considerable time

The patient who is depressed

Neurotic depression (reactive depression) Usually caused by some outside factor such as grief, unemployment or physical disorder. The patient feels 'down', for a prolonged period or deeper than normal. Physical changes include headache, fatigue, insomnia, loss of appetite and constipation. Most patients are treated by their own doctor in the community. Antidepressant drugs and support are usually sufficient.

Psychotic depression (endogenous depression) A serious condition, usually referred to as endogenous implying inner factors rather than outside. The patient has strong delusions of guilt, persecution, feelings of unworthiness and illness. Hallucinations (false perceptions of senses without any outside stimulus) e.g. hearing, seeing, smelling or tasting, may occur.

The patient has a classic sleep pattern – sleeps early part of the night but wakes early in the morning.

There is a serious danger of suicide.

Suggested nursing response

Assessment	Care plan
1 Manifestations of depression – observe for apathy or tiredness and listen for expressions of guilt and unworthiness (often precipitates suicide)	Prevent suicide by careful, vigilant observation. Removal of harmful objects. Prescribed antidepressant drugs. Group therapy sessions.
2 Effects of depression on daily living – lost interest in eating; morbid approach to the environment; lack of conversation, play	Provide a therapeutic environment – bright surroundings; appetizing food in a social setting; nurse involved in conversation, playing games

Electro convulsive therapy may be needed for endogenous depression.
There is a gradual restoration of the patient's self care
If suicide is prevented, and care is given, prognosis is good.

The patient who is excited and over-active – mania and hypomania

Mania
1 Extreme elation, self confidence
2 Extremely active, hypersensitive to noise and space
3 Flitting topics of conversation, 'flights of ideas', using puns, rhymes and bizarre relationships
4 Easily distracted, no time to eat and drink leads to undernourishment
5 May become irritable and aggressive

Hypo mania
1 Extroverted, elated, full of ideas which are not fulfilled
2 Involved in everyone and everything
3 Sees himself as a leader of groups
(Others become irritable and hostile as ideas and leadership lead to nothing.)

Suggested nursing response

Assessment	Care plan
1 Effects of over activity on daily living – dehydration; malnutrition; exhaustion	Provide sedation and tranquilizing drugs. Provide nutrition and rest. Avoid injury to patient and others
2 For switch to deep depressive state	Prevent suicide

An individual nurse–patient relationship is important to channel the patient's energies carefully into short term jobs, avoid irritations leading to aggression.
Electro convulsive therapy may be used effectively.

The patient with schizophrenia

Cause Not known, but there is evidence of
1 Hereditary factors
2 Pre psychotic personality (shy, introverted, day dreamer)
3 Biochemical factors (induced by some drugs)

Types

1 Simple	**3** Catatonic
2 Hebephrenic	**4** Paranoid

Effects

1 Disorders of emotion – little response to events (flattening of affect) or inappropriate response

2 Disorders of self identity – dissociation from his body (depersonalization)

3 Disorders of thinking

   1 Blocking of thoughts – interrupted

   2 Delusions – false fixed beliefs

   3 Inventing and using new words (neologisms)

4 Withdrawal from reality into a fantasy world

5 Hallucinations – false sensory perceptions, such as hearing voices, feeling touch, sensing smells and tastes (less commonly seeing visions)

There is a high risk of suicide in patients with schizophrenia.

The detachment from reality is likely to include an indifference to daily living activities and dehydration, malnutrition and poor personal hygiene will be common.

Suggested nursing response

Assessment	Care
1 Degree of withdrawal from reality	Prevent alienation from human contact
2 Nature of hallucinations or delusions (observed and reported)	Restoration to reality through nurse – patient relationship, establishing points of interest and gradual introduction of activities
3 Thoughts of persecution	Give prescribed tranquilizers. Maintain hygiene and nutrition.
4 Degree of self neglect	Gradually return to self care (avoid institutionalization)

Very careful observation – hallucinatory voices can direct the patient to be aggressive, violent or suicidal.

Expert psychotherapy, electroconvulsive therapy and long term phenothiazine drugs are required. Modecate is the usual long acting phenothiazine drug used.

Chlorpromazine in large doses would be used at the earlier stages of the disorder.

The patient with a personality disorder

Psychopathy refers to a persistent condition of the mind resulting in seriously irresponsible (including aggressive) behaviour.

These patients have no sense of guilt or shame and do not form friendships. Many are criminals requiring long term custody in special hospitals.

Nursing note

The general nurse may encounter personalities like this in general wards, Accident Centres and in the community as well as in mental hospitals.

They need expert psychiatric care. Amateur attempts to 'reform' them can be very traumatic.

The patient who is dependent on alcohol and/or drugs

Psychological dependence The patient uses alcohol or drugs to enable him to cope with stressful or potentially stressful situations rather than think through problems.

Physical dependence As well as seeking the psychological 'support' or 'retreat', the patient will experience physical withdrawal symptoms if the alcohol or drug is withheld. It has been described as 'the cells crying out for morphine instead of food'.

There is serious danger to society from physical dependence as patients will go to criminal extremes in order to obtain their drug and avoid withdrawal symptoms. Daily living is neglected and families are seriously affected socially and financially.

Suggested nursing response

Planned care – aims

1 To stop the intake of alcohol or drugs (in controlled situations – sudden withdrawal can be dangerous)

2 Support the patient while going through withdrawal period. The alcoholic will need multiple vitamins and the heroin dependent may need methadone

3 Restore nutrition, hydration and general health

4 Social support to prevent return to dependence e.g. alcohol – alcoholics anonymous

5 Expert psychotherapy in specialist units may be needed.

The general nurse needs to recognize the physical effects of alcohol abuse too. For example, gastric erosion, cirrhosis of the liver.

The health education role in preventing alcohol and drug dependence should be emphasized too.

Suicide and attempted suicide

Conditions which may lead to suicide

1 Endogenous depression   4 Psycopathic personalities
2 Schizophrenia   5 Physical illness with distressing symptoms
3 Alcoholism and drug dependence   6 Attention-seeking patients

Serious suicide attempts will usually be carried out alone, often without warning and some efforts made to avoid possible rescue.

The 'cri de coeur' (cry of the heart) attempt is often made with a warning and rescue often takes place. It can, of course, go wrong!

The general nurse is often faced with problems in the ward with patients who have attempted suicide a number of times. It is important to recognize that they still have a serious psychological problem and should not be treated as the unpopular patient.

There is a legal obligation as well as a nursing need to prevent suicide in (potential) patients. The law requires every effort to protect the patient from himself.

Nursing note

1 Correct positioning in the ward for observation
2 Remove all sharp objects which could be used
3 Avoid nursing near a high window
4 Ensure that drugs are taken and not hoarded for a later attempt
5 Report any feelings of guilt, evidence of depression deepening or hallucinations

The violent patient

Your own Health Authority has probably laid down guidelines for staff when handling violent patients and the importance of reporting incidents. You are advised to quote these.
The major principles are:

1 Try to pacify but do not attempt to restrain while alone.
2 Send for help. Calmly remove other patients and potential weapons.
3 Apply only reasonable restraint to avoid injury. Hold clothing rather than the body.
4 Report the incident fully, in writing.
5 Discuss with the patient what happened.

2.11 Social problems

The social needs of an individual are concerned with his relationships and life in society.

We will use the five areas in Model B as a foundation for identifying possible problems.

1 **Relating to the family** – includes lovers and pets!
2 **Relating to work**
3 **Economic needs**
4 **Social activities** – recreation, hobbies
5 **Spiritual needs**

Use the nursing process approach again.

1 Family

Assessment

1 Any evidence of family conflicts
2 Patients' anxieties are often for his or her loved ones rather than themselves
3 'Missing' of children can lead to depression in a parent
4 Many elderly patients, particularly, have only a pet as a living companion to relate to at home

Care plan

1 Arrange visiting to enable contact to be maintained
2 Organize privacy for loved ones to communicate sensitively (may be very important just before surgery)
3 Plan visiting for children with care
4 The value of allowing a pet to be brought in, to relieve an old person's anxiety, probably far outweighs any worry of introducing infection, if done wisely
5 Give constant information to patients about their family and pets

2 Work

Assessment
 1 Patients miss the social contact of work mates
 2 They may be anxious about the loss of skill or contracts due to their illness
 3 Long term sickness may seriously affect their future return to work

Care plan
 1 Arrange for visits from work mates
 2 Involvement with the work welfare services
 3 Possible involvement of a disablement retraining officer

Revision note When you have group revision sessions, try to consider the effects of specific conditions on various workers. For example, carcinoma of the bronchus to an actress and diabetes mellitus to a pop star.

3 Economics

Assessment
 1 The patient may have anxieties about paying various bills while in hospital e.g. mortgage, rates, electricity, gas, food, hire purchase payments
 2 There may be worry about future financial burdens with a long term illness
 3 Some businessmen may face serious financial problems – even bankruptcy – requiring expert handling

Care plan
 1 Introduce a medical social worker to help the family over financial aid through sickness – benefits available, visiting allowances, social security help
 2 Provide facilities for discussion with business colleagues, accountants and solicitors as required.
 (The patient may worry far more if he cannot know the facts of his business affairs)

4 Social activities – recreation, hobbies

Assessment
 1 Anxiety about loss of continuity of an interest e.g. TV programme, football team's progress
 2 Feelings of separation from a social group
 3 In children, the stage of intellectual and social development should be noted
 4 In the elderly, an absence of social interest and contact may be part of their normal living
 5 Exaggerated interest in ward activities may hide feelings of isolation and concern about being discharged to loneliness

Care plan
 1 Encourage leisure activities as much as the patient can tolerate – negotiate with him
 2 Allow visiting of social group members
 3 Organize play both individually and in groups for children. Use a skilled play therapist or leader
 4 Group patients with similar social interests in the ward
 5 Discuss the hazards of institutionalization with patients, relatives and friends

5 Spiritual needs

There may be serious religious problems when people are sick. Some groups would consider sickness, even now, to be an indication that 'sin' is the cause and that the individual's relationship with his god is in danger.
 Other problems arise because there is a threat to religious rituals which are seen as essential.

Assessment
 1 Religious beliefs of patients. You should learn the fundamental doctrines of some major ones e.g. Christians (including particular denominations), Moslems, Jews and Hindus
 2 Evidence of anxiety – some 'lapsed' believers feel a need for spiritual help when in hospital

Care plan
 1 Provide facilities for the practice of faiths as far as possible – privacy for prayer, prepare for Communion, welcome for priests, provide special diets, hand washing facilities
 2 Introduce ministers, chaplains and priests as part of the normal ward activity

Some would seek a place for political beliefs within the social domain. The nurse may need to make facilities for patients to exercise their political rights in voting, reading and calm discussion.
 Religion and politics are regarded as taboo subjects for conversation because vehement argument may ensue, but discussion has often proved to be excellent diversional therapy in some wards.

2.12 Drugs and treatments

The main principles in giving drugs and treatments are that they should be given

1 safely	**3 intelligently**
2 accurately	**4 within the law**

You will have been examined on these aspects of drug administration in your ward based practical examination, but you are advised to revise the material again before your written examinations. Eight questions are included in the objective test specifically on *drugs and therapeutic hazards*.

Knowledge of drugs

This should include
1 Methods of administration
2 The carriage of drugs to target sites. This is mainly attached to the plasma proteins of the blood serum, giving a measurable blood level
3 Side effects. Very few drugs have specific target sites and 'side' effects apply to most
4 The methods of excretion of drugs by the liver and the kidneys

Drug calculations

It is not possible to teach arithmetic of drug dosage in a book of this nature. The principles are to calculate every drug dosage and avoid memorizing. Basic formula for the amount to be given is:

$$\frac{\text{Dose prescribed}}{\text{Stock amount}} \times \text{Volume of the stock}$$

Examples

1 Prescribed dose   15 mg
   Stock amount   20 mg in 2 ml
   gives

$$\frac{15 \text{ mg}}{20 \text{ mg}} \times 2 \text{ ml} = 1.5 \text{ ml (to be given)}$$

2 Prescribed dose   200 micro.g/kg
   (Weight of patient = 15 kg)
   Stock amount   10 mg in 1 ml
   gives

$$\frac{200 \text{ micro.g} \times 15}{10 \text{ mg}} \times 1 \text{ ml}$$

you must change milligrams to micrograms (or visa versa)
giving

$$\frac{200 \text{ micro.g} \times 15}{10 \times 1000 \text{ micro.g}} \times 1 \text{ ml} = 0.3 \text{ ml (to be given)}$$

Drugs and the law

Again, the whole of the legislation cannot be given.

Key points
1 Controlled drugs – care and custody of drugs which can cause physical dependence and could have serious social and criminal consequences
2 All other drugs are classified as poisons
3 Classifications on labels
   1 POM – prescription only medicines
   2 P   – may only be sold by a pharmacist or where one is in attendance
   3 GSL – general sales list – small amounts of drugs which may be sold in general stores, supermarkets etc.
4 Drug keys – should be kept on the person in charge of the ward. Local rules apply to trained nurses giving controlled and certain other drugs, but these are Health Authority rules, not in the Misuse of Drugs Act.

Drug groups

A useful 5 point plan for knowledge of specific drugs is
1 The pharmaceutical name
2 The desired effect of the drug

Drug Group	Example	Desired effect	Adult dose			Undesired effects	Contra indications	Nursing notes
			Amount	Route	Frequency			
Antibacterial agent	Benzyl penicillin	Bacteriocidal	600 mg	I.M. or I.V.	6h	Hypersensitivity	Hypersensitivity	Avoid droplet discharge / Self protection – masks and gloves
Try also Ampicillin Chloramphenicol Amoxycillin Cephaloridine	Tetracycline(s)	Bacteriocidal	250–500 mg / 500 mg / 100 mg	Oral / I.V. / I.M.	6h / 12h / 4–12h	Moniliasis – 'Thrush' / Brown staining of growing teeth and bone	Pregnancy / Children under 12	Oral dose should not be given with milk or food
(Sulphonamides)	Sulphadimidine	Bacteriostatic	2 g initially then 0.5–1 g	Oral	6–8h	Allergic reactions / Crystalluria	Renal or hepatic failure / Pregnancy / Infants under 6 weeks / Blood disorders	Plenty of fluids / Observe carefully–for anaemia etc / –for renal problems
	Co-trimoxazole (Sulphamethoxazole 5 pts) (Trimethropin 1 part)	Bacteriocidal	960 mg	Oral / I.M. / I.V.	12h	Bone marrow depression		
Anti-inflammatory agents	Aspirin	Anti-inflammatory / Analgesic / Antipyretic / (Anticoagulant)	300–500 mg	Oral	4–6h	Hypersensitivity / Gastric erosion / (Haematemesis) / Tinnitus / Long-term – thrombocytopenia	Hypersensitivity / Peptic ulcers / Anticoagulant therapy	Watch for combined proprietory drugs / (See also aspirin poisoning)
Cortico steroids	Prednisolone	Anti-inflammatory / Anti-fibrotic / Euphoria	Various preparations			Suppressing signs of infection / Gastric erosion / Cushing's syndrome / Stops ACTH production	Always difficult decision to use them	Careful observations for infection / Oral dose with milk / Careful lifting. Urinalysis / Carry steroid card
Anticoagulants	Heparin	Prevention of thrombus formation	Varies			Haemorrhage / Hypersensitivity	Haemophilia / Peptic ulcer / Severe hypertension	Acts immediately –observe for bleeding / Antidote ready –protamine sulphate
	Warfarin		According to prothrombin times			Haemorrhage	Pregnancy / Severe hypertension / Haemophilia. Peptic ulcer	One dose may take 5 days to be excreted! / Antidote – vitamin K / Carry anticoagulant card
Narcotic	Morphine	Analgesia / Sedation / Relieves L.V. failure	10–12 mg	S.C. / I.M. / I.V.	4h	Physical dependence / Dose tolerance / Nausea. Vomiting. Constipation / Respiratory depression / Retention of urine	Pregnancy / Breast feeding / Respiratory disorder / Liver damage / Raised intracranial pressure	Controlled drug / Often given with anti-emetic / Observe carefully
Tranquilisers – Antipsychotic – Phenothiazine	Chlorpromazine	Tranquillization / Reduces anxiety / Reduces hiccups / Anti-emetic	25 mg / 75 mg / 25–50 mg / 100 mg	Orally / Bed time / Deep I.M. / Suppository	×3 daily / Nightly / 6–8h / 6–8h	Many – see National Formulary	Many cautions –see National Formulary	Causes skin reactions in some handlers – great care with syrups, liquids and suppositories

See also – **Diuretics**, **Digoxin**. Always check the latest edition of the British National Formulary

3 The normal dose – amount, route and frequency
4 The undesired effects of the drug – may include the exaggerated desired effect and side effects
5 Contra indications for giving drugs: pregnancy, liver failure, renal failure for nearly all drugs; others specific (e.g. hypersensitivity to penicillin)

See table for examples of each main group.

Undesired effects of drugs

Anorexia, nausea, vomiting Due to stimulation of the vomiting centre, hence injected drugs can still cause problems.

Hypersensitivity – allergy Drug causes histamine release by acting as an antigen. Histamine causes vasodilation and exudation from blood capillaries. This may give rise to rashes – tingling 'urticaria' (like the nettle rash), asthma or anaphylactic shock – massive vasodilation causing fall of blood pressure.

Blood dyscrasias (see 2.2) may be due to hypersensitive reactions. Very dangerous – aplastic anaemia.

Drug tolerance There is a need to increase the dosage to achieve desired effects.

Drug dependence
1 Psychological – cannot enjoy normal daily living without drugs
2 Physical – withdrawal symptoms if the drug is withheld (see 2.10)

Acute poisoning

Causes
1 Accidental
2 Self poisoning (attention seeking)
3 Suicidal
4 Homicidal

Principles of care

First aid
1 Maintain the airway
2 Medical aid or hospital quickly
3 Do not induce vomiting
4 Give nothing by mouth

Principle aim	Methods used
1 Identify the poison	Questioning. Examination of bottles, evidence, vomit. (May need to be retained for forensic tests)
2 Remove poison before absorption takes place	Oral – induce vomiting; gastric washing (dangerous if semi conscious or unconscious). Skin (snake bites) – apply tourniquet if deadly poison
3 Give antidote if known	*Specific* e.g. desferrioxamine for iron poisoning *General* e.g. anticonvulsant for strychnine poisoning
4 Increase the rate of excretion of the poison	Forced diuresis by giving intravenous fluids and a diuretic (usually frusemide). Catheterization Dialysis – usually peritoneal dialysis
5 Support life until poison is excreted	Care of the unconscious patient. Assisted ventilation. Parenteral nutrition
6 Assess psychiatric needs and start care as soon as possible	Psychiatric opinion. Nursing observations and history

Some specific poisons

Carbon monoxide inhaled exhaust fumes
Dangers
1 Only 1% needed for fatal results
2 Rescuer can easily be overcome too
Care High oxygen and carbon dioxide concentrations are needed although the patient looks pink.

Aspirin popular but unpleasant suicide vehicle!
Effects
1 Severe fluid loss through perspiration leads to dehydration, electrolyte imbalance, headaches, convulsions, mania before late unconsciousness due to acidosis.
2 Acidosis causes over-breathing too (hyperventilation). Note also – roaring or ringing in the ears (tinnitus), gastric erosion and haematemesis

Treatment
1 Forced alkaline diuresis in an intensive care unit. (An alkaline infusion is used for the acidosis, but also increases the rate of excretion of the aspirin.)
2 Fluid and electrolyte balance restored
3 May also need treatment for haematemesis

Iron (very dangerous in children)

Effects
1 Nausea, vomiting, abdominal pain, diarrhoea
2 Haematemesis. Rectal bleeding
3 Coma and death can occur within 4 hours in a young child

Treatment
1 Urgent transfer to hospital
2 Induce vomiting
3 Gastric washing using desferrioxamine solution, leaving 50 ml in the stomach
4 Intra muscular desferrioxamine may also be needed.

For others, see the *British National Formulary* latest edition.

2.13 Operating theatre

The syllabus explains that you should be able to recall:
1 The continuity of care from the anaesthetic room to the operating theatre and recovery room.
   You need to remember here the importance of recognizing the individuality of the patient throughout. *1* Ensure the correct identity of the patient by speech and checking labels, notes and operating theatre lists and addressing by name. *2* Ensure any marking has been done to indicate the correct operation site.
2 The procedures for ensuring the safety for the patient undergoing surgery.

The care of the unconscious patient
1 Maintenance of the airway and oxygenation
2 Maintenance of blood pressure and blood volume
3 Maintenance of hydration and electrolytes

The discipline of asepsis
1 Methods of sterilization used (steam under pressure, hot air, chemicals, irradiation)
2 Strictness of aseptic procedures (scrubbing and hand washing, dressing, instrument handling)
3 Organization of cleaning and preparing operating theatre itself
4 Organization of operating theatre lists to treat infected cases later
5 Principles of air flow to remove micro-organisms

The correct positioning of patients
1 For common operations, the table positions are relevant to care
2 In general, the prevention of pressure sores, diathermy burns and deep vein thrombosis depend on careful positioning of the patient and the equipment used

The checking of drugs, gases and infusions
1 Many are controlled drugs
2 The major gases used are nitrous oxide and halothane. Read the National Formulary for further information. Note especially problems of explosive reactions, operator dependence and danger to the foetus of pregnant staff
3 Note the main anaesthetic agents used and the stages of anaesthesia
4 Problems of spinal and epidural anaesthetics
5 Intravenous infusions may need to be given very quickly

3 The significance of team work in achieving high standards of safe and efficient practice. Learn the roles of the members of the team
   1 the surgeon, the assistant, the table nurse   *4* the recovery room staff
   2 the anaesthetist, the anaesthetic nurse   *5* the theatre sterilizing supply staff
   3 the operating theatre technicians
4 Further knowledge of the post operative needs of patients by observing surgical procedures. Make notes of the operations that you see and the particular problems e.g. finding the appendix; reaching the gall bladder; retropubic approach for prostatectomy

2.14 Children

The syllabus states that you should be able to
1 Demonstrate recognition of the special needs of children in relation to their physical, social, mental and emotional development.
2 Recognize and respect the part played by parents or parent substitutes in the care of a child.
3 Ensure an environment in which the child
 1 is safe,
 2 is enabled to play and
 3 can make social contacts
4 Assess and satisfy the needs of children for
 1 food, hydration, excretion
 2 cleanliness, clothing, comfort
 3 rest and play
5 Make and record observations of a child and take necessary action.
6 Devise and carry out a programme of management for a child
 1 admitted in an emergency   *2* whose admission is planned
7 Recognize and accept your own emotions on the death of a child or such matters as congenital abnormalities.
8 Demonstrate your competence to provide comfort for a distressed child and the parents.

In most text books children are considered in five groups
 1 Infants   **4 School children**
 2 Toddlers   **5 Adolescents**
 3 Pre-school children

Each group will be considered for
 1 their social and emotional development and needs
 2 their psychological (mental) development and needs
 3 their physical development and needs

We will also consider
 4 the observation of children
 5 management of care in an emergency
 6 management of care for a planned admission
 7 special problems – surgery, physical and mental handicap, dying and death of children

1 Infants – the first year

Social/emotional development and needs

The most important social development is that of **bonding** – with the mother first, then with the family. The mother/baby bonding is established by letting the mother hold the baby as soon as possible. Even premature babies or those in incubators need to be held by the mother very early.

Bonding with the family is helped by preparation of father, and brothers and sisters (siblings), before the birth but also in their early holding of the baby and involvement in its care.

The infant's relationships are primarily with the mother but gradually involve the rest of the family. They are essentially egocentric in behaviour, forming centres for attention.

The nurse becomes a parent substitute for an infant and should be aware of possible jealousies from the mother. Mother and infant units help to alleviate this problem. Involvement by the mother in the nursing of the infant is very important to prevent any severance of bonding or jealousy.

Psychological/mental development and needs

The infant learns very rapidly in the first year of life. The learning is known as sensori-motor learning and is essentially by trial and error. There is gradual boundary reaching, learning touch responses, exploring with hands, feet and mouth.

Communication with the mother starts very early with eye contact language, contented gurglings and responses to crying.

Smiling is a very important signal of development. It should occur at about 6–8 weeks.

The nurse needs to be aware of the infant's learning style – toys should be appropriate for their stage of learning – colourful, easily held, comfort giving.

It is also important to recognize the need for safety in infancy – crawling and early steps can lead them to areas of danger – stairs, electrical apparatus, water and poisons. Toys should be safe including safety paint, absence of loose or sharp pieces which could injure the mouth, be swallowed or cause asphyxia by choking.

Physical development

If you have memorized the steps of development then you will be able to consider nursing care in response to each step. For those who have difficulty, some key steps are given.

Head The head is large in comparison to the trunk and limbs at birth. In the first year this ratio changes quite rapidly. Considerable body heat is lost through the head.

Fontanelles – the spaces between the developing cranial bones
1 Posterior fontanelle closes within 3–4 months
2 Anterior fontanelle closes between 10–14 months

Fig. 2.14.1 The foetal skull showing the bones, fontanelles and sutures

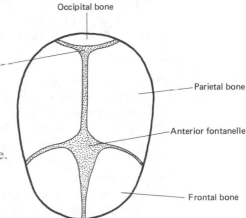

Nursing note
In early infancy, the pulse may be taken at the anterior fontanelle.

Tears arc not present at birth and in the early weeks.

Nursing note
Special care of a baby's eyes when bathing.

Body temperature The control of body temperature is not developed as the hypothalamus is not fully functional at birth and in the early weeks. Heat loss through the head may be considerable. Heat gain in a fever may be difficult to control and convulsions may occur.

Feeding Infant feeding starts with milk – either breast feeding or bottle feeding. You should learn the advantages of the two types of feeding.

Advantages of breast feeding
1 *Bonding* with the mother
2 Immune factors in colostrum and milk – T lymphocytes, B lymphocytes, immunoglobulin A, some disease antibodies
3 Milk at body temperature and does not need to be sterilized
4 Preparation time is minimal and feeding *on demand* can be easily established
5 Release of oxytocin returns uterus to normal size early
6 More economical

Nursing notes
Mothers usually like privacy but some will happily feed their baby in public. The mother needs guidance on maintaining her own fluid and nutrition intake and avoiding foods or drugs which could disturb the baby, e.g. alcohol, onions, rhubarb, sedatives.

Early encouragement for breast feeding is given in ante natal care; active support may be needed at the beginning and guidance on the care of her breasts for comfort and hygiene will be needed.

Advantages of bottle feeding
1 *Bonding* with the mother, but also with the father and other children if they can 'help'
2 No diet restrictions in mother
3 The mother may take drugs if needed
4 Modern prepared feeds give all nutrition requirements
Expressed breast milk is still preferred when possible.

Nursing notes
Feeds must be prepared correctly, using sterile equipment and aseptic technique. Correct measurements of feed and water are necessary and the temperature should be checked carefully before feeding.

Requirement from milk feeding 150 ml per kg body weight in 24 hours – aiming to increase body weight by 200 g per week in the first 3 months

Weaning The introduction of cereals begins from 4–5 months in modern units. (There may be a relationship between early weaning and coeliac disease.) Introduction of tastes should aim at savoury foods before sweet foods. By the end of the first year, the child will usually be able to feed himself, enjoying a minced version of the family meal

Elimination There is no sphincter control and nappy changing is necessary.

Nursing note
Washing and drying carefully should be sufficient care of the nappy area. Nappy rash will occur if faecal matter and urine are next to the skin for too long, due to the action of proteus organisms which convert urea into ammonia.

Activities Note some of the early primitive reflex actions, such as walking/stepping, rooting, grasping and Moro (alarm).

Developments

3 months – kicking, follows with eyes	**9** months – crawling, talking
6 months – full head control, holds objects	**12** months – standing, walking a few steps

Nursing notes

Physical play activities are used to assess developments and reinforce acquired skills. Toys are made available and should be used by nurses as well as parents and play leaders.

It is important to recognize that all so called milestones in child development are phases rather than steps. In many developments the skill may be acquired weeks before or after a 'milestone' time.

Immunity

Very important progress in the development of immunity occurs in the first year of life. Details cannot be covered in this text.

The main components are in the production of

1 antibodies and immunity (humoral) from B lymphocytes
2 sensitized T cells and foreign cell destruction (cell mediated immunity) from T lymphocytes. T indicates migration through the thymus gland which shrinks and becomes redundant.

Types of immunity

Natural – through natural processes e.g. illness itself
Artificial – through artificial processes e.g. immunization
Passive – short acting
Active – long acting

Examples of immunity

Natural passive – in mothers milk
Natural active – invasion by micro-organism
Artificial passive – injecting gamma globulin
Artificial active – immunization

Immunization starts in the first year for diphtheria, tetanus, pertussis and poliomyelitis

1st dose	3 months
2nd dose	3–5 months
3rd dose	9–11 months

Nursing notes

The nurse needs to emphasize the need for immunization to parents – in some areas, the rate of failure to take advantage of the service has risen alarmingly.

Contra indications for immunization are if the child has a fever or known allergic condition (e.g. eczema).

2 Toddlers age 1–3 years (texts vary on ages)

Social/emotional development

The toddler is still very much mother and family centred in his relationships. Play with older brothers and sisters is very acceptable as he is often the centre of attention.
Problems may gradually arise when:

1 another baby arrives, displacing mother attention. Jealousies may arise unless good preparation and involvement are practised.
2 working mothers return to full-time occupations.

Introduction to other toddlers and nursery schools is helpful.

Psychological/mental development

Learning is still sensory-motor, trial and error, but exploration becomes much wider as mobility increases.

The child's vocabulary increases to a thousand words by the age of three and he continually exercises them in talking to himself and asking questions. Repetition of questions is called *echolalia*.

Nursing notes

The child needs repeated opportunities to reinforce his vocabulary. It is an important function to read to a child or tell stories that you know for children.

Clear print books with pictures should enable the three year old to start reading. Toys for helping the child developing handling skills should be available too.

Physical development

Feeding The toddler will be acquiring teeth (sometimes with pain and miserable soreness). Normal food in small portions with small pieces of meat should be given. Patience is needed with earlier attempts at self feeding.

Elimination Toilet training is important. Starts after meals, using the gastrocolonic reflex. Praise for success, ignore accidents and allow time. (Full control is not possible until nerve pathways have matured.) No time schedule should be considered as 'the normal'.

Note that exploration may include the handling of genitalia and even faeces.

Nursing notes
The nurse should be aware that separation from home and illness can lead to regressive behaviour. Patience with toilet habits is needed. The advantage of the mother being there to help is that she may have a good chance of continuing training that she started at home.

Activities The toddler becomes much more physically active–walking, kicking a ball, climbing stairs, handling switches, learning to wash and dress.

By three years, he is gaining stamina too!

Nursing note
The child is in more danger, of course, and awareness of the need to provide a safe environment is very important.

Immunity

Most authorities introduce measles vaccination in the toddler stage of development. Some parents are reluctant to take up the vaccine, but the dangers of measles are serious.

3 Pre-school children

Social/emotional development

Relationships are still essentially based on the family, but more socialization should be developing.

Involvement with play groups, Sunday Schools and 'street groups' is good preparation for day school.

Psychological/mental development

The child has moved into the pre-operational phase of development for learning. Vocabulary rapidly increases, if exercised, to over 2000 words. Reading skills develop rapidly and should be encouraged. Number skills can be reinforced–many teachers think that it is as important as reading. Drawing and painting become more organized but lack real form until a later stage.

Nursing note
Play and involvement with pre-school children is very important. Many of these early skill developments are going to be very important for success at school.

Discipline The toddler and pre-school child may go through phases of 'negativism'–saying 'no', being naughty and generally 'trying' parents and substitutes. Parents have their own views on how this is handled and should be consulted if it happens.

Nursing note
The nurse must be careful in the way she disciplines a child who is naughty. In many cases, it may be ignored, in others the nurse must tell the child. Threats should never be used. Only threats that are actually carried out are effective.

Physical development

The pre-school child is very active in play and leisure. Many can ride tricycles, swim, play vigorous games and sport–but, of course, dangers are still threatening, for example road traffic accidents or falling from trees and play ground apparatus. Exposure to infections is also increased.

It is important that assessments of vision and hearing are carried out before school life. Spectacles or hearing aids may be required.

Feeding Normal diets in increasing amounts. Dental hygiene–teeth cleaning, visits to the dentist should be encouraged.

Elimination Sphincter control is complete before schooling, but illness, anxiety and separation can still lead to the regressive 'accident'. The child may need some treatment and/or reassurance if bed wetting (enuresis) occurs.

Immunity

A booster dose of diphtheria, tetanus and poliomyclitis vaccine is often given before starting school.

4 The school child–up to 11 years

Social/emotional development

The major change from home centred relationships to school is still a major hurdle for some children unless early socialization and preparation has been good. Unfortunately, many parents' negative views of school are sensed by children and this may be the cause of early difficulties.

Soon there are major changes of relationships, with flitting friendships within school, relating to school classes and teachers who begin to develop the child's awareness.

Friends are usually of the same sex. Teachers and nurses may be 'parent' figures.

Psychological/mental development

The child progresses from the pre-operational stage to the concrete operational stage of learning development.

Some significant steps are in the grouping of objects, recognizing that they may be described in different sets e.g. guinea pigs may be brown or belong to the animal kingdom. They learn to discriminate between sizes – first by length, then by mass and finally volume.

Reading skills progress rapidly if nurtured.

Numeracy skills need reinforcement with games, experiments and success (e.g. handling money).

As understanding develops, so does imagination, and fear of the dark, pain and strangers may be increased.

Language development is nearly complete – the child likes to be heard. Some start learning foreign languages at school.

Nursing notes

The nurse should recognize this important period of mental development.

Games and conversations, television programmes and computer activities are helping to expand the awareness even more. Puzzles, books and logic games are popular.

Many paediatric units have a school teacher to enable children to continue with their lessons. Nurses need to show an interest in the child's progress.

Physical development

Activity is vigorous but usually well co-ordinated at this stage. The acquisition of skills is very high during this period – writing becomes ordered, drawing and sewing neater, playing football better. Note the age of some of the gymnasts in world competition.

Feeding Healthy appetite is usual and anorexia is a warning sign of ill health. Dental care remains important as deciduous teeth are replaced by permanent teeth. The school child may develop changes of food likes and dislikes. Some will have the same main meal for days if they like it.

Illness Exposure to infection, possible injury or other factors may lead to loss of school time which can seriously interfere with education. Adequate stimulation and early return to school usually allows the child to 'catch up' but some parents become very concerned and nursing assurance needs to be reinforced by involvement of the school.

5 Adolescents – changing from children to adults

Child care rarely involves those over 16 years.

Social/emotional development

Regarded by many as a most difficult period of social development. There is often rebellion against parental attitudes and a seeking to establish an individual identity.

Relationships are first of all with groups of the same sex (gangs) but eventually with the opposite sex. It should be noted though that some find emotional relationships with the same sex more suited to their personality needs.

There is usually a period of 'idealism' in which the teenager identifies strongly with religious and political dogmas. This may be a cause of serious conflict.

Psychological/mental development

Piaget's description is of 'formal operation' stage of intellectual development.

The child learns to think in the abstract, to see situations from other points of view (hence the idealism). Drawing in three dimensions is developed and imaginary concepts can be portrayed. Learning potential is at its greatest height at this stage.

Preparation for examinations is an important need and again psychological pressures develop. The teenager is at the stage to develop serious psychological problems – see section 2.10.

Physical development

The significant changes are, of course, those of puberty. It should not be necessary to remind you of these but the nurse should be prepared for problems relating to:

 1 teaching for sexual hygiene – vulval care and coping with menstruation for girls, cleansing of the genitalia for boys.
 2 adequacy of sexual education – physical and emotional. Discussion of contraception.
 3 guidance for coping with masturbation, nocturnal ejaculation.

4 coming to terms with the changed body image including: experimenting with clothing; application of make up, shaving; clumsiness; acne; anorexia nervosa (see 2.10); embarrassment about nakedness.

It is also a period of experimentation with a view to impressing. Cigarette smoking and alcohol drinking may commence and eventually become compulsive.

Immunity

Rubella vaccination is offered for girls between 11 and 13 years to avoid foetal rubella syndrome (congenital defects) if the girl later becomes pregnant.

BCG (Bacille Calmette-Guérin) is given between 12–14 years, but follows a Heaf test (6 needles).

Nursing notes
The teenager may well listen to you as a practising nurse about the dangers of missing these two important immunizations.

Legal status of teenagers

16 years – may give legal consent for surgery or medical treatment
        (including contraceptive help)
17 years – may live away from home; may be imprisoned
        (usually starts with Detention Centre or Borstal training)
18 years – may vote, marry without parental consent and assume full adult responsibilities

Observations of children

Remember that observations are necessary for:
1 assessing the existing and changing conditions of the child.
2 determining the nursing responses required to meet the needs of the child.
In examination answers, it is imperative that you indicate:
1 the reasons for the observations
2 the planned frequency that they will be recorded
3 the actions you will take in response to them

Guide lines for observations by using Model B, but it is better to consider the psychological observations first.

Psychological – behaviour observations

The earliest indications of childhood illness are found in behaviour changes
1 becoming quiet and withdrawn, irritable and moody
2 showing evidence of anxiety – facial expression, excessive crying
3 some children with anxiety will show a typical 'rocking' action on their haunches

Children with learning difficulties or learning deficiency may have difficulty communicating in play. Some children who are deprived of love and affection may display attention-seeking behaviour which manifests itself as naughtiness, hurting other children or 'attaching' themselves to nurses. Note also that the anxiety of parents (and substitutes) is easily transmitted to children.

Social observations

Depending on the normal stages of development, relationships with parents, brothers and sisters and other children should be observed for any evidence of difficulty in socialization.

It is difficult to give definitive statements as each child, family and observer is part of the social setting in which observations are made.

Physical observations

– relating to the physiological systems

Skin It is important to observe for
1 colour – paleness, cyanosis and jaundice.
2 rashes – the child is prone to childhood infections where the rash may be the first sign reported. For example, chicken pox – vesicular (blisters containing fluid) and measles – macular (red raised spots).
3 evidence of bruising (but does not necessarily imply child abuse), scratching or wounds.
4 possible infestations e.g. pediculosis capitus (head lice), nits, burrow marks of scabies.

Circulation Normal *pulse rate* is higher in children:
Infants   110–150 per minute
Toddler   100–110 per minute
Pre-school child   80–100 per minute

Temperature regulation is poor in infancy. Although children often show very high temperatures when ill, it is not always reliable to assume that an apparent normal temperature implies that the metabolic rate is not raised – the core temperature may still be very high.

Infants with pyrexia may also have febrile convulsions.

Blood pressure is difficult to record in infancy, but can be recorded normally in the school child. (Check both arm pressures – see coarctation of the aorta)

Respiration Normal rate is higher in children and in early infancy, regularity may not be established.

Infant   20–30 per minute
Toddler   20–30 per minute
Pre-school child 12–20 per minute

It is important to observe the baby's breathing actions in full. Some with hypoxia may have a typical 'flaring of the nostrils'.

Digestion Anorexia is often a first indication of illness in a child. Nausea and vomiting may be indications of toxaemia which may have no relationship with a gastro-intestinal disorder. Projectile vomiting in a little boy may suggest pyloric stenosis.

Diarrhoea along with vomiting in an infant and toddler is serious as fluid depletion (dehydration) may be high in comparison to their total blood volume. Constipation is more often noted by parents. Stool observations are important. Note especially – meconium in the new born baby; cherry red stool for intussusception; fatty, offensive stool for cystic fibrosis.

Abdominal pain is often referred pain in a child and may even be a symptom of tonsillitis. It should always be investigated as the acute abdomen in a child can progress very quickly.

Excretion Urine observation is difficult in the infant and toddler. Special collecting bags may be required for urinalysis specimens. Fluid balance is best measured by weighing.
Burning of micturition may be a cause of unexplained crying.

Neural control The child has difficulty describing pain and may need careful observation. Infants may draw up knees for abdominal pain, bang heads for ear ache or just show abject misery for something like teething pain.

Sleep patterns change significantly throughout childhood. In early infancy, waking appears to be only for feeding and changing of nappies. In fact, some mothers enjoy many more hours of wakefulness with their baby than others.

By adolescence, sleep is as for adults, but varies according to the exercise or developing anxiety.

As children become more imaginative, they may acquire more fear of the dark or 'semi light' with shadows. They may need assurance of this in a children's ward at night time. Many children have a 'comforter' at night.

Changes of observations

Children change notoriously quickly.

Deterioration may be rapid and clinical recordings should be frequent. It is better to think of *continual* observation with scheduled recordings.

Fortunately, the recovery is usually just as dramatic and recordings may not be required frequently for a long period.

Management of a child admitted in an emergency

The nurse should realize that the emergency admission of a child suggests that the condition is serious. It is not undertaken lightly.

There may have been a very sudden interruption to normal daily living. Parents are naturally extremely worried when this happens. They may have feelings of guilt because they feel responsible for all that happens to the child and they may dispel their anxiety or guilt in unexpected reactions, such as aggression towards nursing staff. Every effort should be made to make parents welcome and a room for accommodation should be provided.

There is need for urgent action:
1 Skilled clinical observations
2 Diagnostic investigations e.g. abdominal and rectal examination, lumbar puncture
3 Medical treatment (drug dosage is estimated by the mass of the child in kilograms or body surface area which needs the height measurement too)
4 Surgical treatment

The anxiety and urgency will heighten the fear in the child – the nurse should realize that this fear may be fostered for the remainder of the child's life.

Full nursing history with the child's normal daily living activities (diet, play, sleep) should be completed later in co-operation with parents.

Management of a child admitted as a planned admission

Before admission

It is a great advantage if the out patient clinic is located near to the children's ward. Some authorities have a Childrens' Centre containing clinics, assessment and treatment units and the clinical wards within one site. The child can then be taken to visit the ward and meet staff well in advance of the admission.

Booklets on entering the hospital for children are very helpful.

Parents should have the admission procedure explained in out patients. Advice to bring a favourite toy and usual night comforter will help.

Welcome

The tour of the ward should be relaxed. The nurse should hold hands when the child is ready! The admission interview should be quite formal but in a comfortable, quiet corner of the ward.

The child
1 Speak at eye level and maintain eye contact
2 Phrase questions for them to understand
3 Admit 'teddy' as well!

Parents
1 Discuss daily living activities. For example, food likes and dislikes; words for urinating and defaecation; sleep patterns.
2 Discuss visiting plans. Most units have open visiting for both parents.
3 Negotiate any nursing care that they would like to give to the child.
4 Routine details should be clearly written. Apply discretion when mentioning religion and baptism.

Baptism – some denominations believe very strongly in infant baptism and would require an infant baptized if there was danger of dying.

Some would take a mention of baptism as indication that life was threatened.

Nursing history

In addition to recording the results of your interview for daily living activities, you would make a note of the developmental stage and any factors such as school work.

The nursing care plan would be devised with awareness of all these factors to obtain total patient care.

Special problems of child care

Surgery

Consent can be given by parents or legal guardian (Social Services may be able to give consent for children in care). The surgeon can operate *without consent* to save a child's life.

Children can be made 'wards of court' by magistrates when conflict arises.

Preparation A full explanation, to the child's understanding, should be given, taking great care in avoiding breaches of 'nil by mouth'. Prepare 'teddy' as well.

Some hospitals allow parents to escort their children to theatre.

Physical skin preparation may be needed but shaving only required for teenagers! Examine teeth for loose teeth, dental caries, prostheses. Pre-medication needs careful calculation (according to the child's mass of body surface area).

Example
Doctor's prescription   Trimeprazine 2 mg/kg
Child weighs   11.25 kg
Stock preparation   7.5 mg/5 ml
Using drug calculation formula
$$\frac{\text{Prescribed dose}}{\text{Stock preparation}} \times \text{Volume of stock}$$
$$\frac{2 \text{ mg} \times 11.25}{7.5 \text{ mg}} \times 5 \text{ ml} = 15 \text{ ml}$$

After surgery all care is as for adults in maintaining the airway, observing wounds and drains and preventing vomiting.

Remember that children's perception of pain may not be well established and that post operative analgesia must be carefully calculated.

Physical and mental handicap

The nurse should first of all realize that these do not necessarily go together. It is important that early care for some physically handicapped children is vital to prevent them developing mental handicap.

For example, early cure for deafness will prevent the child lacking educational opportunities (because teachers were not aware).

Parents may have deep psychological difficulty, especially in the early stages, feeling failures or guilty over the child's handicap. They often treat the child as precious – hiding from the need for normal child discipline and even from contact with other children for fear of infection, injury or teasing.

Many have developed great skill in nursing their children and should continue to be involved when the child is admitted for care.

The child may be vulnerable to physical injury or infection (paralysed or deformed limbs may develop pressure sores). They may require movement and exercises performed by nurses, physiotherapists or parents.

Feeding and nutrition should fit in with outside pattern as much as possible.

The child will still like to be involved in social activities – play, television, stories. They should receive teaching and learning stimulation according to individual assessment (this includes the mentally handicapped where learning to eat with a spoon may be a high achievement). Special equipment may be needed.

Other children may need a careful explanation to relate normally with handicapped children. A skilled play leader will be able to integrate them very well. The nurse should develop skills likewise.

Dying and death of children

There is great emotional turmoil for the staff in a childrens' unit over the dying child. Even the most experienced paediatric Sister has difficulty in controlling her emotions to behave professionally towards other children, parents and staff.

Junior nurses need to discuss their emotional feelings and be cared for with sympathy.

Preparation Although parents are told clearly, they often have great difficulty coming to terms with the reality. They may display unexpected reactions initially and may need expert help to guide them through a difficult period.

Care
Physical care Pain relief should be well controlled by skilful awareness of the need to give analgesics regularly, preventing pain developing in severity.

Nursing notes
The nurse needs to be very observant of the effect and length of time that the drug has at changing stages. Dosage and timing will need to be discussed with the Doctor.
Dyspnoea is very distressing both for the child and parents. Oxygen is not always tolerated well.

Nursing note
Careful positioning and changing positions may be helpful.

Rest should be organized. Nursing care should be co-ordinated to give the child good periods without disturbance. Hygiene and nutrition should be maintained as much as the child can tolerate and enjoy.

Psychological care Parents and staff should be made aware of how fear transmits itself to a child.
Older children and adolescents will, of course, have real fear of dying and death

Nursing note
Assurance that pain relief will be maintained, being truthful, discussing feelings, are all important parts of care. Many units consider that the care is not just of the child, but the care of the family.

Social care Open visiting as much as the child can tolerate – parents, brothers and sisters, friends and pets should be allowed. The view from the ward window may be important if children like birds, flowers and scenery. Television is helpful.

Some children have wishes fulfilled, such as meeting their favourite cricketer.

Respect the religious views of the family, involving the family priest, the chaplain or friends.

The death
Informing parents should be in private but friends may be very supportive. It is very difficult over the telephone unless you know that they are not alone. Allow time for early grief.
Last offices A careful choice of staff may be needed, but a junior nurse will often come to terms with the relief from suffering when handling the child at peace.

2.15 Elderly

Your syllabus requires that you should be competent to:
1 Demonstrate your awareness of the normal manifestations of ageing and to recognize deviations from health in the elderly.
2 Promote the maximum degree of dignity for elderly people.
3 Recognize, support and complement the parts played by relatives in the care of the elderly.
4 Practise the nursing care of elderly patients during the acute phases of illness, programmes of rehabilitation and long term care.

We will consider:
1 **The effects of ageing**: physical; psychological; social
2 **The teams involved in care**: the family; the Primary Health Care team; the Hospital teams; Social Services; Voluntary services
3 **Some particular problems of the elderly**: loss of stability and mobility; multiple diagnosis; confusion; incontinence; hypothermia; surgery; drugs

1 The effects of ageing

The cause of the ageing process is not known – it is common to all living organisms.

Physical effects

The rate of cell mitosis is changed as the body ages, with an actual reduction in the number of functioning cells. Many cells do not function as efficiently – fibrocytes tend to produce more collagen fibres than elastic fibres.

Respiratory system As connective tissue becomes less elastic, the lungs tend to 'become more stiff'. There is a decrease in the number of functioning bronchioles and alveoli (without the additional problems of chronic lung disease). Respiratory muscles become progressively weaker.

Nursing notes
Many elderly patients increase their respiratory problems by wearing heavy tight clothing around their chest.
Most find it easier to sleep with extra pillows – either sitting up or high side lying to improve their respiratory volume.

Circulatory system The heart valves tend to become thickened. Cardiac output falls. Blood vessels become 'hardened' as collagen fibre replaces elastic.
Increased peripheral resistance will cause a rise of systolic blood pressure (but do not confuse this with the pathological state of hypertension).

Nursing notes
The lower cardiac output is one of the factors causing the elderly person to slow down. There is no point in 'rushing' old people to do anything.

Digestive system Many have lost teeth and dentures may need replacement as the gums recede.
Peristalsis tends to be slower – constipation is a common problem.
A smaller liver and evidence of reduced insulin production will affect carbohydrate and fat metabolism. Many old people have a depleted glycogen store and one day without nutrition can be very serious – possibly one factor causing confusion in the elderly.

Nursing notes
Dental hygiene and treatment may be needed. Refitting of dentures may need to be arranged. Eating little and often is helpful for the elderly as long as obesity is controlled. Persuasion to eat fibre is not always easy. It is better to reduce fat intake rather than insist on very low carbohydrate intake.

Renal system The kidneys become smaller in size. Bladder capacity is often reduced. Muscles for micturition are less effcient. The prostate enlarges in the older man.

Nursing note
Increased frequency of micturition often disturbs the older person's sleep pattern. They tend to reduce their fluid intake and need gentle persuasion to maintain adequate hydration.

Nervous system Reduction in the number of neurones causes the brain to become smaller. Responses and reaction times are slower.
There are changes of sensory awareness
1 Slower reaction to temperature changes
2 Reduced taste – especially salt (tends to cause them to add more salt to their food)

3 Hearing accuity, especially for high frequency notes is reduced (do not appreciate hi fi)

4 Vision and colour perception are diminished

Nursing notes

It is very important to assess the individual old person's reactions and senses. The rate of change is extremely variable.

Individual sleep patterns should also be assessed, partly because of neurological changes but also because of long established daily living patterns.

Many elderly have reduced pain response too – a factor which is often helpful in controlling drug therapy. It should be noted though that if an older person does complain, the pain is probably very severe indeed.

Locomotor system Most older people are shorter in stature (apart from developing a stoop). Shortening mainly takes place in the vertebral column.

Muscle fibres become smaller and weaker. Joints appear larger and synovial membranes are not so efficient. Cartilage is less smooth. This gives the stiffness of joints.

It is estimated that only 2 out of 1000 reaching the age of 70 will have escaped some form of rheumatism.

Posture is altered and there is more difficulty in maintaining balance (increased sway).

Nursing notes

These factors are again important in the overall slowing of the old person. Patient exercising will maintain activity very well for some, but remember that reduced mobility may have been present for many years.

There is increased danger of falling and advice on home care is important.

Skin Loss of elastic fibres in the areolar tissue leads to the wrinkling of the skin.

Sweat glands become smaller. The hair changes colour and in many there is considerable loss. (The bald head loses more body heat.) Nails become thickened. Blood capillaries are more fragile.

Nursing notes

Many older ladies are still self conscious about wrinkles and they can be encouraged to use make up if they wish to.

Hairdressers are able to maintain not only the looks, but also advise on the health of the hair. Wigs and toupées should be encouraged if they like them.

Nurses should be able to trim most normal nails, but a chiropodist may be needed to deal with thick ones and especially those with a poor peripheral blood circulation.

Observations for bruising from even minor knocks are needed.

Endocrine system The thyroid gland becomes smaller with age and less thyroxine is produced. (It does not follow that all old people get the pathological state of myxoedema though.) Metabolic rate tends to be reduced – see all other systems.

There is a reduction in insulin production – some develop late onset diabetes mellitus.

See 2.8 for *Conditions of the endocrine system.*

Reproductive systems

Men Sperm production decreases with age but is not terminated. Sexual arousal with erection still occurs but is usually slower. Ejaculation force is reduced.

Women The levels of oestrogen fall after the menopause and progesterone ceases completely. The reproductive organs become smaller and the vaginal wall is less elastic. The breasts become smaller (although fat may still be present).

Nursing notes

Many older couples still enjoy an intimate sexuality without intercourse. Privacy should be respected.

Most old people still feel highly embarrassed by their own nakedness and suffer great indignity when being bathed.

Old gentlemen can still enjoy the sight and presence of a pretty girl!

Psychological

There is a changing self perception in the elderly. Loss of work status and family changes, including bereavement, will affect their view of themselves. Nevertheless, they remain individuals with their own personality.

There is a tendency to have a stereotype view of the world due to limitations of movement and experience, but some are remarkably adaptable.

Nursing notes

It is most important that older patients are treated as individuals with integrity – using their correct name, allowing personal dress likes and dislikes and respecting their views and experiences.

Feelings of insecurity and fear can arise in many circumstances:

1 Fear of injury and assault   *2* Fear of terminal illness and death   *3* Embarrassment if exposed

Nursing notes
Observations for indications of fear and insecurity are important. Behavioural as well as clinical observations should be reported. They may appear over-active, withdrawn and quiet or even show defence mechanisms such as aggression or regression.

Learning is generally more difficult for elderly people as memory patterns change. The usual picture is that long term memory circuits are functioning well (they remember, vividly, incidents from thirty years ago) but short term memory circuits are faulty (cannot remember what they did yesterday). Nevertheless, some old people do enjoy learning and reading. Many develop new creative skills in retirement.

Nursing note
Again, the important point is to assess the individual's capacity. An awareness of events in modern history may in fact prove to be a good point of communication with the elderly.

Communication for the elderly is often affected by their health problems. Deafness and loss of vision will create problems.
Remember also that some old people have lived alone for many more years than you have lived.

Nursing note
The nurse needs to consider her use of words and body language in communicating with the elderly. Speaking at eye level, clearly and in language that makes sense (but not infantile talk!).

Social effects

The family changes are significant for the elderly. As their children develop their own families, many elderly people feel isolated. The accumulation of conflict over grandchildren's behaviour sometimes increases the isolation.
Grandparents may sometimes become very possessive over their grandchildren. Many, however, enjoy a special relationship which should be recognized.
Some authorities are trying 'adopt a grandparent' schemes for integration of elderly, lonely people with youngsters.

Nursing note
Visiting by families is important. Open visiting (including grandchildren) helps younger people to maintain visiting.
Loneliness is the major problem facing elderly patients and is inclined to become worse as isolation develops. There are often serious problems for the elderly patient before being discharged home to their loneliness.
Retirement can be a great hurdle for elderly people. Their role in society changes and social contacts may be broken.
Many authorities help with preparation-for-retirement courses, running retirement clubs, using retired workers as guides to their works. Some pensioner's clubs are either run or supported by various unions.

Nursing note
Awareness of the past occupation helps in communicating and may indeed be a guide to a diagnosis. Conversely, it may be necessary to reinforce their integrity by referring to their skills as gardeners, cooks or seamstresses which they have developed since retirement.

Economic factors have a serious effect on many elderly patients. Loss of earnings, small pensions and limitations on economic spending can affect their diet, their housing and heating and also the comfort and fashion of their clothing.

Nursing note
Many elderly patients are not aware of the financial help that is available. Introduction to a social worker will often help in finding ways to assist them.

Social life for the elderly is dependent on their mobility and the local services available. Many still enjoy bingo and many go dancing and enjoy social outings with other people.

Nursing note
Many geriatric units organize excellent social activities for their patients. The nurse's role in organizing them is part of her total patient care for individual patients and groups.

Many elderly people are deeply religious and enjoy a very active and devout church life. Their faith is often strong and impressive. Even those who have had little interest earlier in life often find support in their later years. Bereavement for some is borne through their faith.

Nursing note
The nurse should be prepared to listen openly to the spiritual needs and views of older patients. Provision for rituals such as Holy Communion is again an important part of total patient care.
In terminal illness, many would need the support of a Minister or Priest.

Grief Of course, the major social change occurs with the loss of a spouse through death. Grief may be summarized in three phases:

1 – shock and incomprehension, followed by
2 – depression with occasional tearful outbursts, and gradually,
3 – adjustment and acceptance.

Some use different phases to describe the grieving process. Most agree that it can take 2–3 years for 'recovery', and, of course, some never do 'accept'. Very often, in a devoted couple, the one may die soon after the other.

Emotional upset may cause physical symptoms (see diabetes mellitus).

Nursing notes

Recognition of the deep effects of grief in elderly patients will help the nurse to make a realistic and sensitive care plan for them. Note again how very individual the reactions can be.

2 The teams involved in the care of the elderly

The family

Most younger people do feel a great sense of responsibility for their elderly relatives. There are serious problems of modern living that make it difficult to translate that responsibility into practical care.

Geography Many families live far away from elderly relatives. Although cars make contact seem possible, the ease of visiting is not always fulfilled.

Some have a grandparent living with them or in very close proximity, but this can lead to conflict.

Work Many families have both the man and wife working, both for economic and social fulfilment. This limits the time they can spend with grandparents and also increases the tiredness (and frustration) of 'doing things' for them.

Morals and ethics There is often a conflict of the older person's view of 'right and wrong' behaviour compared with the younger generation – the 'generation gap'.

Surprisingly, many young people find that they can, with effort, bridge the gap and enjoy discussing moral issues with older people.

The primary health care team

This is the medical based team caring for the community and many have developed special services in their care of the elderly. You should have some experience of them from your allocated Community Care experience.

The team consists of: the General Practitioners, the Health Visitors and Community trained nurses (with possible help from auxiliaries and bath attendants). You should make or review your notes of the roles and functions of each of these members of the team.

The Primary team can refer patients for other medical care – chiropody, optical and dental care, and some would employ para medical workers themselves. Some authorities have domiciliary physiotherapy and occupational therapy services too.

The hospital team

You are no doubt well aware of the hospital team, but again you are reminded to revise your notes on the roles and functions of:

1 The Geriatrician
2 The Nursing team
3 The Ancillary team; physiotherapists; occupational therapists; speech therapists
4 The Medical social workers

You should consider also the important stages of nursing the elderly sick patient.

1 Assessment and acute care
2 Rehabilitation for daily living
3 Long stay care or Continuing care
4 Day hospital provisions

The social services team

Local authorities and social workers make special provisions for the care of vulnerable groups in society – including the elderly. These provisions include direct care and information.

Care in the home Help is provided for cleaning and shopping by home care assistants (or home helps). The service may be free or provided on an 'ability to pay' scale of charges.

Meals on wheels are provided at a nominal cost by authorities (usually delivered by voluntary workers).

Care in the community Some authorities make provision for luncheon clubs and day centres. Many are actually run by voluntary workers and the elderly themselves.

Residential care Local authorities provide accommodation for those who are old and infirm enough to require care and attention. There is not usually the provision for full nursing care however. The accommodation is known as Part 3 (from Part III of the 1948 National Assistance Act).

Some authorities pay for the elderly to be cared for in private homes.

Sheltered housing Many authorities have built special houses (often bungalows) for elderly people with warden supervision. Many wardens have nursing qualifications, but it is not intended that a full nursing service be given.

There is great effort in some communities to integrate the residences and sheltered houses with the younger elements of society. Many new estates are built with the concept of the old being near to the young.

Voluntary services

You should make yourself familiar with the role and functions of some voluntary organizations. The main ones for the services to the elderly are: **Help the Aged; Age Concern; Women's Royal Voluntary Service; Red Cross.**
Note also the services provided from local churches and schools.

3 Nursing the elderly patient with particular problems

Loss of stability and mobility

Assessment – factors causing instability are:
1 Many older people naturally sway much more
2 Physical disorders include
    1 Cardiovascular conditions, particularly with low blood pressure, anaemia and cardiac rhythm changes
    2 Neurological conditions such as Parkinson's disease, cerebro-vascular accidents and confusion
    3 Locomotor conditions with osteo-arthrosis and muscle weakness
    4 Endocrine conditions such as hypothyroidism, diabetes mellitus (hypoglycaemia especially)
    5 Drugs may affect stability in the elderly
3 Psychological problems – increased fear and anxiety
4 Social problems. For example, poor housing conditions with bad lighting; obstructions and hazards which cause a fall, which in turn creates more fear.

Immobility is caused by instability and fear of falling but other factors as well as those above include:
1 Pain – particularly joint pain; chest pain in angina
2 Weakness – due to anaemia, muscle wasting and neurological conditions
3 Depression and social isolation

Planned care should include an awareness of the vulnerability of the elderly and mobility cannot be hastened.

Care may need to be negotiated with medical staff for the treatment or adjustment of treatment for physical factors. Expert help from physiotherapists and occupational therapists needs to be co-ordinated and continued by nursing staff. Psychological assurance needs to be reinforced by providing reliable aids for stability (e.g. Zimmer frames).

The environment needs to be planned in a geriatric unit and in the patient's home for clear and safe movements.

Pain relief by intelligent administration of prescribed analgesia will help in mobilization. Weakness may be helped by treatment and nutrition, but where paralysis occurs, support braces may be required.

Hazards of immobilization
Physical problems
1 Pressure sores (see 2.7)   4 Urinary tract infection (see 2.4)
2 Deep vein thrombosis (see 2.2)   5 Constipation and diverticulitis (see 2.3)
3 Pneumonia (see 2.1)

Psychological problems
1 Even more depression
2 Resignation

Social problems
1 Increased loneliness and isolation
2 Economic difficulty (shopping)

Multiple diagnosis

Many patients are admitted to geriatric units with more than one condition. Some may have three or more and also be suffering from combination effects of the treatment prescribed.

The role of the nurse in helping the doctor with diagnosis may be quite difficult. Observations need to be accurate and clearly recorded.

Factors which may affect test results should be identified – careful nursing history taking.

Confusion

Two states of confusion are recognized in the elderly – acute confusional state and dementia.

Acute confusional state

Assessment – factors causing confusion include
1 Physical conditions
  1 Hypoxia of brain cells due to: anaemia, heart failure, respiratory disease
  2 Lack of glucose and nutrition to brain cells due to: malnutrition, starvation
  3 Fluid and electrolyte imbalance e.g. intestinal obstruction, diabetes mellitus
  4 Toxaemia due to infection
  5 Head injury
  6 Drugs and alcohol (or alcohol withdrawal)
2 Psychological conditions
  1 Loss of intellectual and concentration powers
  2 Changing memory states
3 Social conditions – removal from familiar environment
In many patients, there will be combinations of factors leading to confusion.

Planned care should include the assistance in removing physical factors
  1 Giving of oxygen or just fresh air, deep breathing and coughing
  2 Ensuring adequate nutrition, particularly of glucose. Many emergency admission patients have used up their glycogen reserves while ill at home
  3 Restoring fluid and electrolyte balance
  4 Removing drugs to avoid self dosing
  5 Possible giving or withholding of alcohol
  6 Care of infection

Psychological factors are more difficult and gentle re-orientation using expert communication skills and patience is required. Individual nursing care is stressed.

Any planned change of environment should be carefully thought through and discussed.

Sedation tends to exacerbate confusional states. Remember that relatives are distressed by the acute confusional state in their loved ones. They will need support and guidance too.

Dementia Is a progressive pathological state in which brain cells become seriously depleted and malfunctioning. There is a gradual breakdown of personality with irreversible confusion. The combination of behavioural disorder and often physical deterioration also, leads to hospitalization in a psycho-geriatric unit. Total nursing care by skilled psycho-geriatric nurses is required. Families need much support and care again.

Incontinence

Urinary incontinence

Assessment – factors causing urinary incontinence include
1 Physical conditions
  1 Urinary tract infection
  2 Enlarged prostate gland
  3 Vaginitis, prolapsed uterus
  4 Neurological damage to brain cells or spinal cord
  5 Unconsciousness
  6 Drugs, e.g. diuretics; sedatives
2 Psychological conditions
  1 Anxiety
  2 Depression
3 Social conditions
  1 Poor toilet facilities (including the cold, outside toilet)
  2 Change of environment with anticipated loss of privacy
  3 Isolation

Planned care should include assisting in the diagnosis and treatment of physical factors.
1 Establishing a habit training, by using continence charts, timing of providing bottles, bed pans, commodes or escorting to the toilet.
2 Maintain the cleanliness and comfort of the genital area.
3 Giving prescribed emepronium bromide to increase the bladder capacity.
4 Psychological assurance and reforming the patient's self-identity will help to overcome depression and isolation.

5 Care should be exercised on admission of elderly patients to prevent loss of continence due to the changed environment.

6 Local authorities may need to be involved in improving toilet facilities if the patient is not to be discharged home to become incontinent again.

7 Incontinence may be impossible to control by the above. Appliances are then employed but must be used as the manufacturer recommends. Learn the main ones used in your unit currently as fashions change quite frequently.

8 Permanent indwelling catheters do have a place in the care of incontinence. The special catheters for long term care must be used. Some authorities organize regular irrigation and the catheter will need to be changed according to local practice (3 monthly is a reasonable régime). The patient will need to be encouraged to maintain a good fluid intake – up to 2 or 3 litres per day may be needed.

Faecal incontinence

Assessment – the factors causing faecal incontinence include:

1 Faecal impaction, which may be a consequence of constipation. Constipation may be due to:
  1 Physical factors – insufficient dietary fibre; drugs slowing down peristalsis; anal strictures; immobility
  2 Psychological factors – depression
  3 Social factors – poor toilet facilities or loss of bowel habit
2 Dietary indiscretion, e.g. excess alcohol
3 Rectal condition, e.g. carcinoma
4 Neurological condition – brain or spinal cord damage
5 Drugs, e.g. excessive aperients, antibacterial agents

Planned care should include assistance in the diagnosis and treatment of the physical conditions.

1 Removal of impacted faeces – first by softening with warm olive oil or glycerin rectally, followed by digital evacuation if impaction remains.
2 Re-establish good fibre diet and fluid intake.
3 Habit training and education to avoid recurrence. Medical staff may review drug régime.

Hypothermia See Section 2.8 – Myxoedema

Hypothermia is also a problem of the elderly patients with normal thyroid function. Assessment and care is as in 2.8.

Prevention needs to be exercised both in the community and hospital wards.

1 Adequate heating – may be quite difficult for elderly patients because of expense and immobility.
2 Warm clothing should include covering for hands and feet. The head may need extra covering too as thinning hair allows extra heat loss.
3 Adequate nutrition – may again be difficult with immobility for shopping and cooking and inability to chew food.
4 Maintained activity – again a problem with immobility and instability.

Surgery

Before surgery

1 Assessment and preparation for surgery may take longer for elderly patients.
2 Orientation and physical assessment of all systems may take time.
3 Patient preparation with physiotherapy will minimize anaesthetic risks.
4 Explanations for surgery may need to be repeated often before understanding is clear. Communication will need to be maintained until anaesthesia – remember to send hearing aid to theatre.

Anaesthesia Age alone is not a contra indication for general anaesthetic. Local or epidural anaesthetics may be used for patients who are risks because of a respiratory condition.

After surgery The main specific problems facing elderly patients after surgery are:

1 Increased risk of respiratory difficulty – good physiotherapy and nursing guidance should help
2 Different pain perceptions. The nurse may have to elicit a pain complaint from some elderly patients. If they do complain, the pain is probably very severe.
  Post operative analgesia depresses breathing but intelligent use of them to enable the older patient to sit up sooner, to cough and expectorate sputum may in fact improve the ventilation and oxygenation
3 Mobilization to prevent deep vein thrombosis and chest infection needs to be sensitively aware of the patients limitations. Many surgeons prescribe prophylactic anticoagulants.

Drugs

Some elderly patients, particularly with multiple diagnoses, are prescribed a multiplicity of drugs. In addition, they are inclined to indulge in self medication.

Many of their health problems arise out of the effects of indiscriminate taking of drugs.

Although the correction of this is mainly the work of the physician, the nurse may be able to help by taking a careful history and noting any bottles brought in. Observation for undesired effects needs great awareness and experience.

Names Patients will often refer to 'my heart tablet' rather than a named drug.

Doses Prescribers usually order reduced amounts for elderly patients. Changes in blood volume, liver and renal functions tend to increase the potency of drugs.

There is often confusion on the timing of drugs and many devices are used to help them to take their tablets at the right time.

Effects Many elderly patients have increased effects and side effects from even small doses of drugs. In some cases, the effect is quite different from that intended. For example, barbiturates can occasionally cause increased activity.

Effects of drugs are often prolonged. Some night sedations cause drowsiness well into the following day.

See the British National Formulary for information to prescribers for the elderly and for specific drug effects.

Section 3
The nurse as a manager, teacher, health educationalist and professional person

You can use variations of the nursing process to analyse your roles as manager and teacher.

Manager

Use five elements of the nursing management process to help in deciding routine functions and problem solving.

1 *Assess*

   Routine
   1 The actual work – patient care needed
   2 The priority care which is needed
   3 The skills of the staff available to do the work
   4 The amount of time available
   5 Equipment and supplies needed
   6 Staff development needs – it is important to remember that all staff need stimulus and their interest maintained for job satisfaction
   7 The legal requirements in your work.
   8 Problems or incidents – What actually happened? What the complaint is (you will need to know your own authority's policy on complaints. Complaints should be dealt with positively – it is an absolute right of individuals to complain).

2 *Organize*

   Routines
   1 The allocation of work – staff to patients
   2 The availability of equipment e.g. for medicine rounds, for meal times

   Priority care It is good preparation for management to write down lists of priorities for almost anything you do. *What should be done first? What is the most important work to be done?* It also helps you with evaluation questions on objective tests (see Section 5)

   Problems or incidents Organization would be part of your investigations of the problem or incident. You will need to plan, for instance:
   1 how you would carry out a search for a missing patient
   2 how you are going to deal with a complaint
   In most cases, you will need to show that you are organizing the collection of more information.

3 *Supervise* In some cases you will be 'doing' the work yourself, but when you are in charge, it is most important that you can oversee what your team is doing – delegating and supervising.

   Routines
   1 Standards of care being given by your team
   2 Teaching and development of team members
   3 Meeting of priorities

   Problems or incidents
   Having organized a search, you will need to supervise that it is being done correctly. For example, if you arranged for an injured member of the staff to visit the Accident Centre or Occupational Health Service, you would need to check that it had been carried out.

4 *Evaluate*
   As well as developing your own critical approach, you need to stimulate this within your staff also.

   Routines
   1 Hold evaluation sessions where you decide if the work has gone well or not so well
   2 Could our performance have been improved?
   3 When work has gone well, evaluation must include praise and thanks

   Problems or incidents
   1 Has the problem been resolved or not?   2 Could the incident be repeated?

5 *Report*
Management is not something carried out in isolation. Managerial teams, including Senior nurses, need the information to be able to organize support. This is why communication in reports is so important.

It should also be recognized that litigation is possible, sometimes many years after the original incident. The accuracy of nurses' reports is then very critical.

Reports should be:
1 Written as well as given by mouth.
2 Written in English that can be clearly understood–no abbreviations.
3 Factual–you must only state what actually happened as witnessed e.g. 'the lady was found at the side of her bed', rather than 'the lady fell out of bed' (unless she was seen to fall). You must record the time that incidents took place. It is wise to write a report as soon as possible after the event–timing will be more accurate and witnesses will still be available.
4 Treated as legal documents and kept secure.

Legal requirements It is not possible to cover all legal responsibilities in detail but in your revision periods you should spend some time in your School of Nursing library and with your tutorial staff to make yourselves fully aware of the law as applied to a Registered General Nurse.

Criminal law You have no special privileges in criminal law and would be required to help police in enquiries into crime. However, your authority will probably have a policy on how this should be done on hospital premises, especially involving patients in your care.

Nurses are exempt from the Rehabilitation of Offenders Act. Any criminal offence in your past may be communicated to your employing authority.

Breaches of the criminal law by registered nurses will be referred to the English National Board to determine if professional misconduct has occurred. If so, disciplinary action may be taken by the United Kingdom Central Council for Nursing, Midwifery and Health Visiting.

Criminal cases are referred to the police.

Civil law Check on the law concerning:
1 Consent for treatment or operation
2 Detention of patients against their will
3 Health and safety at work
4 Compensation for injury by negligence
5 Protection of patients' property and its disposal
6 Witnessing of legal documents–especially wills
7 Coroners' inquests

You should make yourself familiar with the main principles of:
1 The Misuse of Drugs Act   4 The 1983 Mental Health Act
2 The Abortion Act   5 The Human Tissues Act
3 The Health and Safety at Work Act

Teacher and health educationalist

Many examination questions will ask you to describe 'how' or 'what' you will teach junior nurses. They will also ask you to show your awareness of your role in health education.

You need to be aware of
1 the process of teaching   2 the importance of research

The process of teaching

Using a model similar to nursing and our management process.

1 *Assessment*
   1 The present awareness of the learner   *2* How motivated they are to learn

   This is done by question and answers first.

   Motivation may be high in nurse learners but not so good in a group of school children listening to you on positive health!

2 *Organizing learning*
   This is a better expression than teaching in that teaching is often seen as in one direction. The important activity is learning.

   Knowledge learning
   1 Presentation of material in logical order. Your teaching cards (see Section 1) are very helpful.
   2 Reinforcement by testing. Remember the need to test again within 24 hours, if possible, for memory.
   3 Use visual aids and books–but of course in the clinical setting, patient centred teaching is ideal.

   Skill learning
   1 Demonstration at normal speed. It is best for the learner to see the quality of skill that she is aiming for.

2 Demonstrate slower (but maintain safety) with a commentary, breaking down the skill into parts.

3 Allow the learner to practise under supervision.

4 Organize plenty of practice.

5 Test and reinforce high quality skill with praise.

Attitude learning

1 Organize work with sensitive staff.

2 Encourage discussion of nurses' own feelings and reactions.

3 Reinforce by praise.

Of course, the organization of learning includes creating an atmosphere where learning and teaching can flourish. Your own learning and research will be most influential.

3 *Supervise learning*

1 Observe how much learning is being fostered

2 Make books, visual aids and patients' notes available

3 Encourage completion of work sheets

4 Prepare for practical assessments

4 *Evaluate learning*

1 Testing of required knowledge, skills and attitudes

2 Correction of misunderstandings as quickly as possible (unlearning and relearning are very difficult)

3 Reinforce by praise and credit

Team teaching All trained nurses are teachers – indeed many first year nurses become teachers as timid new learners ask for help.

You need to discuss the team approach with your School of Nursing. Tutors and Clinical Teachers will help in the development of teaching skills throughout training. It is important to recognize their special expertize.

Health Education You will need to keep up to date through the nursing and daily press on current issues. You may be called upon to teach, advise or organize learning on some of the following:

1 Wise eating and nutrition	**6** Hygiene
2 Exercise	**7** Sexual awareness
3 Accidents	– responsible sex education
4 Alcohol	– sexually transmitted disease
5 Smoking	

Nursing research

There is a rapidly expanding volume of nursing research available now. Much is American (but is often still valid for this country) but there is lot of research into British nursing too. More recent research findings may be found in your nursing journals. No doubt your Tutor will have introduced you to some. When you can quote in your essays, the examiner will give you credit for it.

Two classic studies that you should be aware of are

1 Norton, D., McLaren, R., Exton-Smith, A. N., *An investigation of Geriatric Nursing Problems in Hospital* (Churchill Livingstone) – contains the important research on pressure area care.

2 Jones, D., *Food for thought* (RCN Research Publication) – contains important research into nasogastric feeding of patients

Professional person

Only a limited number of specific questions relate to the professional role, but you would be expected to demonstrate a professional approach in your essays. The elements of a profession may be summarized as:

1 Clients should have confidence that the practitioner has the knowledge and skill to help them.

2 The public can have confidence in the conduct and discipline of members of the profession.
You should then be aware of your position (when registered) within such a profession.

The Nursing profession is now controlled by the United Kingdom Central Council for Nursing, Midwifery and Health Visiting.

The Council is responsible for:

1 The development of standards of nursing care

2 The maintenance of a register of professional Nurses, Midwives and Health Visitors

3 The maintenance of professional conduct of Nurses, Midwives and Health Visitors through internal discipline. See Code of Professional Conduct

The Code of Professional Conduct is included, but you should note that it is rewritten annually. You must check the latest edition available.

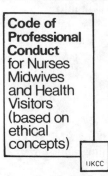

Code of Professional Conduct for Nurses Midwives and Health Visitors (based on ethical concepts)

UKCC

United Kingdom Central Council for Nursing, Midwifery and Health Visiting

Each registered nurse, midwife and health visitor shall act, at all times, in such a manner as to justify public trust and confidence, to uphold and enhance the good standing and reputation of the profession, to serve the interests of society, and above all to safeguard the interests of individual patients and clients.

Each registered nurse, midwife and health visitor is accountable for his or her practice, and, in the exercise of professional accountability shall:

1 Act always in such a way as to promote and safeguard the well being and interests of patients/clients.

2 Ensure that no action or omission on his/her part or within his/her sphere of influence is detrimental to the condition or safety of patients/clients.

3 Take every reasonable opportunity to maintain and improve professional knowledge and competence.

4 Acknowledge any limitations of competence and refuse in such cases to accept delegated functions without first having received instruction in regard to those functions and having been assessed as competent.

5 Work in a collaborative and co-operative manner with other health care professionals and recognise and respect their particular contributions within the health care team.

6 Take account of the customs, values and spiritual beliefs of patients/clients.

7 Make known to an appropriate person or authority any conscientious objection which may be relevant to professional practice.

8 Avoid any abuse of the privileged relationship which exists with patients/clients and of the privileged access allowed to their property, residence or workplace.

9 Respect confidential information obtained in the course of professional practice and refrain from disclosing such information without the consent of the patient/client, or a person entitled to act on his/her behalf, except where disclosure is required by law or by the order of a court or is necessary in the public interest.

10 Have regard to the environment of care and its physical, psychological and social effects on patients/clients, and also to the adequacy of resources, and make known to appropriate persons or authorities any circumstances which could place patients/clients in jeopardy or which militate against safe standards of practice.

11 Have regard to the workload of and the pressures on professional colleagues and subordinates and take appropriate action if these are seen to be such as to constitute abuse of the individual practitioner and/or to jeopardise safe standards of practice.

12 In the context of the individual's own knowledge, experience, and sphere of authority, assist peers and subordinates to develop professional competence in accordance with their needs.

13 Refuse to accept any gift, favour or hospitality which might be interpreted as seeking to exert undue influence to obtain preferential consideration.

14 Avoid the use of professional qualifications in the promotion of commercial products in order not to compromise the independence of professional judgement on which patients/clients rely.

Notice to all Registered Nurses, Midwives and Health Visitors

This Code of Professional Conduct is issued by the United Kingdom Central Council for Nursing, Midwifery and Health Visiting.

It is issued for the guidance and advice of all registered nurses, midwives and health visitors.

Further explanatory notes, discussion papers or comments on specific points in the Code of Professional Conduct may be issued by the Council from time to time.

The Code will be subject to periodic review by the Council.

The Council expects members of the profession to recognise it as their responsibility (as well as the Council's) to re-appraise the relevance of the Code to the professional and social context in which they practice.

The Council will welcome suggestions and comments for consideration in its periodic review of the Code of Professional Conduct. Such suggestions and comments should be sent to:

The Council delegates the education and training of Nurses, Midwives and Health Visitors to the National Boards, within the Council's policies.

The National Boards also *investigate* possible breaches of professional conduct and refer cases to the Council.

As a registered nurse, you are obliged to:

1 Take part in elections of the Boards
2 Maintain your own professional standards (see Code of Practice)
3 Report misconduct for investigation

You should also check that you are aware of the structure, functions and your own relationship with:

1 The National Health Service
    1 the Department of Health and Social Security
    2 Regional Authorities
    3 District Authorities
    4 Nursing functions and posts

2 The Professional organizations and Unions e.g.
    1 Royal College of Nursing of the United Kingdom
    2 Confederation of Health Service Employees
    3 National Union of Public Employees

3 The International Congress of Nursing
4 The European Economic Community

Section 4
Examination questions analysis

Introduction to essay questions

The following are a collection of final examination questions, taken from old papers set by the General Nursing Council and used with permission.

Read the questions **carefully** before looking at the analysis and plan. The important point is to **read** and **answer** the actual question on the paper. The analysis and plan is to enable you to think of the **timing** and **planning** of your writing during the examination. As stated in Section 1, **planning** is extremely important. Some candidates plan each question as they come to it, others plan all five before starting to write. Do scribble your pencilled plan on the answer book if you wish, but then cross it through before you start to answer formally in ink. The plans given are very brief and will not necessarily cover all the points you might think of.

When you write essays ask your Tutor to mark them; it is important that you gain experience in having your answers marked. The English National Board issue answer guides to the School of Nursing and your Tutor will be able to discuss your answer against the key points that examiners are looking for. Your Tutor will also be able to ensure that you are composing logical answers and adequately projecting your own caring attitude on paper.

Respiratory system

Mr Watts is a 60-year-old postman who shares a basement flat with his wife. He has developed an acute exacerbation of chronic bronchitis.

(a) *With particular reference to his dyspnoea*, describe the nursing care which should be given to relieve Mr Watts discomfort on admission and during his first three days in hospital. (80%)

(b) What is the nurses' rôle in preparing Mr Watts for his return to work. (20%)

Analysis

You are asked to focus your attention here to the specific problems related to his dyspnoea. You have limited time to work in and a total patient care plan would not only be irrelevant (there are no marks for irrelevant material), it would be almost impossible.

Part (a)   Concentrate on the cause factors of his dyspnoea
  ▶ airways obstruction due to bronchitis and sputum
  ▶ bronchospasm due to acute inflammation
  ▶ hypoxia due to involvement of alveoli
  ▶ retention of carbon dioxide depressing respirations by narcotic effect
  ▶ breathing affected by fear and anxiety
Then apply your nursing care in a logical way.

Part (b)   Think of your management and teaching role
  ▶ assessment of problems facing his work
  ▶ organizing discharge, care at home and rehabilitation
  ▶ supervising breathing exercises; advising

Plan could include:

Part (a)   Immediate care and for three days
  ▶ antibacterial drugs for infection
  ▶ antispasmodic drugs for bronchospasm
  ▶ oxygen therapy for hypoxia and observe
  ▶ nursing position and physiotherapy for good ventilation, and expectoration
  ▶ reassurance to relieve fear and anxiety
  ▶ give fluids and energy foods for strength to breathe
(Notice the importance of relating your care to the breathing problems)

Part (b) 1 Assess
  ▶ his exercise tolerance
  ▶ his motivation to work
  ▶ his wife's co-operation

2 Organize
  ▶ continual physiotherapy
  ▶ drugs to take home

3 Advise
  ▶ avoid smoking, dampness, mixing in crowds

Respiratory system

Mr Bond, a 45-year-old sports commentator, is married and has a teenage son. He has been admitted for laryngectomy.

(a) *Using a problem solving approach*, describe the responsibilities of the nursing team for maintaining Mr Bond's airway during the first 48 hours following his surgery.   (70%)

(b) In what ways may Mr Bond be prepared for and assisted with post operative communication? (30%)

Analysis

Part (a)   Questions asking you to use a problem solving approach require you to analyse as many possible problems as you can, assess how data will help you to solve them and then organize care to deal with them.

Notice also that this question refers to the responsibilities of the nursing team. You need to regard yourself as the leader of that team for these examinations.

Try to avoid generalizing on this question – it is specifically about maintaining the airway. All the care needs to be related directly to that.

Part (b)   Read this part of the question very carefully – the key words are . . . *be prepared for* as well as *assisted*. Much of this would be pre-operative care.

Plan could include:

Part (a) 1 Problems relating to the airway would be
- ▶ haemorrhage
- ▶ oedema
- ▶ blockage of tracheostomy tube
- ▶ infection in the trachea and bronchi leading to sputum
- ▶ communication fears

2 Identification data would come from
- ▶ constant observation and supervision
- ▶ co-operation of the patient

3 Problems dealt with by
- ▶ return to theatre for haemorrhage
- ▶ change of tracheostomy tubes if blocked
- ▶ aseptic suction technique
- ▶ possible use of antibacterial drugs for infection
- ▶ clear guidance on communication

Part (b) 1 Development of
 – non verbal communication and
 – oesophageal speech

2 Techniques involve guidance of speech therapist, help from a 'laryngectomy' patient

3 Encourage early practice

4 Involve the family, especially his son

Cardiovascular system

Ian, a 19 year-old student, collapsed on the rugby field following a fierce tackle. On admission, he is in a shocked condition and a ruptured spleen is diagnosed.

(a) Describe the nursing care and management that Ian will require from his admission until he arrives in theatre.   (70%)

(b) What are the hazards of blood transfusion and what measures should be taken to avoid them? (30%)

Analysis

Part (a)   Notice that you are asked to describe the nursing care and management. You should, therefore, consider yourself as the nurse in charge of his care. Assessment, planning and the carrying out of care should be included.

Note the timing is before surgery, but needs to be taken right up to the anaesthetic room to fulfil the criteria of the question.

Part (b)   This may be treated as two questions, but it may be better to consider each hazard in turn with the measures required for avoidance applied to that hazard. Do not worry if you have to repeat yourself in 'measures to avoid'. Watch the timing here, you will only have about 10 to 12 minutes to answer this part of the question. The wording would allow you to write brief notes, but a list would not be enough.

Plan could include:

Part (a) 1 Assessment and planned care for a *shocked* patient (must take priority)
- ▶ hypovolaemic and neurogenic shock
- ▶ blood replacement, analgesia, reassurance

2 Assessment and planned care for a patient with bleeding into the abdominal cavity
- ▶ pain, distension, reduced peristalsis

3 Assessment and planned care for a patient who is to have abdominal surgery
  ▶ skin care, nasogastric aspiration, intravenous infusion, anxiety, consent, explanation, reassurance, pre-medication, informing relatives

Part (b) 1 Hazards should include
  ▶ agglutination
  ▶ immune reactions
  ▶ over transfusion
  ▶ perhaps embolism or hazards of any other infusions but watch the time

2 Measures to avoid should include
  ▶ careful cross matching and checking of blood
  ▶ strict observations during infusion for reactions
  ▶ strict control of infusion flow rate

Cardiovascular system

Mrs Baker, a 70-year-old widow who lives in sheltered accommodation, has been admitted to the ward with severe congestive cardiac failure.

(a) Using a problem solving approach, describe in detail a plan of care to meet Mrs Baker's needs in relation to her cardiac condition during her stay in hospital.   (80%)

(b) What advice should be given to her on discharge to enable her to minimize her symptoms?   (20%)

Analysis

Part (a)   The key wordings in this question relates to the *problem solving approach, describe in detail, cardiac condition, during her stay in hospital.* Your first activity is to identify the problems – thinking of your model of nursing or through the effects of congestive cardiac failure. A detailed nursing care plan would include observations relating to the problems and care in response. Reasons should be included where possible. For example, observations of dyspnoea, respiratory rate and sputum would direct your care to careful positioning, oxygen therapy and assisting with physiotherapy.
It is doubtful if you would have the time to cover all her problems, therefore, think of the major ones.

Part (b)   Remember when stating your advice to confine it to relate to her symptoms.

Plan could include:

Part (a)   Observations and care required for a patient with
  ▶ breathlessness
  ▶ poor cardiac output
  ▶ poor renal flow
  ▶ fluid retention and oedema
  ▶ indigestion, liver engorgement
  ▶ anxiety about her survival in heart failure

Part (b)   Advice relating to
  ▶ breathlessness, cough, sputum
  ▶ postural oedema
  ▶ difficulty sleeping
  ▶ difficulty digesting food

Digestive system

Ann Clarke aged 11 years and the eldest of four children, is admitted to the paediatric ward with a perforated appendix. She is accompanied by her parents and is anxious, pyrexial and nauseated.

(a) How should Ann be admitted and prepared for surgery?   (50%)

(b) Describe Ann's specific post operative care during the first 48 hours following her operation.   (50%)

Analysis

Part (a)   Notice first of all that the weighting on this question is even between the two parts.
The word *How* implies a description but also invites you to include wording to show your attitude – observations would be done *carefully*, washing would need to be done *sensitively*, recognizing her pain and growing self consciousness.

Part (b)   The word *specific* often disturbs candidates in this type of question. The important point is to relate your planned care *directly* to her *appendicectomy, peritonitis* and the fact that she is an *eleven year old girl.*

Plan could include:

Part (a)   Position in the ward and in bed
Care to relieve her anxiety (and that of her parents)
Care to control her metabolic rate which is high
Care to protect her from vomiting – likelihood of a paralytic ileus
Preparations for surgery – rehydration, electrolyte balance,
antibacterial agents, as well as general care of a child for surgery.

Part (b) 1 Post operative care related to surgery for perforated appendix
  ▶ still has peritonitis – nasogastric aspiration; intravenous fluids; nutrition and drugs
  ▶ maintain the airway
  ▶ wound and drains
  ▶ assessment for complications – abscesses

2 Care of an eleven-year-old
  ▶ school – importance of reading development
  ▶ eldest of four – relationships with siblings (visiting)
  ▶ possibly early puberty

Digestive system

Miss Susan Small, an air hostess aged 27 years, has been admitted to a medical ward with a provisional diagnosis of ulcerative colitis.

(a) List the problems which may have led Miss Small to consult her General Practitioner. (15%)

(b) Give an account of the care Miss Small will require during the period of investigation until her diagnosis has been confirmed. (85%)

Analysis

Part (a) This question asks for a list of problems. There is no need to elaborate on a list and note the limited number of marks available. It is a sign of intelligent thinking if you can put your list in groupings.
E.g. Problems relating to her diarrhoea
Problems relating to her loss of weight

Part (b) *Give an account of* . . . means write a description with explanations or reasons. Read carefully the time factor here – it is up to the confirmation of diagnosis, therefore, an account of treatment is not required, but it does include investigations. Observations should be included also.

Plan could include:

Part (a) 1 Problems relating to diarrhoea
  ▶ frequency of bowel action
  ▶ nature of faeces
  ▶ presence of blood and mucus

2 Problems relating to loss of weight (nutrition)
  ▶ increasing fatigue
  ▶ changed body image

3 Psychological problems
  ▶ anxiety
  ▶ depression

Part (b) 1 Planned observations and care relating to her signs and symptoms
  ▶ bed position
  ▶ stool chart
  ▶ weighing
  ▶ diet, fluids

2 Planned preparation and care for investigations – sigmoidoscopy, barium enema, blood analysis

3 Planned observation for evidence of complications
  ▶ perforation
  ▶ severe haemorrhage

4 Planned assessment and care of her psychological state

Renal system

Mr Turner's pyelogram shows a right staghorn calculus and he is admitted for a right nephrectomy.

(a) Explain the effects of a staghorn calculus on renal function (25%)

(b) Giving reasons, describe in detail the post operative care and management Mr Turner will require up until he is discharged home. (75%)

Analysis

This type of question is frequently avoided by candidates because of the applied physiology involved, although their awareness of the post operative care for a patient following nephrectomy may be very good.
Try to look at both parts of the question and weighting of the marks. You could, in fact, do the two parts in reverse order but you would need to make it very clear to the examiner.

Part (a) *Explain the effects* . . . some try to use a diagram, but you really do not have time. By all means use a rough pencil one to help you trace the effects back through the pelvis of the kidney, collecting tubules and nephrons, but only as rough work.

Part (b) Challenging – you must give reasons and reasonable detail for your post operative care and management until discharge. It would be sensible to consider about five major factors, rather than minor ones, as details are required.

Plan could include:

Part (a)   Effects on renal function
      ► glomerular filtration – back pressure will ....
      ► selective reabsorption – damaged nephrons will ....
      ► formation of urine and drainage – the stone will ....

Part (b) 1 Management of
      ► breathing – immediate and subsequent care
      ► pain control
      ► wounds and drains
      ► hydration
      ► nutrition
      ► mobilization

        2 Identifying and care of complications
      ► infection
      ► thrombosis

        3 Advice before discharge home

Renal system

Mrs Jones, aged 34 years, is admitted to the ward with acute pyelonephritis. On admission, she has loin pain and a temperature of 39.6°C.

(a) State the cause and list the possible predisposing factors of this condition   (20%)

(b) Describe the nurses' rôle in the care and treatment Mrs Jones will need during her stay in hospital
    (60%)

(c) Outline the possible complications that could occur with this condition   (20%)

Analysis

Part (a)   The word *state* obviously requires a clear statement and *list* means a collection of factors. Try to group them though as if you were teaching a junior nurse.

Part (b)   Remember your rôles as a nurse
      ► Assessor of needs
      ► Planner of care
      ► Practitioner of care
      ► Evaluator of care plans
      Notice that nurses' is in the plural, meaning that you are organizing a group of nurses.

Part (c)   *Outline* means to give a summary – requires more information than a list.

Plan could include:

Part (a)   The cause of acute pyelonephritis is infection by micro-organisms. (You could then given examples of the main ones)
      Your list of factors could be grouped into
      1 Vulnerable groups (elderly, promiscuous)
      2 Pathological factors (congenital disorder)
      3 Introduction through catheters

Part (b) 1 Assessment, care given and the patient reaction to
      increased fluid intake
      antibacterial drug therapy (prolonged)
      bed rest, controlling body temperature, diet

        2 Advice for completion of treatment

Part (c)   1 Chronic pyelonephritis may develop because ....
      2 Ureteric calculi are associated with infection
      3 Chronic renal failure may follow chronic pyelonephritis

Nervous system

Dr Stephanie Potter, a medical registrar aged 40 years, is admitted to your ward conscious but drowsy following a suspected sub-arachnoid haemorrhage.

(a) Explain the importance of the observations the nurse should make of Dr Potter's condition during her first 24 hours in hospital   (60%)

(b) Assuming Dr Potter is to have a lumbar puncture, describe the nurses' responsibilities before, during and after the procedure   (40%)

Analysis

Part (a)   The key words are obviously *the importance of the observations*. A list of observations and charts would not be sufficient here.
      You may also see questions asking for *the significance* of observations.
      There are two important points to remember about observations:
        1 They tell you about the patient's condition, diagnosis and progress.
        2 Your nursing management and the medical treatment should be related to them as they are part of the assessment phase of nursing process.

Part (b) Describe means *giving an account with reasons* and notice the three time factors – *before, during and after*.

You can choose whether to write about each of the responsibilities and relate to the times or the other way round. Assume that you are the nurse in charge.

Plan could include:

Part (a) 1 Observations relating to *rising* intracranial pressure
- ► *changing* conscious levels, pupils
- ► *rising* blood pressure, *slowing* pulse rate
- ► vomiting

2 Observations relating to meningism
- ► photophobia, headache (or pain in head)
- ► neck stiffness

3 Observations of anxiety state

Part (b) Nurses' responsibilities (notice that nurses' is in the plural)
1 Assessment
- ► equipment, staff, environment, staff learning needs

2 Planning or organizing
- ► preparation of Dr Potter
- ► preparation of trolley and bed space
- ► nurses' participation and observations
- ► observations after the procedure

3 Practising assistance and observations (2 nurses)
- ► helping the doctor
- ► correct position during and after the procedure
- ► observing for danger of 'coning'
- ► increasing headache

4 Evaluating
- ► the safety of procedures
- ► if any learning by the nurses

5 Reporting
- ► visual observations
- ► pressure of cerebro spinal fluid
- ► patients reactions

Nervous system

Mr Rees, a building contractor, aged 30 years has been admitted with recurrence of a cerebral tumour. Mr Rees is married, has two children aged 5 years and 2 years, and his wife feels unable to cope with him at home.

(a) Identify difficulties which may have developed within the family during recent months. (30%)

(b) Outline a plan of care for a period of 24 hours which would meet Mr Rees' physical and psychological needs. (70%)

Analysis

There is a considerable amount of information given to you in this patient setting. Use as much of it as possible in your answers. Try to avoid a 'stock' answer about cerebral tumours.

Part (a) There are only 30% of the marks here and you would only have about 10 minutes to identify the difficulties. An extended list would be acceptable but it might be better to concentrate on some major difficulties and express your sensitive awareness in your answer.

Part (b) *Outline a plan* would require more than a plan list. Some reasons for your inclusions into the plan would be needed. You would be expected to give quite a full plan though, covering as many of his needs as you can imagine. Remember that a 24 hour plan must include night care also.

Plan could include:

Part (a) 1 Psychological difficulties
- ► behavioural changes – moodiness, irrational behaviour, irritability with the children
- ► loss of self esteem without work
- ► altered body image

2 Social difficulties
- ► wife having to give physical and psychological care to children as well as husband
- ► five-year-old needs to go to school

3 Physical difficulties
- ► increasing fatigue for man and wife
- ► Mr Rees – loss of weight, vomiting, possibly incontinence
  - – increasing headaches and pain
  - – pressure sores developing

Part (b)   Your plan of care could be in the terms given
    1 For physical needs
- assessment and care for headache
- assessment and care of pressure sores
- assessment and care of malnutrition
- assessment and care of vomiting
- assessment and care for incontinence
- assessment and care for insomnia

    2 For psychological needs
- assurance and care concerning lost esteem
- care of depression and anxiety
- possible anxiety concerning his approaching death
- recognition of possible guilt feelings in Mrs Rees

It would be wise to include spiritual care here also.

You would not need to write a time schedule out but your plan would need to give indication of the frequency at which observations and care would be carried out.

Locomotor system

Mr James, a 50-year-old bank manager, is admitted to hospital for possible surgery to remedy a prolapsed lumbar intervertebral disc.

(a) Describe how you would explain to Mr James how a myelogram will demonstrate a disc lesion and how such a procedure may affect him.   (30%)

(b) Describe the nursing management required to meet Mr James's needs during the first week following an operation on his lumbar spine.   (70%)

Analysis

Although the information about Mr James is minimal, there is sufficient for you to realize that he is a man of esteem and intelligence.

Part (a)   A description should include reasons for statements, but in the short time available you cannot go into detail.
Remember you need to describe:
    1 How you would explain (testing your own teaching skill)
    2 (to the examiner) that you know how a myelogram will demonstrate a disc lesion and its possible effects on Mr James.

You really only have time for very brief descriptions. Some nurses were afraid of this question because, although they could answer most of it, they were unsure of how a myelogram works, but you should realize by analysis that, in fact, it is only a small part of the whole question.

Part (b)   *Describe the nursing management . . .*
is asking you to be the nurse in charge, organizing assessment and care to meet Mr James's needs.

Plan could include:

Part (a)   Ensure Mr James's understanding by discussing the anatomy and physiology with the aid of a diagram. (You would not need to include a diagram in your answer though).
Give him clear information that 'a dye opaque to X-rays is injected into the arachnoid space under local anaesthetic. Obstruction to its movement would occur if a disc lesion was present'.
Explain possible effects – for example a headache, (without alarming him).

Part (b) 1 Physical
- assessment and care of the airway and breathing
- assessment and care of the wound for haemorrhage, leakage of cerebrospinal fluid, inflammation and infection
- assessment and care for pain
- planned mobilization with physiotherapist
- planned care for nutrition, hygiene, elimination, rest and sleep

    2 Psychological and Social
- care to avoid boredom – reading, radio, television
- negotiated visiting arrangements – wife and business colleagues

Locomotor system (also child care)

Simon, aged nine months and the youngest of three children, has been admitted to the children's ward with a fractured shaft of femur. Gallow's (Bryant's) traction has been applied.

(a) Describe Simon's total nursing care whilst he is in hospital   (70%)

(b) How should the nurse in charge ensure that the needs of Simon's family are met whilst he is in hospital?
                                                                                                      (30%)

Analysis

Although the setting is clear, the actual information given about Simon and the family is very limited. When you look at the two parts of the question – one asking for total nursing care and the other concerning the needs of the family, you will have to rely on your assessment model to give a full answer.

Part (a)   *Describe* means give a fairly detailed account with reasons.
Whilst he is in hospital does not expect you to know a magical time of how long he should be in. It does, of course, mean that you need to think of care plans going on for some days or weeks rather than 24 hours.

Part (b)   *How* means that you need to describe *the way* in which *you* will ensure the needs are met, using adjectives to show your attitude towards them.

Plan could include:

Part (a)   Applying assessment model A from Section 1 p 2.

   1 Assessment and care to ensure that Simon is safe
      ► cot, care of the traction equipment
      ► avoiding twisting, correct alignment and ensuring counter traction

   2 Assessment and care of Simon's breathing

   3 Assessment and care of Simon's nutrition, elimination, skin hygiene, dressing, body temperature, sleeping

   4 Communication is important, remembering the need for a nine month old child to practise words and sounds

   5 Remember also his psychological learning needs for play

As you are going to deal with the family needs in (b), there is no need to include the social care in this part but it might be wise to point out to the examiner what you are doing.

Part (b)   You will need to use a management process model here.

   1 Assess
      ► the family needs to maintain bonding, mother, father, brothers and sisters
      ► any constraints

   2 Organize
      ► open visiting arrangements
      ► facilities for mother or father to be there as required
      ► visiting by other children

   3 Supervise
      ► observe family relationships
      ► allow and encourage participation in care of Simon
      ► counsel learners on needs for the family

You could extend thoughts to Health Visitor calling at home to ensure that the family was coping, but watch the limitation on time.

Skin

Miss Gray, aged 75 years, is a very independent lady who lives alone. She has recently been neglecting herself and has a large varicose (gravitational) ulcer. She has very reluctantly agreed to be admitted to hospital.

(a) What problems may be encountered in caring for Miss Gray during the first 12 hours in hospital, and how should these problems be dealt with?   (60%)

(b) Outline the explanation that should be given to a junior nurse on the principles of management of Miss Gray's varicose (gravitational) ulcer.   (40%)

Analysis

This question needs to be read very carefully before attempting an answer. It is not a simple question about the care of varicose ulcers. You need to imagine this lady and realize that part (a) in particular is about her full needs. Even part (b) is about the *principles* of management, not details of dressings etc.

Part (a)   *What problems . . . and how they should be dealt with.* You need to consider the physical, psychological and social problems and then decide on *priorities* in order to deal with the first 12 hours in hospital!

Part (b)   *Outline the explanation to a junior nurse* – you need to think of the teaching model here. Careful wording of your answer should indicate your awareness of the principles *and* how you transmit them to the junior nurse.

Plan could include:

Part (a) 1 Psychological and social problems
      ► fear of hospital
      ► depression about loss of independence
      ► possible guilt if she has contaminated the ulcer or ignored community nurse advice!
      ► change of environment may cause confusion

2 Physical problems
  ▶ poor venous drainage and varicose veins
  ▶ the ulcer crater
  ▶ eczema – irritation around the ulcer
  ▶ probably long term immobility
  ▶ very likely unstable on her feet
Think then of the care plans to deal with all these in the first 12 hours. You could, in fact, delay looking at the ulcer until she has settled down and accepted the nurse assigned to care for her.

Part (b) Principles of management of the ulcer
  1 Treat any infection and prevent further infection
  2 Promote better venous drainage
  3 Prevent eczema irritation
You could say a little of how the principles would be achieved by practice but it would make sense to include that in your explanation to the nurse. There are two possibile ways:
  1 *Promotion of better venous drainage* is achieved by support bandaging and useful positioning of legs
  2 You apply support bandaging and position the legs carefully in order to *promote venous return*.

Skin

Pressure sores are a cause of discomfort to the patient and of protracted and expensive hospitalization.

(a) How may a nurse working in an acute geriatric ward assess her patients' risk of developing pressure sores?
(30%)

(b) Discuss the ways in which good nursing team-work may contribute to a reduction in the incidence of this problem
(70%)

Analysis

This is a generalized question as you will realize. The statement at the beginning sets the scene for you instead of a patient profile. You should make use of ideas from the statement when you come to part (b) of the question.

Part (a) *'How may a nurse . . . assess her patients' risk.'* Notice that patients' is in the plural.
You obviously need to apply your skills of assessment here. The most important one is observation. Correct application of the *Norton scale* is bound to influence the examiner.

Part (b) *'Discuss the ways . . .'* – you will need to do a lot of planning here. Discuss means to view from differing view points or as many areas as possible.
You will need to have thoughts on team-work that you can apply.

Plan could include:

Part (a) A nurse would assess her patients' risk of developing pressure sores by observing the patients'
  ▶ physical conditions
  ▶ mental conditions
  ▶ activity
  ▶ mobility
  ▶ incontinence

Part (b) For good team-work, by applying the management model in 2.16.
Senior nurse will
  ▶ assess – using Norton scale
  ▶ assess learners and auxiliaries awareness of the *cost* of pressure sores
  ▶ organize
    – regular change of position
    – pressure relief apparatus
    – nutritional requirements
    – aseptic dressings to broken skin
    – good lifting and moving technique
  ▶ supervise the team in carrying out the organized care
  ▶ evaluate by reviewing practise regularly
  ▶ praise staff and informing them of reduced incidence
  ▶ report and ensuring that others report and communicate well

Endocrine system

Paul, aged 10 years, has recently been diagnosed as having diabetes mellitus. He has been admitted for stabilization of his condition and is keen to learn about his treatment.

(a) Describe how the nurse should teach Paul and his parents to prepare and give his insulin injections.
(40%)

(b) Identify the problems which Paul and his parents could encounter as they come to terms with his condition and suggest how these may be overcome.
(60%)

Analysis

The amount of information about Paul is very limited and you must assume that he is an 'average' ten year old – that is an active, inquisitive and occasionally mischevious school boy.

Part (a) Note the wording – describe *how* the nurse should teach. You would be required to show your teaching skills first. Obviously, the examiner would like you to say *what* you would teach but you must describe that within your teaching method.

Part (b) *Identify the problems* means that you will need to use a full assessment model to cover the physical, psychological and social ones.

Don't forget the second part of this question – suggest *how* these may be overcome. It would be quite time consuming to deal with all the problems in this way. You could let the examiner know that you are giving examples in more detail but brief notes on some of the others.

Plan could include:

Part (a) The nurse would teach Paul and his parents to give insulin by
1 demonstrating or asking another diabetic youngster to demonstrate.
2 demonstrating the different parts of the skill – measuring, handling the syringe, checking the insulin, cleaning skin, the injection, the sterilization and maintenance of equipment.
3 letting Paul try under supervision – may be better for Paul to learn before his parents but depends on individuals.
4 letting Paul practise frequently and encourage him with praise.

Part (b) 1 Physical problems – could be related to body systems or daily living activities. You must mention
  ▶ understanding and acceptance of diet control
  ▶ balancing of exercise with diet and insulin
  ▶ prone to infection
  ▶ delayed healing of wounds
  ▶ hypoglycaemia
  ▶ keto acidosis

2 Psychological problems
  ▶ altered self image
  ▶ problems with schooling
  ▶ parents may suppress activity and play because of fear of injury and illness

3 Social problems
  ▶ feeling different in the family
  ▶ work prospects
  ▶ parents' anxieties about marriage later?

Endocrine system

Mrs Goodwin, aged 30 years and married with two small children, has had a partial thyroidectomy following medical treatment for thyrotoxicosis.

(a) Describe *how you would recognize* five major post-operative complications and the action which should be taken if they occur. (60%)

(b) What other post-operative care will Mrs Goodwin require whilst she is in hospital? (40%)

Analysis

Note the weighting of the two parts of this question. You will only have eighteen minutes to deal with five complications and twelve minutes to cover the other care required.

Part (a) Note the wording in italics – *how you would recognize*.
The question is more about your observations for complications than a detailed knowledge of physiology changes. The other important point is to state what action should be taken – this opens it up to what the surgeon may do as well as the nursing staff.

Part (b) Obviously, you could only cover general post-operative care to a limited extent, but you must make particular mention of Mrs Goodwin's husband and children.

Plan could include:

Part (a) Observations and planned action for five of the following:
  ▶ haemorrhage
  ▶ airway obstruction
  ▶ recurrent laryngeal nerve pressure
  ▶ thyroid crisis
  ▶ tetany (carpopedal spasm)
  ▶ infection
  ▶ (later) evidence of hypothyroidism
  ▶ cosmetic effect leading to stress and anxiety

Part (b) **1** Care of the lady's
- ► hygiene, mobilization, dressing
- ► wound (sutures, clips, drains)

  2 Care of visiting arrangements for her husband

  3 Information about the children if visiting is not possible

Reproductive system

Mrs Jane Grant, aged 20 years, a primigravida, is admitted directly to the ward in a collapsed state due to a ruptured tubal pregnancy. She is accompanied by her husband.

(a) Describe the nursing care Jane should receive until her transfer to the operating theatre.   (60%)

(b) What explanations should you give to a junior nurse about the reasons for Jane's condition and need for surgery?   (40%)

Analysis

The information is quite full here – you need to make use of as much of it as possible in your answers. Notice the weighting of the questions – part (b) is going to need a fair amount of work for 40% of the marks.

Part (a)   *Describe* – means that you need to give a quite clear explanation of what should be done. It also invites you to show your sensitivity though.

  1 It is an acute emergency – so use words like *quickly* and *immediately* in your description.
  2 Husband and wife are both distraught – use words like *carefully* and *gently* in your physical and psychological handling of the situation.

Part (b)   Aim your explanations to a *junior nurse* all through the answer. (Some candidates did not even mention her!)

  Notice that you need to explain *both* the reasons for Jane's condition *and* the need for surgery.

Plan could include:

Part (a)   Immediate
- ► assessment and care of *shocked* patient
- ► replace blood volume – IV infusion
- ► give analgesia – with premedication
- ► give reassurance
- ► quick preparation and transfer for surgery – minimal requirements

  Psychological care of Jane and her husband. (One candidate, in the midst of all the crisis gave time for Jane and husband to have a *'just together'* period! Examiners are human!)

Part (b)   Junior nurse needs to understand

  1 Pregnancy
  - ► the physiology and anatomy
  - ► the significance of primigravida
  - ► the psychology of parenthood

  2 Ruptured tubal pregnancy (ectopic)
  - ► possible causes
  - ► local and general effects
  - ► urgency of haemorrhage and peritonitis
  - ► psychological stresses

  3 Urgent treatment
  - ► blood replacement
  - ► surgery to ligate blood vessels, evacuate the peritoneal cavity of blood and the blastocyst and resection of the tube

Reproductive system

Mrs Ann Young, a 35-year-old fashion model, has been admitted to hospital with a painless swelling in her left breast. The possibility of left simple mastectomy has been discussed with her.

(a) Describe how Mrs Young's needs will be met during the pre-operative period   (40%)

(b) What special aspects of post-operative nursing care, up to and including discharge, would need to be considered if Mrs Young requires a left simple mastectomy?   (60%)

Analysis

The introduction gives you a good profile of the patient. The potential factors of her relationship with her husband and her body image for work are clear, in addition to the anxieties about cancer.

Part (a)   The emphasis is to *describe* how Mrs Young's needs will be met. It would not be sufficient to give a list of problems or potential problems.

  You realize, of course, that the wording enables you to co-ordinate the work of other members of the team – physiotherapists and breast care nurse in particular.

  Note that in 12 minutes you need to mention physical, psychological and social needs. You would have to concentrate on major specific factors.

Part (b)   Pick your way carefully through the wording of this question. Key words – *'special aspects'* – must relate *directly* to Mrs Young and her left simple *mastectomy*.
Again, you need to include physical, psychological and social aspects.

Plan could include:

Part (a)   Care and preparation for surgery
    1 Physical needs
        ▶ skin preparation
        ▶ arm exercises, with physiotherapy

    2 Social and psychological needs
        ▶ assurance about body image, sexuality, survival
        ▶ husband must be involved

Breast care nurse may help with counselling and introducing successful patients as well as fittings for prosthesis or implants.
Note: If you do include the work of a specialist nurse like this, you must indicate to the examiner that you know what she does.

Part (b)   Special aspects
    ▶ observations and care of the wound and drains
    ▶ positioning of the left arm and exercises
    ▶ maintaining posture
    ▶ psychological acceptance of the wound
    ▶ early prosthesis and bra application
        Note: If your surgeons are using implants then you could explain so to the examiner

    ▶ early support for husband
    ▶ wearing of clothes is important to this lady so help with dressing
    ▶ preparation for discharge may include explanations about radiotherapy to follow

Psychological problem

(a) Outline the general features of depressive illnesses.   (40%)
    Mary Brand, 22 years old, has been treated by her General Practitioner for depression since the breakdown of her marriage eight months ago.
    She has been admitted to the medical unit after taking a large quantity of tricyclic antidepressant tablets. On admission she is conscious but very drowsy and unco-operative.

(b) Describe the specific nursing care Mary will need during her first 48 hours in hospital.   (60%)

Analysis

It is important to read through this question carefully before you commit pen to paper. Note the weighting.

Part (a)   Is a generalized question and, in fact, is about depressive *illnesses*. You need to have a good working knowledge to do justice to it in the time available.
Outline means *give an extended list* – that is a list with brief notes.

Part (b)   Notice, describe the *specific* nursing care must relate directly to: Mary; the drugs taken; her drowsiness and non co-operation; and her attempted suicide.

Plan could include:

Part (a) 1 Mood
        ▶ sadness, hopelessness
        ▶ lethargic, anorexia
        ▶ flattening of personality
        ▶ loss of concentration and memory

    2 Appearance
        ▶ unkempt, sitting motionless, agitated
        ▶ miserable

    3 Physical
        ▶ constipation, weight loss due to anorexia
        ▶ loss of libido
        ▶ altered sleep patterns

    4 Talk
        ▶ flat, disinterested
        ▶ chat to hide despair
        ▶ threatening suicide

Part (b) 1 Physical observations and care for:
        ▶ prevention of further suicide attempts
        ▶ effects of tricyclic drugs
        (specific – need cardiac monitoring for arrhythmias)

▶ increased excretion – encourage fluids
(forced diuresis is *not* indicated)
▶ note effects of drowsiness if prolonged or possible loss of consciousness

2 Psychiatric observations and care:
▶ establishing relationship
▶ listening to feelings
▶ continue observations of behaviour
▶ professional psychiatric opinion

Drugs

Describe the nurses' responsibilities to patients, whilst they are in hospital and on their discharge, who are receiving the following drugs:

(a) anticoagulants   (35%)
(b) steroids   (35%)
(c) antibiotics   (30%)

Analysis

The words *describe* implies that a fair amount of detail is required. Notice that the question is about nurses' (plural) responsibilities to patients.

Your study of drugs, their effects and undesired effects should all be directed to patient care. Pure theoretical knowledge of pharmacology is useful but do not stray in your answers to this question.

From the weighting, you will have 8–12 minutes for each one.

Plan could include

1 Assessment
▶ the correct drug (names)
▶ the desired effects
▶ the dose, route and frequency with any special precautions
▶ undesired effects
▶ contra indications that should be reported

2 Organize and supervise
▶ taking of drugs correctly
▶ giving safely
▶ drugs to take home
▶ any cards to be carried

3 Evaluate
▶ patients reaction and co-operation

Part (a)   Anticoagulants

1 Heparin
▶ immediate effect
▶ need for antidote – protamine sulphate
▶ injection routes

2 Warfarin
▶ according to prothrombin time
▶ importance of accuracy due to very long excretion time
▶ antidote – vitamin K
▶ no aspirin or derivatives
▶ carrying of anticoagulant card

Part (b)   Steroids

1 Hydrocortisone injections; ACTH gel injections
▶ psychosis
▶ Cushing's syndrome (long term) – protein catabolism (muscle wasting, pathological fractures); diabetes mellitus; fatness of face and shoulders; fluid retention (moon face); sexuality changes

2 Prednisolone (various preparations)
▶ gastric erosion if taken orally
You would probably only have time to give brief notes
Steroid card – danger if stress, injury, illness or surgery

Part (c) Antibiotics

1 Examples – penicillin, tetracycline(s), chloramphenicol

2 Careful observations for:
▶ anaphylactic reactions
▶ aplastic anaemia
▶ candida infections

3 Importance of timing and completion of course to prevent organisms becoming resistant

There is a lot of information to be given in this question. Many are tempted to rush in and start writing immediately. In fact, you will write much more if you spend five minutes planning and thirty minutes very fast writing.

Operating theatre

Mrs Williams is to have a laparotomy under a general anaesthetic. What safety precautions should be taken:

(a) in the ward and operating theatre to ensure that she has the correct operation;   (30%)

(b) in the operating theatre to prevent
    1 infection   (45%)
    2 any other hazards to Mrs Williams   (25%)

Analysis

Although there is the name of the patient, this is, in fact, a general question. Notice that the wording *What safety precautions . . .* applies to all three parts of the question. You need to concentrate on those precautions, but, of course, you would be expected to give reasons and explanations.

Note the weighting gives most marks to (b) *1* concerning infection in the operating theatre.

Plan could include:

Safety precautions – could be in your nursing process model for management
- assessment
- organization
- supervision

Part (a)   Correct operation

Assess, organize and supervise
- nursing staff awareness
- operating theatre list
- that markings have been carried out
- correct labelling of the patient
- correct notes and X-rays with the patient
- house officer is undisturbed while admitting and marking the patient's skin

Part (b) *1* Prevent infection in the operating theatre

Assess, organize and supervise
- the correct operating order for infected patients late on the list if possible
- scrupulous cleaning of the theatre itself
- hygiene of theatre staff and surgical teams
- sterilization of instruments, dressings and sutures
- correct handling of equipment
- air flow extracting contaminated air

2 Prevention of other hazards

Strict procedures to avoid
- hazards from drugs and gases
- diathermy burns
- deep vein thrombosis
- pressure sores
- swabs and instruments left in

You would only have time to give statements – little detail could be given but do remember that it is the precautions that are being asked for.

Children

Helen, aged 3 years, is admitted from the waiting list for minor eye surgery. She is accompanied by her mother who has left Helen's 4 year old sister at play school.

(a) What behaviour may be expected from Helen during her first 24 hours in hospital.   (25%)

(b) Describe how details obtained on admission would help the nurse in her care of Helen during this 24 hour period.   (40%)

(c) How should the nurse provide the reassurance that both Helen and her mother require.   (35%)

Analysis

This question needs very careful reading. The only reference to Helen's eye surgery is in the introduction. The actual questions are about child care, not ophthalmic surgery.

The information is quite full apart from no reference to the father.

You will need to time yourself carefully. After planning time, you only have about 7½ minutes for part (a), 12 minutes for part (b) and 10½ minutes for part (c).

Part (a)   *What behaviour may be expected . . .*
    You can only refer to your awareness of normal 3-year-olds.

Part (b)   *Note:* the details described must be related to her care. You would only have time for examples.

Part (c)   *How* invites you to describe with a chance of showing your attitudes to Helen and her mother. Some examiners would give you credit for involving father as well.

Plans could include:

Part (a)   Self centred behaviour
▶ crying for mother and father
▶ may be difficult for feeding
▶ may regress and wet the bed
▶ bewildered by strange environment and people
Do not be tempted to go into your nursing response at this stage – it is not asked for yet and time is precious.

Part (b)   Admission details relevant for care
▶ names, home, relationship with her sister
▶ food likes and dislikes
▶ aids for rest and sleep – comforter and teddy bear
▶ own washing and toilet habits (name for the toilet)
▶ favourite toys
Each of these would need to be related to your care plan
e.g. food likes and dislikes – careful selection of food (especially the first meal)

Part (c)   Establish good relationships with Helen and mother
Listen to anxieties and fears
Encourage open visiting for mother and father
Careful explanations of preparation before and care after surgery
Physical handling – cuddling, holding hands
Encourage mother to help as she feels able.

Elderly

(a) Outline a suitable diet for an elderly person, justifying your choice with reference to the principles of a balanced diet.   (60%)

(b) Discuss the responsibilities of the nurse in charge at meal times in a Rehabilitation Ward for the elderly.   (40%)

Analysis

A general question on the care of the elderly which, at first, seems to be based on elementary knowledge. It is important to read through to the second part of the question and realize that nearly half the marks are contained in a nursing management element.

Part (a)   *Outline* – means to give a list but with brief notes in support. The questioner actually gives you the lead there to refer to principles of a balanced diet.
Notice that it asks for a diet, not a menu!
The elderly person could be at home.

Part (b)   *Discuss the responsibilities* – quite a demanding task in the time available. To discuss means to see from differing points of view. You could use the management model for these. Try to convey a sensitive approach.

Plan could include:

Part (a)   Principles of a balanced diet
▶ adequate protein – need to find easily chewable and digestible proteins e.g. chicken, vegetable proteins
▶ carbohydrate – controlled amounts to avoid obesity, but adequate for ill patients
▶ fat – controlled amounts to avoid obesity. Usually reduced
▶ minerals – note especially iron, potassium, sodium contents
▶ vitamins – care with cooking to avoid loss of vitamins from food
▶ fibre – careful explanations and encouragement to promote peristalsis (e.g. prevent diverticulitis)
▶ fluids – for good renal and bowel function

Part (b)   Responsibilities of the nurse in charge
1 Assess
▶ individual patients nutritional needs, likes and dislikes
▶ need for making meals a social event
▶ training needs of learners

2 Organize and supervise
▶ serving of meals
▶ feeding of patients (encouraging self help)
▶ teaching learners to help with meals

3 Evaluate
▶ check that food has been eaten
▶ control wastage
▶ praise for all!

Health educationalist

You are invited back to your old school to join with others in a series of debates on health matters. Discuss the points that could be made, so that a positive approach to health will result from a debate on:

either (a) Excessive drinking   (100%)
or   (b) Smoking   (100%)

Analysis

Many nurses do not like 100% questions for some reason. In fact, as long as you can devise a plan to work to, they are potentially very good questions to do. You only have to worry about one plan and if you remember to persuade the examiner that you have benefited from three years' reading and experience, you should get enough points to score well.

Beware of just putting down your own opinion. You need to give supporting evidence from your own reading and experience (although you will not have to remember exactly where you read it!).

This particular question should be read carefully. The main element is for you to discuss points for a positive approach to health. It is tempting to emphasize the diseases without stressing the positive benefits of avoiding the problem.

Plan could include:

(using a physical, psychological and social model)

    (a) Excessive drinking

1 Physical	*positive*	►	enjoy taste of controlled drinking
	negative	►	gastric erosion
		►	liver damage
		►	alcohol physical dependence
		►	withdrawal symptoms
2 Psychological	*positive*	►	feeling of well being
	negative	►	psychological dependence
3 Social	*positive*	►	family and pub life
	negative	►	family breakdown, loss of work, social outcast
		►	financial problems

    (b) Smoking

1 Physical	*positive*	►	free and easy breathing
		►	able to run, dance, play
	negative	►	bronchial carcinoma
		►	chronic obstructive airways disease
		►	coronary artery disease
2 Psychological	*positive*	►	'security' without cigarettes
	negative	►	psychological dependence
3 Social	*positive*	►	free to go anywhere
		►	enjoy interaction – kissing!
		►	economical
	negative	►	smoking areas only
		►	coughing in bed
		►	financial difficulty

Manager

Discuss the nursing responsibilities and actions which should be taken in the following situations:

(a) a long stay orthopaedic patient who has become aggressive and demanding   (33%)

(b) a patient who falls out of bed during visiting time but appears to be unhurt   (33%)

(c) a retired nurse, whose mother is a patient in the ward, complains that her mother is being neglected.
                                                                                              (34%)

Analysis

Many management questions start with *discuss the responsibilities*. You need to have a clear idea of your management rôle as a staff nurse.

This one has three parts, approximately equal in weighting. Plan carefully to give as much effort to part (a) as part (c).

Additional wording to watch for – *actions which should be taken* – could include actions by other staff.

Plan could include:

(using the management model – assess, organize, supervise, evaluate, report)

Part (a) 1 Assess
           ► the reasons and pattern of his behaviour
           ► possible pathological cause including anxiety state
           ► possible inter personal clash with next patient or the nurse allocated to care for him

2 Organize
► visit by doctor, relatives, social worker

3 Supervise
► possible move in the ward
► tactful change of nurse
► care to avoid over dependence

Part (b)   Priorities
► patient back to bed, reassurance
► calm visitors down
► medical examination by doctor
► completion of accident/incident report form with witnesses
► assess whether the patient needs cot sides for further safety

Part (c)   Assess
► the basis of the lady's complaint
► any anxiety on her part
► information from nurses allocated to care for her mother (later)

Establish a relationship if possible. Inform the lady of the complaints procedure and assure her of full investigation. You may quote your own authority's procedure – e.g. some would state that it must be referred to a senior member of the staff and that liability must not be admitted.

Staff shortage would not excuse neglect.

Written statements from nurses involved in the care may be required.

Section 5
Multiple choice questions

Introduction to multiple choice questions

The following are a series of multiple choice questions based upon brief 'story lines' of patients with conditions. They have been compiled by the author with guidance from the Professional Adviser (Examinations) at the English National Board.

They have not been pre-tested and are, therefore, not necessarily of the degree of difficulty (or ease) that you would expect in the examination.

Before reaching the final examination, they would be edited and pre-tested against groups of finalist nurses and then analysed. If they were too difficult or too easy, they would either be eliminated or rewritten for further pre-testing. This is an important safeguard to ensure the fairness of questions set. You should feel assured that if you have read widely and studied the questions carefully, then the test gives a good indication of your knowledge of facts, terms, processes and your ability to use judgement and understanding, justifying your admission to the Register.

The analyses will be at the end of each series of questions. They are designed to show you, not just the **right** answer, but how to read carefully **all** the information and wording of the questions.

It is advisable to read all through the series of questions before answering. You will see the progression of questions through the nursing process and/or the chronology of the patient's needs.

Take your time. Although your first thought is probably right, check that you have not been misled by the question. Initially, look for what you expect the **right** answer to be. Elimination of the **wrong** answers is time consuming, but is an acceptable way of reassuring yourself.

The present balance is that half the questions are in this 'story' form, and the remainder are general questions taken from the whole spectrum of nursing. The latter selection emphasizes again the need for wide reading.

Respiratory condition

John Adams is a fifteen-year-old schoolboy who has been admitted to the ward in status asthmaticus. He is an only child and his mother is quite distraught. John is due to take his 'O' levels in two months time.

1 Which of the following should be the nurse's *first* action on admitting John to the ward? Inform the doctor and:
   A give John oxygen at 24–28%
   B divert Mr and Mrs Adams to a sitting room
   C take a nursing history from Mrs Adams
   D sit with John and gain his confidence

2 Which of the following is the *best* description of John's condition? Wheezing and:
   A spasmodic attack, frothy sputum
   B persistent attack, viscous sputum
   C nocturnal attack, mucoid sputum
   D anxiety attack, muco purulent sputum

3 Which one of the following actions should the nurse take to help relieve Mrs Adams' immediate anxiety:
   A encourage her to stay with John as long as she likes
   B arrange an early discussion with John's consultant
   C give early advice about controlling allergens
   D assure her that psychological factors are not the only cause

4 Which one of the following should Mrs Adams be advised, if she asks what she should bring in for John to do:
   A only light reading while he is in hospital
   B a mixture of light reading and his study books
   C he should be able to resume concentrated revision within 24 hours
   D his aircraft modelling kit as diversion therapy

5 Which one of the following should the nurse encourage to help John's breathing? That he:
   A uses an armchair and makes an effort on inspiration
   B uses an armchair bed and makes an effort to cough up sputum
   C adopts a high pillow arrangement and makes an effort on expiration
   D adopts the orthopnoeic position and makes an effort to use his sodium cromoglycate inhaler

6 Which one of the following nursing observations would indicate that John was showing an undesired response to his prescribed treatment? That:
   A he was becoming drowsy and unresponsive
   B his breathing was becoming quieter and more shallow
   C there was an increasing amount of sputum expectorated
   D there was an increasing redness of his facial colour

Cardiovascular condition

Miss Amelia Johnstone is an eighty-year-old lady who lives alone in a first floor flat. She has been very independent. She has been found at the side of her bed, pale and confused. Her general practitioner suspects that she may have pernicious anaemia.

1 Which one of the following is likely to have contributed *most* to Miss Johnstone's anaemia:
   A lack of green vegetables and indigestion
   B her inability to buy red meat and achlorhydria
   C lack of fresh fruit and constipation
   D her dislike of dairy foods and recent diarrhoea

2 Which one of the following facts, obtained during the nursing assessment, will help to confirm Miss Johnstone's provisional diagnosis? The she has:
   A been on long-term aspirin treatment for arthritis
   B refused to have meals-on-wheels
   C an unsteady gait and paraesthesia in her feet
   D thinning of her hair and is intolerant of the cold

3 Which one of the following pairs of actions would it be *best* to include in the nursing orders to minimize Miss Johnstone's confusion on her first night? That the night nurses:
   A talk to her about her past and give her sweet tea
   B make sure that the ward is dark and avoid giving her any stimulants
   C put her in a light part of the ward and ensure she has night sedation
   D repeat explanations of what is happening and give her milky drinks

4 For which of the following reasons is it better to wait until Miss Johnstone is no longer confused before giving her a Schilling test? Because:
   A fear of radioactive substances may increase her confusion
   B her confusion would affect the results of the test
   C her co-operation is needed for taking gastric washings
   D she needs to be able to complete a 24 h urine specimen

5 Which one of the following amounts should be drawn up into a syringe from an ampoule containing 250 microgram/ml in order to give Miss Johnstone her prescribed dose of 0.75 mg of hydroxocobalamin:
   A 0.30 ml
   B 0.75 ml
   C 1.50 ml
   D 3.00 ml

6 Which of the following is *most important* when planning Miss Johnstone's discharge? To:
   A arrange a home help and meals on wheels
   B ask a dietician to advise her about buying and cooking food
   C arrange a continuity of care by the community nurse
   D arrange for sheltered accommodation with warden supervision

Digestive condition

Ms Jacqueline Smart is a 23-year-old fashion model. She travels widely and eats her meals at infrequent intervals. Recently she has been losing weight and has had attacks of diarrhoea and abdominal pain. She has been admitted to the ward for investigations for Crohn's disease.

1 Which one of the following assessments, taken during the nursing history, would be *most* helpful in confirming Ms Smart's diagnosis:
   A the colour and consistency of her faeces
   B her food likes and dislikes
   C the colour and texture of her skin
   D her previous and present weight

2 For which of the following investigations would the nurse be asked to prepare Ms Smart:
   A barium meal and follow through
   B barium meal and gastroscopy
   C barium enema and sigmoidoscopy
   D barium enema and colonoscopy

3 Which of the following explanations should be given to a junior nurse who asks for the *main* cause of Ms Smart's weight loss? It is due to:
   A loss of nutrients, because of her diarrhoea
   B poor digestion of nutrients, due to inflammation
   C poor absorption of nutrients, due to inflammation
   D repeated anorexia, because of the abdominal pain

4 Which one of the following diets should the nurse advise Ms Smart to follow? One that contains:
   A increased animal protein
   B increased vegetable protein
   C controlled carbohydrate
   D low residue and fat

5 Which one of the following should the nurse take into account when advising Ms Smart about her daily living activities? That:

A her career is likely to be affected by her deteriorating health

B her body image is likely to change with her new diet regime

C she needs to be aware of the possible complications and surgery

D she will need to have regular work schedules for her eating regime

6 Which of the following actions should a nurse take *first* if Ms Smart develops an intestinal obstruction? Send for the Doctor and:

A measure her waist for a base-line girth dimension

B pass a flatus tube to decompress the bowel

C pass a nasogastric tube to aspirate the stomach

D place her in a semiprone position to prevent inhalation of vomit

Renal condition

Ruth Jones, aged 16 years, has been admitted with a temperature of 40°C and a diagnosis of glomerulonephritis. She is accompanied by her mother and has a brother, aged 4 years, who is at home with father.

1 Which one of the following facts, obtained whilst taking the nursing history, would contribute to the confirmation of Ruth's diagnosis:

A a friend at school has rubella

B her brother has a urinary tract infection

C she had vomiting and diarrhoea a week ago

D she had scarlet fever three weeks ago

2 Which one of the following groups of signs and symptoms would the nurse expect to observe:

A polyuria, dehydration, pyuria

B oliguria, haematuria, facial oedema

C oliguria, dehydration, pyuria

D polyuria, haematuria, facial oedema

3 Which one of the following should be included in Ruth's care plan in order to reduce and control her body temperature? To:

A nurse her unclothed with one sheet and apply fan cooling

B nurse her in a cotton nightdress with one sheet and apply fan cooling

C carry out sponging with water at 20°C

D carry out sponging with water at 30°C

4 For which one of the following reasons should Ruth's fluid intake be controlled initially? To:

A correct her dehydration

B maintain her metabolic rate

C prevent her blood pressure rising

D avoid undesired drug reactions

5 Which of the following pairs of observations of Ruth would need *most* urgent attention:

A temperature 39°C, pulse rate of 112 beats per minute

B proteinuria, thirst and dry mouth

C urine output 10 ml in 4 hours, blood pressure 130/95 mm Hg

D quiet and withdrawn behaviour, loin tenderness

6 Which of the following is it *most* important to assess before explaining the principles of peritoneal dialysis to a junior nurse? She understands that:

A the peritoneal membrane allows small molecules to cross it

B the peritoneal cavity can hold 2 litres of dialysate fluid

C the dialysate fluid is sterilized before use

D fluid returned will be the same volume as that introduced

Nervous condition

Sarah Taylor, aged 10 years, was knocked down while cycling home from school. She has been admitted to the ward from the Accident and Emergency Department with head injuries. She is conscious but has a little blood in her left ear.

1 Which of the following would be the *main* reason for nursing Sarah in a semi-prone position? To:

A prevent hypostatic pneumonia

B prevent inhalation pneumonitis

C drain the discharge from her ear

D increase blood flow to her brain cells

2 Which one of the following brain surroundings will *always* be damaged in a fracture of the skull:

A dura mater

B arachnoid mater

C pia mater

D cranial periosteum

3 Which of the following would be the *best* advice that the nurse could give to Sarah's parents? That:
  A sitting by Sarah's bed would be helpful for her recovery
  B they will be contacted by telephone if there is any change
  C most young people recover from head injuries without brain damage
  D the bleeding from the ear is unlikely to lead to deafness

4 Which one of the following groups of signs and symptoms would indicate that Sarah's intracranial pressure was rising? She was:
  A becoming sleepy, feeling nauseated and her pulse rate was increasing
  B unable to remember the accident, her pulse rate was decreasing and her pupils constricting
  C slower to respond to questions, her pupils were dilating and she was vomiting
  D becoming irritable, her blood pressure was falling and her skin was becoming hot and dry

5 At which one of the following rates should the infusion set, delivering 15 drops/ml, be fixed in order for Sarah to receive 500 ml of Mannitol 10% over the next 6 hours:
  A 15 drops per minute
  B 20 drops per minute
  C 25 drops per minute
  D 30 drops per minute

6 Which one of the following nursing actions would be needed as specific care to prepare Sarah for a craniotomy:
  A maintaining neurological observations
  B introducing a urinary catheter
  C washing Sarah's hair carefully
  D helping with neurological tests

Locomotor condition

Mrs Prudence Moss is a 38-year-old housewife. Her husband is a policeman and they have two teenage daughters. She has recently been diagnosed as having rheumatoid arthritis and has been admitted this morning in an acute phase of the disease.

1 Which of the following household tasks is likely to have proved *most* difficult for Mrs Moss:
  A gardening
  B ironing clothes
  C knitting
  D washing dishes

2 Which of the following pairs of changes is likely to have caused Mrs Moss to visit her doctor:
  A increased tiredness and stiffness in her knees after walking
  B palpitations and hot swollen knuckles on waking
  C restlessness and neck stiffness in the mornings
  D listlessness and aching muscles in the evening

3 For which of the following reasons will it be necessary for the nurse to include keeping Mrs Moss's hands and feet warm in her plan of care? Because:
  A they will feel cold due to her raised core temperature
  B anaemia associated with arthritis lowers the temperature
  C swollen arterial walls limit the blood supply to hands and feet
  D warming always relieves the painful joints

4 Which one of the following principle aims of physiotherapy should the nurse be continuing in her care plan for Mrs Moss:
  A immobilizing painful joints, warming muscles
  B exercising muscles to strengthen joints, preventing dislocation
  C using wax baths to relieve pain when exercising
  D applying heat to counteract the inflammation of joints

5 For which of the following prescribed pairs of treatment is it necessary for the nurse to test Mrs Moss's urine daily:
  A phenylbutazone and physiotherapy
  B prednisolone and strict bed rest
  C salicylates and fan cooling
  D indomethacin and occupational therapy

6 Which one of the following instructions should be given to a junior nurse before she tests Mrs Moss's urine:
  A test for glucose using an early morning specimen
  B using a multi-test strip on a fresh specimen
  C use a urinometer on a catheter specimen
  D test for nitrates on a mid-stream specimen

Skin condition

Mrs Read, aged 50 years, is secretary to the managing director of a local business. She is divorced and lives with her daughter, an unemployed teacher. Mrs Read has tripped over a trailing cable and fallen against an electric fire. She has burns to her right hand and arm.

1 For which one of the following reasons should Mrs Read's arm be cooled as a first aid measure? Because:
   A cooling inhibits the reproduction of all bacteria
   B cold tissues limit the extent of inflammation
   C cooling deactivates the metabolites in burnt tissue
   D cold tissues are less likely to bleed profusely

2 Which one of the following pairs of symptoms would Mrs Read experience early if the deep tissues of her hand were burnt:
   A increasing severity of pain and feeling more thirsty
   B decreasing severity of pain and feeling faint
   C weakness in her finger movements and drying of the mouth
   D contraction deformity and a moist forehead

3 Which of the following is the *main* principle of care that the nurse should follow when planning the application of dressings to Mrs Read's burns:
   A reducing the pain by excluding air from the tissues
   B preventing infection by controlling bacterial growth
   C preventing disfigurement by support bandaging
   D killing bacteria by using a strict aseptic technique

4 With which of the following is Mrs Read *most* likely to need the nurses' assistance as she becomes more convalescent:
   A putting her out-door clothes on
   B going to the toilet and washing
   C applying make up and hair dressing
   D eating her lunch at the dinner table

5 Which of the following, in addition to eliminating infection, would be *most* important for Mrs Read's rehabilitation? That she is:
   A assured that she will be able to use an electronic typewriter
   B taught about the use of camouflage cosmetics for her scars
   C taught about wearing gloves for washing up
   D encouraged to exercise the hand and arm for full movement

6 Which one of the following actions should the nurse take in regard to the prevention of similar incidents in the future? Arrange for:
   A the hospital safety officer to speak to Mrs Read and her daughter
   B Mrs Read and her daughter to meet the Health Visitor
   C a discussion with Mrs Read's daughter at visiting time
   D safety in the home leaflets to be left on Mrs Read's locker

Endocrine condition

Mrs Margaret Tiler is seventy-five years old. She is a widow, lives alone and used to be a music teacher. Recently, she has been 'slowing down' and finding it difficult to concentrate. Her doctor suspects that she may have myxoedema and she has been admitted for investigations and commencement of treatment.

1 Which of the following pairs of effects of Mrs Tiler's condition is likely to have caused her distress:
   A difficulty combing her hair and feeling cold
   B increasing deafness and dry skin
   C decreased appetite and gaining weight
   D lethargy and a slow pulse rate

2 Which one of the following should be included in the nursing plan in order to care for Mrs Tiler's skin:
   A a nurse to escort her for a daily shower
   B a daily blanket bath using a soft soap
   C washing and application of lanolin cream
   D sponging down with warm water only

3 For which one of the following reasons would the nurse need to reassure Mrs Tiler about her progress after two weeks in hospital? Because:
   A progress is usually very slow in the first month
   B an increase in the dose of thyroxine does not mean that she is worse
   C there is a rapid loss of weight in the early period of care
   D she may be more self conscious of her appearance

4 For which one of the following reasons will the nurse need to discuss with Mrs Tiler her home heating arrangements before she is discharged? Because Mrs Tiler will:
  A feel the cold weather more
  B feel that her rooms are warmer
  C be less active than previously
  D not be able to tolerate warm clothing

5 Which of the following would be the *main* reason for the Community Nurse visiting Mrs Tiler when she had been discharged home? To:
  A give her injections
  B supervise her taking her tablets
  C assess her coping with daily living
  D ensure that any home alterations had been done

6 Which of the following would be *most* important for Mrs Tiler to report to her doctor after her discharge home? That she:
  A feels hungry and nauseated before meals
  B is losing weight and eating between meals
  C has developed shiny skin and perspires freely at night
  D has palpitations when sitting watching television

Reproductive condition

Mr James Tarr is a 35-year-old man who works on an oil rig. Although married, he tends to 'sleep around' when he is ashore. He has been referred to the Special Clinic with a diagnosis of gonorrhoea.

1 Which of the following is the *main* cause of the spread of gonorrhoea:
  A poor genital hygiene
  B direct contact
  C indirect contact
  D promiscuous living

2 Which of the following is the *most* likely reason for Mr Tarr seeking help:
  A his raised metabolic rate
  B frequency of micturition
  C a yellow purulent urethral discharge
  D scalding sensation on micturition

3 Which of the following amounts of procaine penicillin would the nurse need to give Mr Tarr if the prescription was for 2.4 g and the stock contained 300 mg/ml:
  A 8.0 ml
  B 7.2 ml
  C 1.3 ml
  D 0.8 ml

4 Which of the following is the *main* reason for the contact nurse needing to know Mr Tarr's sexual partners? Because:
  A there is a legal requirement to notify cases
  B female patients are more reluctant to attend clinics
  C early signs of gonorrhoea are often painless in women
  D prognosis is good if early treatment is given

5 Which of the following is the advice that Mr Tarr should be given regarding intercourse with his wife? He should:
  A wear a contraceptive sheath
  B abstain until both have completed treatment
  C abstain for a minimum of three weeks
  D apply an antibacterial cream

6 Which of the following would have the *most* serious effects if Mrs Tarr became infected:
  A salpingitis
  B endometriosis
  C cervical irritation
  D Bartholin's abscess

Answers to multiple choice questions

Respiratory condition

Key points
1 Status asthmaticus
2 Studying for O levels
3 Distraught mother

Question 1 Correct Answer is **D**
The nurse would calm John and Mrs Adams by gaining his confidence through a calm approach

Question 2 Correct answer is **B**
A straight forward knowledge question about the effects of status asthmaticus.

Question 3 Correct answer is **B**
The consultant would be able to give information and also gain understanding of factors leading to John's condition.
Staying with John as long as *she* likes may in fact convey anxiety to him.
Until the cause of John's asthmas is established, advice on allergens and psychological factors is not justified.

Question 4 Correct answer is **B**
The O levels are important, but he would not be ready for concentrated work.
The modelling kit probably contains glue!

Question 5 Correct answer is **C**
Whenever there are two factors in an answer, both must be right. Although the exact nature of the high pillow arrangement is not there, it could apply to orthopnoea or high side lying. Effort on expiration is required for *breathing*, to overcome the airway narrowing.
Note: Armchair beds do not always give good posture for patients with respiratory difficulty.

Question 6 Correct answer is **A**
Both are indications of carbon dioxide narcosis due to oxygen therapy.

Cardiovascular condition

Key points
1 *Miss* Johnstone
2 Independent 80-year-old
3 Pale, confused
4 Pernicious anaemia

Question 1 Correct answer is **B**
The red meat is not so specific to pernicious anaemia but the achlorhydria is.

Question 2 Correct answer is **C**
Read carefully through the wording of the question. The unsteady gait and paraesthesia are due to sub acute combined degeneration of the cord – a specific complication of pernicious anaemia.

Question 3 Correct answer is **A**
Relating to her past helps to establish a relationship and gradually she can be orientated. The sweet tea (you may assume that she takes sugar) helps to maintain her glucose levels.
Option **D** may be tempting, but the achlorhydria would make it difficult for her to digest milk.

Question 4 Correct answer is **D**
Concentrate on what you know about the test before going into the options. It then becomes obvious.

Question 5 Correct answer is **D**
There may be a few calculations included on final papers. There is no option but to learn the correct technique. Numbers are usually given in an ascending or descending order. Don't panic – just look at them carefully.

Question 6 Correct answer is **C**
All the options in this one are possibly important. You need to use your judgement of the *most*. This is called an evaluation type question. The reason why **C** is considered to be the *most* important is that Miss Johnstone must continue to have:
1 assessment of her daily living ability
2 injections of hydroxocobalamin
3 evaluation of her progress at home

Digestive condition

Key points
1 23-year-old fashion model
2 Life style
3 Symptoms so far
4 Crohn's disease

Question 1 Correct answer is **A**
This is an evaluation question in which all options are right. Judgement that **A** is *most* helpful is that it relates *directly* to Crohn's disease.

Question 2 Correct answer is **A**
Of the options given to you, it is the only one that will show up the small intestine (although Crohn's disease may also affect the stomach and colon of course!).

Question 3 Correct answer is **C**
Relating again to the main area of damage in the ileum and physiology.

Question 4 Correct answer is **B**
It may be argued that this is a dietician's role, but the nurse should also be able to give advice on nutrition. Vegetable protein will add fibre and control the fat intake – both would be acceptable for Ms Smart.

Question 5 Correct answer is **C**
This question is, in fact, an obscure one. The nurse would, of course, take *all* the points into account. Although, in a small sample, most students went for **C** and it fulfilled testing criteria, it would possibly be re-written. The argument is that in saying 'which *one*', you may only use one of the options, in which case, **C** was most popular.

Question 6 Correct answer is **D**
An evaluation question in which all four may be done. Inhalation of vomit is life-threatening.
Option **C** is tempting, but the patient needs to be examined first. Passing a nasogastric tube into a grossly distended stomach can be very hazardous.

Renal condition

Key points
1 16 years old
2 Temperature 40°C
3 Glomerulo nephritis

Question 1 Correct answer is **D**
Most people are wary of the 'sore throat'. The point is a 'haemolytic streptococcal infection' and scarlet fever fits.

Question 2 Correct answer is **B**
There may be a number of questions with 'groups' or 'pairs' of options. You must ensure that they *all* fit, by elimination process if necessary.

Question 3 Correct answer is **B**
Note the words are to reduce *and control* the body temperature. She would be very self conscious about being unclothed but that could be your next option. 20°C is cold sponging, 30°C is tepid sponging. Both would reduce the temperature but could be tiring, embarrassing and would not *control* the temperature.

Question 4 Correct answer is **C**
Note the word 'initially', indicating that she is in the oliguric phase and has retention of fluid with rising blood volume.

Question 5 Correct answer is **C**
An evaluation question. All are important, but severe oliguria and rising blood pressure indicate danger of acute renal failure.

Question 6 Correct answer is **A**
Remember, it is about *principles*, and **A** describes the action of a *semi permeable* membrane in *dialysis*.

Nervous condition

Key points
1 Age 10 years
2 Head injuries
3 Conscious
4 Blood in left ear

Question 1 Correct answer is **B**
Inhalation of even a small amount of vomit may cause pneumonitis.

Question 2 Correct answer is **D**
A straightforward question relating to the anatomy of the cranium.
Remember that cranial periosteum is on the outside of the skull as well as the inside.

Question 3 Correct answer is **A**
Apart from being the best advice anyway, your reading through the rest of the questions may alert you to the possibility that she may deteriorate and it may be delaying to have to contact by telephone.
Both **C** and **D** are indirectly suggesting the possibility of brain damage or deafness.

Question 4 Correct answer is **C**
Groups of signs and symptoms for you to pick your way through carefully. Many leave these questions until later to give themselves time to think.
C is the only one in which *all* are indicators of rising intracranial pressure.

Question 5 Correct answer is **B**

Don't be fooled by all the numbers. The 10% has no part of the calculation here. If you can memorize the answer, don't waste time. If you want to be sure, it is:

$$\frac{500 \text{ ml} \times 15}{6 \times 60} \text{ drops per minute} = 20.833$$

Question 6 Correct answer is **C**

Don't be put off by the obvious. All the others would be continued if Sarah was *not* to have a craniotomy. Some would say that it should include shaving too, but it is not absolutely necessary *within this question*. It merely says 'which of the following. . . .'

Locomotor condition

The information about her husband and daughters is not used in these questions. (Perhaps you would like to write out some questions of your own, using this system to test against each other in groups.)

Information that is used

1 Housewife, aged 38 years
2 Rheumatoid arthritis
3 Acute phase

Question 1 Correct answer is **C**

Not all evaluation questions are difficult. This one refers, of course, to her problems of fine finger movements. Maybe there is an assumption that she has a husband and daughters to do the gardening, ironing and washing of dishes!

Question 2 Correct answer is **B**

Remember that both of a pair must fit. It is often missed that these patients do get palpitations, which are often quite frightening.

Question 3 Correct answer is **C**

An understanding question of the effects of associated conditions of the disease. The arteritis will give her cold hands and feet.

Question 4 Correct answer is **B**

Strengthening joints and preventing dislocation are both principle aims of physiotherapy.

Question 5 Correct answer is **B**

Remember that both of a pair should be relevant. Prednisolone may cause glycosuria. Bed rest may cause stagnation and urinary tract inflammation.

Question 6 Correct answer is **B**

Tests for urinalysis should all be done on fresh specimens. The multi-test strip would indicate other abnormalities *in addition* to glycosuria.

Skin condition

Key points

1 50-year-old lady, divorced, secretary
2 Daughter – teacher
3 Burns

Question 1 Correct answer is **B**

Straightforward understanding of the reasons for the first aid. One cannot stress enough that you need to be aware of the reasons for any care that you give. 'Why' is the most important question in training.

Question 2 Correct answer is **B**

Deep tissue burns destroy nerve endings, reducing the pain. Falling blood pressure in shock causes the faintness. Remember, both of the factors must be correct.

Question 3 Correct answer is **B**

Try to identify *principles* of care – the intent behind the care. There will be other questions based on principles. The principle is *always* applicable, the local practice may be different.

Note that we have three correct answers which are all **B**. Some candidates have been put off by this in an examination, but it can happen and you should not be alarmed.

Question 4 Correct answer is **A**

An evaluation question which needs a little imagination. **A** is suggested as presenting most problems as she will need the fingers of *both* hands for buttons, zips and fasteners.

Question 5 Correct answer is **D**

Another evaluation question. All options are possible but the advantage of **D** is that it is relevant for *all* daily living activities.

Question 6 Correct answer is **C**

You are then respecting the daughter's intelligence and making sure that the subject is covered. Meeting the Health Visitor would be a reasonable alternative. Pre-testing would show if it was too strong a distractor. If it was, the question would be re-written.

Endocrine condition

Key points
1 75 years old
2 Widow. Lives alone
3 Music
4 Indications of hypothyroidism

Question 1 Correct answer is **B**

An evaluation question and some would say, obscure in that it is subjective to other aspects of Mrs Tiler's personality. In fact, most learners appreciate the distress that deafness would cause to a music teacher.

Question 2 Correct answer is **C**

The washing could, of course, include bathing. The main point is the lanolin cream to soften the coarse dry skin – particularly for a lady.

It could be that the answer to *question 2* gives you a strong clue to *question 1*. This would show up on pre-testing. If it did, the questions would be re-written.

Question 3 Correct answer is **B**

It is common to increase the dose of thyroxine after two weeks. She will need to be aware of dosage and could well be concerned at a 'doubling' of the dose.

Question 4 Correct answer is **B**

This is a question for you to show understanding of the effects of her treatment with thyroxine. The increase in metabolic rate would make her feel warmer and the question specifically refers to her home heating. Although **D** is probably true, it is not specific to the wording of the question.

Question 5 Correct answer is **C**

One of the main reasons for the Community Nurse to visit any patient who is discharged home. **B** is tempting, but this intelligent lady would not need direct supervision. Of course, the Community Nurse would include a discussion about taking tablets.

This is not an evaluation question because not all options are correct.

Question 6 Correct answer is **D**

This one *is* an evaluation question. All options are possible. Palpitations are a clear indication of thyroxine toxicity.

Reproductive condition

Key points
1 Married
2 Special clinic
3 Gonorrhoea

Question 1 Correct answer is **B**

Straightforward knowledge question – probably too easy and likely to be eliminated on pre-testing.

Question 2 Correct answer is **C**

An evaluation question in which all are possible. Most judge that the discharge would be most alarming and, of course, is specific to gonorrhoea.

Question 3 Correct answer is **A**

Again, a calculation which needs sorting out. The amount may seem alarming to you – trust your ability to calculate and, in fact, it is a reasonable *single* dose treatment for the condition.

Question 4 Correct answer is **D**

An important emphasis on the positive approach to this area of nursing care.

Question 5 Correct answer is **B**

Intercourse would only be safe when treatment was completed in the sense that both were free from infection. None of the others would be absolutely safe.

Question 6 Correct answer is **A**

An important recognition of the danger of salpingitis both initially and later in causing ectopic pregnancy.

Section 6
Examination papers

Introduction

With the kind permission of the English National Board for Nursing, Midwifery and Health Visiting, the following two examination papers are included for you to attempt.

1 Read the instructions at the beginning very carefully.
2 You may try to answer single questions, a series of questions or even a whole paper but it is vital that you time yourself carefully. Try to recreate classroom conditions and, most important, have them marked by your tutor.

You may like to study and analyse first. If you do, you should delay attempting the essays until at least two nights have elapsed, to ensure that you have remembered the material.

MORNING PAPER

ALL ASPECTS OF NURSING CARE AND TREATMENT OF PATIENTS
(included in the Syllabus of Training)

Time allowed 3 hours

IMPORTANT. – *Read* the questions *carefully, and* **answer only what is asked** *in the sections as indicated, as no credit will be given for irrelevant matter. The percentages shown on the right of this paper denote the weighting allocated to each section of the question.*

NOTE. – Candidates MUST answer FIVE questions.

1 Mr Dodds, aged 60 years, has been admitted to hospital with a diagnosis of myocardial infarction. He has severe central chest pain and is cold and clammy. He is accompanied by his wife who is extremely anxious and upset.
   (a) Describe the nurse's role during the period of Mr Dodds' admission. 60%
   (b) Discuss the means by which the major risk factors involved in the development of coronary artery disease may be reduced in society. 40%

2 Mr Walters, a 60-year-old widower, who lives alone, is admitted to a surgical ward with acute abdominal pain. He is accompanied by his son and daughter-in law and is to have an emergency resection of colon for a perforated diverticulum.
   (a) Describe the nurse's role in the care and management that Mr Walters will require in preparation for his operation. 70%
   (b) What advice would Mr Walters be given on discharge from hospital to help prevent a recurrence of his diverticulitis? 30%

3 Mrs Biffin, aged 85 years, who lives with a married daughter and her family of five, is admitted to an assessment ward for the elderly. She is found to have impacted faeces and has a history of chronic constipation.
   (a) What are the possible pre-disposing factors which may cause chronic constipation in the elderly? 20%
   (b) What *immediate* nursing measures would be taken to relieve Mrs Biffin's discomfort and to encourage a normal bowel movement pattern? 45%
   (c) Describe the help and advice which might be given to Mrs Biffin and her daughter before discharge home. 35%

4 Tommy, aged 3½ years, has been admitted to the ward in a tired and distressed condition. He was found wandering in a wood six hours after his loss had been reported to the Police by his parents.
   (a) What information should be obtained about Tommy's physical, emotional and social needs? 65%
   (b) Indicate how this information should be used in planning his care during his hospital stay. 35%

5 John, aged 17 years, is brought to the Accident and Emergency Department with extensive burns to the trunk and legs after an explosion at his place of work.
   (a) Describe how fluid is lost and the importance of fluid replacement in this situation. 60%
   (b) What are the other priorities in the management of John's condition in the Accident and Emergency Department? 40%

6 *Mrs Elsie White, aged 55 years, is married to a retired postman and lives in a Council house. She has had rheumatoid arthritis for the past five years and is admitted to the ward with an acute exacerbation of her condition.*

(*a*) Identify Mrs White's most likely problems and describe the nursing care and management she will require during her first 48 hours in hospital.   80%

(*b*) List the facilities which will be available to her in the community.   20%

7 Mr Jones, a 30-year-old teacher, is accompanied to the ward by his wife. He is conscious and very anxious. A diagnosis of viral meningitis has been made.

(*a*) With reference to Mr Jones' probable physical problems, describe his total care for the first 24 hours in hospital.   75%

(*b*) In what ways may the nursing staff provide reassurance to Mr Jones and his wife?   25%

8 Mrs Sonia Gibbs, aged 45 years and married with three children, has asked to be discharged home. She has been treated for carcinoma of the lung and now has secondary deposits in the lumbar spine.

(*a*) What nursing problems may develop as the disease progresses?   45%

(*b*) How may the nurse in charge of the ward facilitate continuity of care following Mrs Gibbs' discharge?   55%

9 Mrs Lewis, aged 28 years, is expecting her first baby.

(*a*) What may have led Mrs Lewis to suspect that she was pregnant?   20%

(*b*) Discuss the importance of her first visit to the ante-natal clinic.   80%

MORNING PAPER

ALL ASPECTS OF NURSING CARE AND TREATMENT OF PATIENTS
(included in the Syllabus of Training)

Time allowed 3 hours

IMPORTANT. – *Read the questions **carefully**, and **answer only what is asked** in the sections as indicated, as no credit will be given for irrelevant matter. The percentages shown on the right of this paper denote the weighting allocated to each section of the question.*

NOTE. – Candidates MUST answer FIVE questions.

1 Mr James, a 44-year-old bus driver, has been admitted to the ward for vagotomy and pyloroplasty.

(*a*) Identify the physical problems Mr James may have experienced prior to his admission to hospital.   15%

(*b*) Plan the care to meet Mr James' needs for the first 48 hours following his transfer from the recovery area to the ward.   85%

2 Miss Charlotte Long, a recently retired domestic assistant, is recovering from a mild, right cerebro-vascular accident but is still occasionally incontinent of urine. She
is soon to return home to her small house where she lives with her elder sister.

(*a*) Describe the nursing measures that may have been taken to resolve the problem of incontinence during Miss Long's stay in a medical ward.   70%

(*b*) What is the purpose of a home visit prior to Miss Long's discharge?   15%

(*c*) List the various services which could be called upon to support Miss Long and her sister.   15%

3 Miss Timson, a 35-year-old civil servant, has been admitted to the medical ward to have steroid therapy for a chronic disorder.

(*a*) Identify the possible side-effects which Miss Timson may experience and outline the baseline observations, both physical and psychological, which would enable them to be assessed.   35%

(*b*) What advice should be given and what actions may be taken to reduce the side-effects identified in part (*a*)?   65%

4 Mr Davis, aged 65 years, is admitted to a medical ward with cor pulmonale. He is extremely dyspnoeic, agitated and has a productive cough.
Using a problem-solving approach, describe how the nursing staff should care for Mr Davies during the next 72 hours.   100%

5 (*a*) Outline the means which may be used to aid the early detection of breast cancer.
                                                                                              30%
Mrs Watson, a 55-year-old widow, lives with her daughter. She has been admitted to hospital for mastectomy and is extremely anxious.
   (*b*) Describe the pre-operative preparation Mrs Watson will require prior to mastectomy.   70%

6 Paul Mason, a 4-year-old only child, has been admitted to hospital for the first time. He is fretful and unco-operative whilst being nursed. Paul's mother works as a part-time shop assistant and his father is a night foreman.
   (*a*) How may Paul's co-operation and trust be gained when carrying out his general nursing care?   65%
   (*b*) Describe the ways in which Mrs Mason's anxiety may be lessened during Paul's hospital stay.   35%

7 Mr Eric Cox, a 55-year-old writer who lives alone, has been admitted to the ward for terminal care. He has inoperable carcinoma of the pancreas with liver metastases and is anxious, emaciated and jaundiced. Mr Cox's ascites is to be relieved by paracentesis abdominis.
   (*a*) What is the nurse's role in the care of Mr Cox throughout the paracentesis procedure?   25%
   (*b*) Describe the nursing care that Mr Cox will require during the last stages of his illness.   75%

8 (*a*) Give a brief account of the ways in which the body limits haemorrhage.   20%
Ann Jones, a 17-year-old schoolgirl, has been admitted to hospital following repeated heavy nosebleeds. The current episode is being controlled with ice packs. She has been received into a 4-bedded bay.
   (*b*) Outline a plan of care, for a period of 24 hours, with particular reference to Ann's
      (i) bleeding;   40%
      (ii) discomfort;   25%
      (iii) anxiety.   15%

9 Mrs Samuels, an 80-year-old slightly confused lady, is confined to bed. She is occasionally incontinent of faeces and reluctant to eat or drink.
With reference to the actual and potential problems identified when undertaking Mrs Samuels' nursing assessment, describe the role of the nurse in the prevention and detection of pressure sores.   100%

Index

tonsillitis, 9-10
tooth decay, 56
toxic shock, 21
tracheostomy, 12
traction (nursing response), 131
treatment, drugs and, 182-5
tuberculosis, pulmonary, 22-3
tumours
  bladder, 94
  bone, 128-9
  brain, 112
  breast, 174
  kidney, 88
  medulla, 153
  nervous system, 112-3
  ovaries, 162
  pituitary gland, 145-6
  skin, 141
  testes, 159
  uterus/cervix, 166
typhoid, 68-9

ulcerative colitis, 73-4
ulcers, 39, 63-5, 141-3
uraemia (chronic renal failure), 90-1
ureters, 84, 92-3

urethra, 84, 96-9
urinary incontinence, 200-1
urinary tract, 84, 92-9
urine retention, 97-8
uterine (fallopian) tubes, 163-5
uterus, 165-8
uveitis, 120

vagina, 168-70
varicocele, 159
varicose ulcers, 39, 142
varicose veins, 38-9
vas deferens, 159-60
vasectomy, 160
veins, 38-40
violent behaviour, 180
visual defects, 118-9
voluntary services, 199
vulva, 168-70

Wilms tumour, 88
work (social problems), 181